Marine Natural Products as Anticancer Agents

Marine Natural Products as Anticancer Agents

Editors

Celso Alves
Marc Diederich

MDPI • Basel • Beijing • Wuhan • Barcelona • Belgrade • Manchester • Tokyo • Cluj • Tianjin

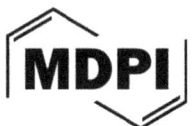

Editors
Celso Alves
MARE - Marine and
Environmental Sciences Centre
Polytechnic of Leiria
Peniche
Portugal

Marc Diederich
Department of Pharmacy,
College of Pharmacy
Seoul National University
Seoul
Korea, South

Editorial Office
MDPI
St. Alban-Anlage 66
4052 Basel, Switzerland

This is a reprint of articles from the Special Issue published online in the open access journal *Marine Drugs* (ISSN 1660-3397) (available at: www.mdpi.com/journal/marinedrugs/special_issues/AnticancerAgents).

For citation purposes, cite each article independently as indicated on the article page online and as indicated below:

LastName, A.A.; LastName, B.B.; LastName, C.C. Article Title. *Journal Name* **Year**, *Volume Number*, Page Range.

ISBN 978-3-0365-1820-6 (Hbk)
ISBN 978-3-0365-1819-0 (PDF)

© 2021 by the authors. Articles in this book are Open Access and distributed under the Creative Commons Attribution (CC BY) license, which allows users to download, copy and build upon published articles, as long as the author and publisher are properly credited, which ensures maximum dissemination and a wider impact of our publications.

The book as a whole is distributed by MDPI under the terms and conditions of the Creative Commons license CC BY-NC-ND.

Contents

About the Editors vii

Celso Alves and Marc Diederich
Marine Natural Products as Anticancer Agents
Reprinted from: *Marine Drugs* **2021**, *19*, 447, doi:10.3390/md19080447 1

Mariarosaria Conte, Elisabetta Fontana, Angela Nebbioso and Lucia Altucci
Marine-Derived Secondary Metabolites as Promising Epigenetic Bio-Compounds for Anticancer Therapy
Reprinted from: *Marine Drugs* **2020**, *19*, 15, doi:10.3390/md19010015 5

Sungmi Song, Sua Kim, Eslam R. El-Sawy, Claudia Cerella, Barbora Orlikova-Boyer, Gilbert Kirsch, Christo Christov, Mario Dicato and Marc Diederich
Anti-Leukemic Properties of Aplysinopsin Derivative EE-84 Alone and Combined to BH3 Mimetic A-1210477
Reprinted from: *Marine Drugs* **2021**, *19*, 285, doi:10.3390/md19060285 33

Yong Tae Ahn, Min Sung Kim, Youn Sook Kim and Won Gun An
Astaxanthin Reduces Stemness Markers in BT20 and T47D Breast Cancer Stem Cells by Inhibiting Expression of Pontin and Mutant p53
Reprinted from: *Marine Drugs* **2020**, *18*, 577, doi:10.3390/md18110577 63

Shao-Qian Sun, You-Xi Zhao, Si-Yu Li, Jing-Wen Qiang and Yi-Zhi Ji
Anti-Tumor Effects of Astaxanthin by Inhibition of the Expression of STAT3 in Prostate Cancer
Reprinted from: *Marine Drugs* **2020**, *18*, 415, doi:10.3390/md18080415 77

Yu-Jen Wu, Wen-Chi Wei, Guo-Fong Dai, Jui-Hsin Su, Yu-Hwei Tseng and Tsung-Chang Tsai
Exploring the Mechanism of Flaccidoxide-13-Acetate in Suppressing Cell Metastasis of Hepatocellular Carcinoma
Reprinted from: *Marine Drugs* **2020**, *18*, 314, doi:10.3390/md18060314 91

Amanda Mara Teles, Leticia Prince Pereira Pontes, Sulayne Janayna Araújo Guimarães, Ana Luiza Butarelli, Gabriel Xavier Silva, Flavia Raquel Fernandes do Nascimento, Geusa Felipa de Barros Bezerra, Carla Junqueira Moragas-Tellis, Rui Miguel Gil da Costa, Marcos Antonio Custódio Neto da Silva, Fernando Almeida-Souza, Kátia da Silva Calabrese, Ana Paula Silva Azevedo-Santos and Maria do Desterro Soares Brandão Nascimento
Marine-Derived *Penicillium purpurogenum* Reduces Tumor Size and Ameliorates Inflammation in an Erlich Mice Model
Reprinted from: *Marine Drugs* **2020**, *18*, 541, doi:10.3390/md18110541 103

Lin-Lin Jiang, Jin-Xiu Tang, Yong-Heng Bo, You-Zhi Li, Tao Feng, Hong-Wei Zhu, Xin Yu, Xing-Xiao Zhang, Jian-Long Zhang and Weiyi Wang
Cytotoxic Secondary Metabolites Isolated from the Marine Alga-Associated Fungus *Penicillium chrysogenum* LD-201810
Reprinted from: *Marine Drugs* **2020**, *18*, 276, doi:10.3390/md18050276 123

Tzu-Yin Huang, Chiung-Yao Huang, Chih-Hua Chao, Chi-Chien Lin, Chang-Feng Dai, Jui-Hsin Su, Ping-Jyun Sung, Shih-Hsiung Wu and Jyh-Horng Sheu
New Biscembranoids Sardigitolides A–D and Known Cembranoid-Related Compounds from *Sarcophyton digitatum*: Isolation, Structure Elucidation, and Bioactivities
Reprinted from: *Marine Drugs* **2020**, *18*, 452, doi:10.3390/md18090452 133

Tingrong Zhang, Shaojie Miao, Mingxiao Zhang, Wenjie Liu, Liang Wang and Yue Chen
Optimization of Two Steps in Scale-Up Synthesis of Nannocystin A
Reprinted from: *Marine Drugs* **2021**, *19*, 198, doi:10.3390/md19040198 . . . . **147**

About the Editors

Celso Alves

Dr. Celso Alves holds a PhD in Marine Science, Technology, and Sea Management (Do*Mar) in 2019 from the University of Aveiro, Portugal. He is a Researcher at the Marine and Environmental Sciences Centre in the Polytechnic of Leiria and invited assistant Professor at the Polytechnic of Leiria. His scientific work has been focused on the study of plants and marine organisms (e.g., seaweeds, bacteria, fungi, jellyfish, sponges, etc) as sources of new natural bioactive compounds with potential for biotechnological and therapeutic applications.

Marc Diederich

Dr. Marc Diederich earned his PhD in molecular pharmacology in 1994 from the University Henri Poincaré Nancy 1, France. After training at the University of Cincinnati, USA, he focused his research on cancer and leukemia cell signaling pathways and gene expression mechanisms triggered by natural compounds with epigenetic, anti-inflammatory, and cell-death-inducing potential. He directs the Laboratory for molecular and cellular biology of cancer (LBMCC) at Kirchberg Hospital in Luxemburg. He was appointed associate Professor of Biochemistry at the College of Pharmacy of Seoul National University in 2012. In 2017, he was tenured and promoted to full professor at SNU. Since 1998, he has been the organizer of the "Signal Transduction" meetings in Luxembourg.

Prof. Diederich's research focuses on the development of novel anticancer drugs. As an example, natural marine compounds represent an interesting source of novel leads with potent chemotherapeutic or chemo-preventive properties.

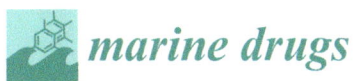

Editorial

Marine Natural Products as Anticancer Agents

Celso Alves [1],* and Marc Diederich [2],*

1. MARE—Marine and Environmental Sciences Centre, Polytechnic of Leiria, 2520-630 Peniche, Portugal
2. Department of Pharmacy, College of Pharmacy, Seoul National University, 1 Gwanak-ro, Gwanak-gu, Seoul 08826, Korea
* Correspondence: celso.alves@ipleiria.pt (C.A.); marcdiederich@snu.ac.kr (M.D.)

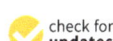

Citation: Alves, C.; Diederich, M. Marine Natural Products as Anticancer Agents. *Mar. Drugs* **2021**, *19*, 447. https://doi.org/10.3390/md19080447

Received: 23 July 2021
Accepted: 30 July 2021
Published: 4 August 2021

Publisher's Note: MDPI stays neutral with regard to jurisdictional claims in published maps and institutional affiliations.

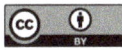

Copyright: © 2021 by the authors. Licensee MDPI, Basel, Switzerland. This article is an open access article distributed under the terms and conditions of the Creative Commons Attribution (CC BY) license (https://creativecommons.org/licenses/by/4.0/).

Cancer remains one of the major threats to human health and one of the deadliest diseases worldwide [1]. Therapy failure and consequent cancer relapse are the main factors contributing to high cancer mortality, making it crucial to find and develop new therapeutic options. Over the last few decades, natural products became one of the key drivers in the drug development of innovative cancer treatments [2]. In opposition to drug development from terrestrial resources, the marine environment only recently emerged as a prolific source of unparalleled structurally active metabolites [3]. Due to their excellent scaffold diversity, structural complexity, and ability to act on multiple cell signaling networks involved in carcinogenesis, marine natural products are ideal candidates to inspire the development of novel anticancer medicines [4,5].

The Special Issue "Marine Natural Products as Anticancer Agents" (https://www.mdpi.com/journal/marinedrugs/special_issues/AnticancerAgents (accessed on 15 June 2021)), gathered nine publications, including a review, a communication, and seven research articles, providing an excellent overview of the chemical richness offered by different marine organisms. Indeed, sponges, myxobacteria, fungi, and soft corals, provide essential scaffolds at the origin of the synthesis and molecular modeling of new anticancer drugs. Marine natural compounds or derived products described in this Special Issue belong to distinct chemical classes, including terpenoids, alkaloids, cyclodepsipeptides, polyketides, and hydroxyphenylacetic acid derivatives. These compounds modulate cancer cell mechanisms in vitro and in vivo in chronic myeloid leukemia, breast adenocarcinoma, prostate carcinoma, and hepatocellular carcinoma cell types. These compounds exhibited high specificity and great affinity to interact with distinct biological targets linked to specific intracellular signaling pathways, including mitochondrial dysfunction, autophagy, endoplasmic reticulum (ER) stress induction, apoptosis, inflammation, migration, and invasion.

Conte and collaborators [6] provide a critical review focused on the ability of marine natural products and their synthetic derivatives to act as epigenetic modulators, discussing advantages, limitations, and potential strategies to improve cancer treatment.

Song and co-workers [7] studied the pharmacological potential of four newly synthesized aplysinopsin derivatives to treat chronic myeloid leukemia, identifying the EE-84 analog as a promising novel drug candidate. EE-84 induces a cytostatic effect, leading to mitochondrial dysfunction, the induction of a senescent-like phenotype, autophagy, and ER stress. Its co-administration with the BH3 mimetic A-1210477 promoted a significant synergistic effect on cancer cell death.

Astaxanthin, a xanthophyll carotenoid that can be found in several marine organisms, including microalgae, bacteria, fungi, sea snails, and sea urchins, among others [8], demonstrated the capacity to decrease the levels of stemness markers (Oct4 and Nanog) in breast carcinoma cells, negatively modulating the expression of pontin and mutant p53 proteins [9]. Furthermore, this carotenoid also inhibited the proliferation of aggressive prostate cancer DU145 cells, triggering apoptotic cell death and decreasing invasion and migration capabilities. From a mechanistic point of view, cell death was triggered by a down-regulation of STAT3 mRNA and protein levels, accompanied by an up-regulation of pro-apoptotic (BAX, caspase3, and caspase9) and a down-regulation of pro-survival (JAK2, BCL-2, and NF-κB) proteins [10].

Wu and co-workers [11] studied the therapeutic effects of flaccidoxide-13-acetate diterpenoid, previously isolated from the marine soft coral *Sinularia gibberosa*, on hepatocellular carcinoma (HCC). The authors focused on tumor metastasis formation as this compound decreased the viability, migration, and invasion capability of HCC cells. These effects were mediated by a decrease in the expression levels of matrix metalloproteinases MMP-2, MMP-9, and MMP-13, the suppression of PI3K/Akt/mTOR signaling, the down-regulation of Snail and the up-regulation of E-cadherin protein expression. The modulation of these signaling pathways eventually suppressed the epithelial–mesenchymal transition, invasion, and migration of HCC cells.

Teles and collaborators [12] reported the antitumor properties of a *Penicillium purpurogenum* ethyl acetate extracellular extract, rich in meroterpenoids, using an Erlich mouse model. The extract decreased tumor-associated inflammation and necrosis without causing weight loss nor renal and hepatic toxicity.

The isolation of new marine natural products with cytotoxic activities was also reported in this Special Issue. Jiang and co-workers [13] described the isolation of three new molecules from *Penicillium chrysogenum* LD-201810, a marine alga-associated fungus: a pentaketide derivative, penilactonol A, and two new hydroxyphenylacetic acid derivatives, (2′R)-stachyline B and (2′R)-westerdijkin A. (2′R)-westerdijkin A was significantly cytotoxic to the hepatocellular carcinoma cell line HepG2.

One of the biggest challenges associated with bioprospecting and the pharmacological application of marine natural products is the low yield of extraction, which can compromise the supply chain to accomplish pre-clinical and clinical trials and thus develop a new drug. Several strategies were developed to overcome these limitations, such as genetic engineering, aquaculture/cultivation, chemical modification, semi-synthesis, and synthesis [14]. Some of those approaches were addressed in this Special Issue. Huang and collaborators [15] reported the isolation of four new biscembranoidal metabolites, sardigitolides A–D (1–4), from the cultured soft coral *Sarcophyton digitatum*. The new biscembranoid, sardigitolide B, significantly reduced the cell viability of breast adenocarcinoma cell lines, MCF-7, and MDA-MB-231.

On the other hand, Zhang and co-workers [16] communicated the optimization of two critical steps in the scale-up synthesis of nannocystin A, a 21-membered cyclodepsipeptide with remarkable anticancer properties, achieving a synthesis at a four hundred milligram scale.

Altogether, the nine publications included in this volume provide an exciting overview of marine natural products as potential therapeutic agents for cancer treatment.

Funding: M.D. was supported by the National Research Foundation (NRF) (grant number 019R1A2C-1009231). Support from Brain Korea (BK21) FOUR and the Creative-Pioneering Researchers Program at Seoul National University (funding number: 370C-20160062) are acknowledged. M.D. also acknowledges support by the "Recherche Cancer et Sang" Foundation (Luxembourg), "Recherches Scientifiques Luxembourg" (Luxembourg), "Een Häerz fir kriibskrank Kanner" (Luxembourg), Action Lions "Vaincre le Cancer" (Luxembourg), and Télévie Luxembourg. C.A. acknowledges the support by the Portuguese Foundation for Science and Technology (FCT) through the strategic project UIDB/04292/2020 and UIDP/04292/2020 granted to MARE—Marine and Environmental Sciences Centre and through the CROSS-ATLANTIC project (PTDC/BIA-OUT/29250/2017).

Acknowledgments: As guest editors, we would like to sincerely acknowledge the efforts provided by all authors that participated in this Special Issue with their scientific outputs, all reviewers that carefully reviewed the manuscripts, the editorial board, and the *Marine Drugs* editorial office for their support and assistance, with special thanks to Grace Qu.

Conflicts of Interest: The authors declare no conflict of interest.

References

1. Sung, H.; Ferlay, J.; Siegel, R.L.; Laversanne, M.; Soerjomataram, I.; Jemal, A.; Bray, F. Global Cancer Statistics 2020: GLOBOCAN Estimates of Incidence and Mortality Worldwide for 36 Cancers in 185 Countries. *CA Cancer J. Clin.* **2021**, *71*, 209–249. [CrossRef] [PubMed]
2. Florean, C.; Dicato, M.; Diederich, M. Immune-modulating and anti-inflammatory marine compounds against cancer. *Semin. Cancer Biol.* **2020**. [CrossRef] [PubMed]
3. Schumacher, M.; Kelkel, M.; Dicato, M.; Diederich, M. Gold from the sea: Marine compounds as inhibitors of the hallmarks of cancer. *Biotechnol. Adv.* **2011**, *29*, 531–547. [CrossRef] [PubMed]
4. Harvey, A.L. Natural products as a screening resource. *Curr. Opin. Chem. Biol.* **2007**, *11*, 480–484. [CrossRef] [PubMed]
5. Alves, C.; Silva, J.; Pinteus, S.; Gaspar, H.; Alpoim, M.C.; Botana, L.M.; Pedrosa, R. From Marine Origin to Therapeutics: The Antitumor Potential of Marine Algae-Derived Compounds. *Front. Pharmacol.* **2018**, *9*, 777. [CrossRef]
6. Conte, M.; Fontana, E.; Nebbioso, A.; Altucci, L. Marine-Derived Secondary Metabolites as Promising Epigenetic Bio-Compounds for Anticancer Therapy. *Mar. Drugs* **2020**, *19*, 15. [CrossRef] [PubMed]
7. Song, S.; Kim, S.; El-Sawy, E.R.; Cerella, C.; Orlikova-Boyer, B.; Kirsch, G.; Christov, C.; Dicato, M.; Diederich, M. Anti-Leukemic Properties of Aplysinopsin Derivative EE-84 Alone and Combined to BH3 Mimetic A-1210477. *Mar. Drugs* **2021**, *19*, 285. [CrossRef] [PubMed]
8. Galasso, C.; Corinaldesi, C.; Sansone, C. Carotenoids from Marine Organisms: Biological Functions and Industrial Applications. *Antioxidants* **2017**, *6*, 96. [CrossRef] [PubMed]
9. Ahn, Y.T.; Kim, M.S.; Kim, Y.S.; An, W.G. Astaxanthin Reduces Stemness Markers in BT20 and T47D Breast Cancer Stem Cells by Inhibiting Expression of Pontin and Mutant p53. *Mar. Drugs* **2020**, *18*, 577. [CrossRef] [PubMed]
10. Sun, S.Q.; Zhao, Y.X.; Li, S.Y.; Qiang, J.W.; Ji, Y.Z. Anti-Tumor Effects of Astaxanthin by Inhibition of the Expression of STAT3 in Prostate Cancer. *Mar. Drugs* **2020**, *18*, 415. [CrossRef] [PubMed]
11. Wu, Y.-J.; Wei, W.-C.; Dai, G.-F.; Su, J.-H.; Tseng, Y.-H.; Tsai, T.-C. Exploring the Mechanism of Flaccidoxide-13-Acetate in Suppressing Cell Metastasis of Hepatocellular Carcinoma. *Mar. Drugs* **2020**, *18*, 314. [CrossRef]
12. Teles, A.M.; Pontes, L.P.P.; Guimarães, S.J.A.; Butarelli, A.L.; Silva, G.X.; do Nascimento, F.R.F.; de Barros Bezerra, G.F.; Moragas-Tellis, C.J.; de Costa, R.M.G.; da Silva, M.A.C.N.; et al. Marine-Derived *Penicillium purpurogenum* Reduces Tumor Size and Ameliorates Inflammation in an Erlich Mice Model. *Mar. Drugs* **2020**, *18*, 541. [CrossRef]
13. Jiang, L.-L.; Tang, J.-X.; Bo, Y.-H.; Li, Y.-Z.; Feng, T.; Zhu, H.-W.; Yu, X.; Zhang, X.-X.; Zhang, J.-L.; Wang, W. Cytotoxic Secondary Metabolites Isolated from the Marine Alga-Associated Fungus *Penicillium chrysogenum* LD-201810. *Mar. Drugs* **2020**, *18*, 276. [CrossRef] [PubMed]
14. Lindequist, U. Marine-Derived Pharmaceuticals—Challenges and Opportunities. *Biomol. Ther.* **2016**, *24*, 561–571. [CrossRef] [PubMed]
15. Huang, T.Y.; Huang, C.Y.; Chao, C.H.; Lin, C.C.; Dai, C.F.; Su, J.H.; Sung, P.J.; Wu, S.H.; Sheu, J.H. New Biscembranoids Sardigitolides A-D and Known Cembranoid-Related Compounds from *Sarcophyton digitatum*: Isolation, Structure Elucidation, and Bioactivities. *Mar. Drugs* **2020**, *18*, 452. [CrossRef] [PubMed]
16. Zhang, T.; Miao, S.; Zhang, M.; Liu, W.; Wang, L.; Chen, Y. Optimization of Two Steps in Scale-Up Synthesis of Nannocystin A. *Mar. Drugs* **2021**, *19*, 198. [CrossRef] [PubMed]

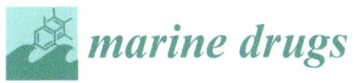

Review

Marine-Derived Secondary Metabolites as Promising Epigenetic Bio-Compounds for Anticancer Therapy

Mariarosaria Conte *,†, Elisabetta Fontana †, Angela Nebbioso and Lucia Altucci *

Department of Precision Medicine, University of Campania 'Luigi Vanvitelli', Via L. De Crecchio 7, 80138 Naples, Italy; elisabetta.fontana@unicampania.it (E.F.); angela.nebbioso@unicampania.it (A.N.)
* Correspondence: mariarosaria.conte@unicampania.it (M.C.); lucia.altucci@unicampania.it (L.A.)
† Co-first authors.

Abstract: Sessile organisms such as seaweeds, corals, and sponges continuously adapt to both abiotic and biotic components of the ecosystem. This extremely complex and dynamic process often results in different forms of competition to ensure the maintenance of an ecological niche suitable for survival. A high percentage of marine species have evolved to synthesize biologically active molecules, termed secondary metabolites, as a defense mechanism against the external environment. These natural products and their derivatives may play modulatory roles in the epigenome and in disease-associated epigenetic machinery. Epigenetic modifications also represent a form of adaptation to the environment and confer a competitive advantage to marine species by mediating the production of complex chemical molecules with potential clinical implications. Bioactive compounds are able to interfere with epigenetic targets by regulating key transcriptional factors involved in the hallmarks of cancer through orchestrated molecular mechanisms, which also establish signaling interactions of the tumor microenvironment crucial to cancer phenotypes. In this review, we discuss the current understanding of secondary metabolites derived from marine organisms and their synthetic derivatives as epigenetic modulators, highlighting advantages and limitations, as well as potential strategies to improve cancer treatment.

Keywords: secondary metabolites; epigenome; epigenetic signaling; bioactive compounds; cancer therapy; marine species; environment

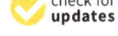

Citation: Conte, M.; Fontana, E.; Nebbioso, A.; Altucci, L. Marine-Derived Secondary Metabolites as Promising Epigenetic Bio-Compounds for Anticancer Therapy. *Mar. Drugs* **2021**, *19*, 15. https://doi.org/10.3390/md19010015

Received: 15 December 2020
Accepted: 28 December 2020
Published: 31 December 2020

Publisher's Note: MDPI stays neutral with regard to jurisdictional claims in published maps and institutional affiliations.

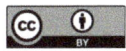

Copyright: © 2020 by the authors. Licensee MDPI, Basel, Switzerland. This article is an open access article distributed under the terms and conditions of the Creative Commons Attribution (CC BY) license (https://creativecommons.org/licenses/by/4.0/).

1. Introduction

Marine habitats are an extraordinary source of new and structurally complex bioactive metabolites naturally produced by different organisms and characterized by unique functions with marked biological activities. These features can be attributed to extreme environmental conditions such as lack of light, high pressure, ionic concentration, pH and temperature changes, scarcity of nutrients, and restricted living spaces [1]. The high concentration of coexisting organisms in a limited area also makes them very competitive and complex, resulting in the development of adaptations and behaviors aimed at safeguarding the species, such as the adoption of chemical strategies exploiting the wealth of bioactive molecules produced by the secondary metabolism [2,3]. Marine-derived metabolites originate from different signal transduction pathways activated as a consequence of epigenome changes in the organisms that produce them. Phenotypic/genotypic alterations of marine organisms are characterized by an intricate network of interactions that influence each other. Such interplay is further complicated by epigenetic modifications, which can trigger adaptive biochemical processes in the species [4]. The marine environment (characterized by biotic and abiotic factors), in turn, plays an essentially selective role in intrinsically changing organisms, exerting an inductive function on epigenetic, genetic, and phenotypic changes with transgenerational effects on the species [5,6] (Figure 1). Since the reprogramming of epigenetic states can be induced by environmental exposures in the marine habitat, secondary metabolites produced by a large number of organisms might represent good candidates as novel natural molecules with potential pharmacological activity for cancer treatment [7]. Cutting-edge chromatographic isolation and purification techniques, pharmacological screening methods, and numerous spectroscopic approaches for structural investigation such as mass spectroscopy and nuclear magnetic resonance (NMR) were used to isolate and characterize several new marine-derived compounds [8–10], some of which have potential anticancer activities. The chemical composition of isolated molecules has a major impact on both the epigenome of the organism [11] and any potential epigenetic effects produced, reflecting a complex and interconnected machinery of information exchange. In this review, we describe the therapeutic potential of marine-derived secondary metabolites and their synthetic derivatives in cancer, focusing on their importance as epigenetic modulators generating posttranscriptional, inductive (produced by the metabolism of the organism), and induced (produced by alterations in marine environment) modifications. We also discuss the challenges involved in discovering new natural and synthetic marine bio-compounds with anticancer activity in light of the enormous variability that characterizes the organisms themselves and the environment that surrounds them. This review also highlights sustainable use of marine resources as producers of high yields of value added bio-molecules for pharmaceutical field towards a more sustainability of economic growth in terms of development, research and transmissibility of marine technology in terms of development, research, and transmissibility of marine technology.

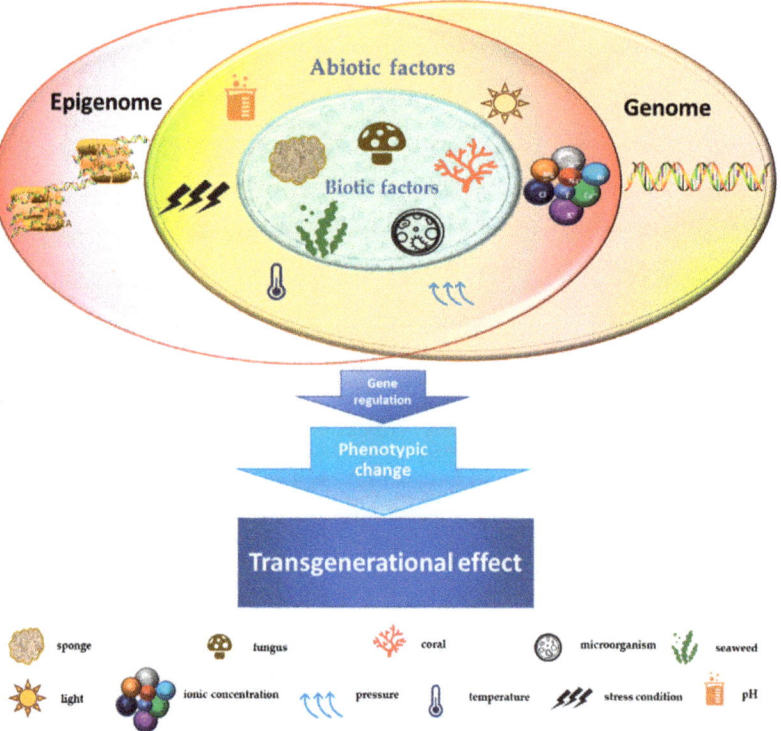

Figure 1. Schematic representation of the crosstalk between biotic/abiotic factors and transgenerational genetic/epigenetic effects.

2. Anticancer Activities of Marine-Derived Secondary Metabolites with Inductive and Induced Epigenetic Modifications

Epigenetics belongs to a branch of genetics based on the concomitance of complex biomolecular mechanisms, which coordinate genetic information in the nucleus, culminating in control of gene expression [12], which in turn propagates in subsequent generations. All this information is further conditioned by perturbations from the external environment. Epigenetic alterations in gene activity are mitotically stable in the absence of changes in DNA sequence [13]. Generally, mechanisms of environmental perception act through alterations in chemical tags that normally exist in the genome. In cancer, "epigenetic markers" [14] serve as a sort of barcode of DNA function, indicating whether genes are active or silent. The alteration and reprogramming of epi-signals can lead to changes in gene expression and also directly influence transcriptional regulator function, with downstream effects on the way cells and tissues work. In addition to genetic alterations, a hallmark of various types of cancer, epigenetic dysregulations affecting DNA methylation, histone modifications, and microRNAs introduce another layer of complexity, contributing to tumor progression and changes in the phenotypic state. These epi-alterations are further regulated by so-called chromatin writers, readers, and erasers, which constitute specialized protein machinery able to modulate and reversibly influence the epigenome. DNA methyltransferases (DNMTs), histone acetyltransferases (HATs), histone methyltransferases (HMTs), and lysine/arginine methyltransferases (KMTs/RMTs) are all writers, due to their ability to add a modification on DNA and histones; readers, able to "read" and thus interpret covalent modifications include: bromodomains, specific for acetylation site recognition; chromodomains, recognized by methyl-readers; methyl-lysine readers such as ATRX-DNMT3-DNMT3L (ADD), ankyrin, bromo-adjacent homology, chromobarrel, WD40, and zinc finger CW domains, as well as double chromodomain, and tandem Tudor domain. In addition, plant homeodomains bind to methylated histone H3, while the PWWP domain can bind DNA and methylated histones. Erasers include TET proteins, which remove modifications from DNA and histones, as well as histone demethylases (HDMs), histone deacetylases (HDACs), protein phosphatases, and deubiquitinating enzymes, which remove methyl, acetyl, phosphate, and ubiquitin groups from histones and other proteins, respectively [15–17]. Since modern medical approaches are based on the personalization of human healthcare, bioactive molecules with epigenetic activity isolated from marine sources represent a valid alternative to conventional therapies for use in extensive preclinical assessments and the advanced phases of clinical studies. Furthermore, given the resistance developed by some pathogens to pharmacological treatments and the inefficacy of traditional chemotherapies, efforts are being made to identify more biologically active and effective molecules [18]. In marine ecosystems, sessile organisms are much more susceptible to changes in the external environment [19] and adopt complex survival strategies. Moreover, the set of biotic and abiotic components in these organisms are extremely predominant, determining the production of secondary metabolites with almost unique chemical-physical characteristics. A further level of complexity is added by the intricate relationship between secondary metabolites and epigenetic functions, which in turn contribute to the development of defense mechanisms by the species that are transmitted across generations [20]. Secondary metabolites can harbor several beneficial properties for human health such as antioxidant, antibacterial, antivirus, anticoagulant, antidiabetic, anti-inflammatory, antihypertensive, and antitumor activities [21]. Furthermore, their natural biological functions are strongly influenced by the surrounding environment, including conditions of climatic stress or attack by predators. Computational programs using knowledge-based algorithms or sequence-based prediction [22] have identified genes responsible for the production of these natural products, but only for some species. These genes are usually located in specific biosynthetic gene clusters (BGCs) in the genome [23] that contain the required enzymes responsible for synthesis of secondary metabolites and regulatory structures. Considering the enormous genetic and epigenetic variability among marine species, it is not always possible to predict their BGCs and therefore their association with the production of secondary metabolites. For example, under certain conditions chromatin remodeling factors can switch on or switch off specific genes continuously over time. Cutting-edge technologies such as those involved in triggering the activation of silent BGCs, which include changes in growth conditions (e.g., temperature and pH) or genetic engineering-based approaches [24,25] are emerging to better study the interaction between the production of metabolites and the genes that produce them. One of the goals of anticancer research is to extract and select biomolecules from these organisms in order to exploit their properties and generate synthetic analogues (Figure 2). To date, the U.S. Food and Drug Administration (FDA) has approved several marine-derived therapeutic compounds such as cytarabine, vidarabine, ziconotide, omega-3 acid ethyl esters, eribulin mesylate, brentuximab vedotin, and iota-carrageenan [26–32] (Figure 3) and further studies aimed at characterizing and developing new drugs are ongoing. The following section describes the epigenetic role of well-known marine-derived secondary metabolites, classified according to their biosynthetic pathways and subdivided into three major families: phenolic compounds, cyclic peptides, and alkaloids. Their mechanism of action as potential epigenetic bio-compounds for the treatment of different type of cancers is also discussed.

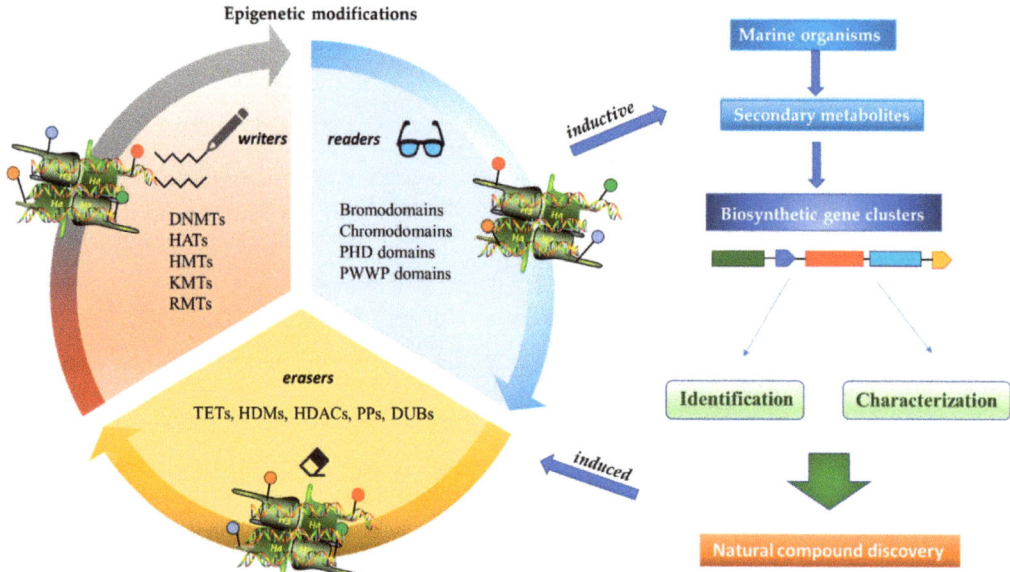

Figure 2. Inductive and induced epigenetic modifications by secondary metabolites produced by marine organisms. Epigenetic writers, readers, and erasers regulate production of secondary metabolites, which in turn induce epi-modifications.

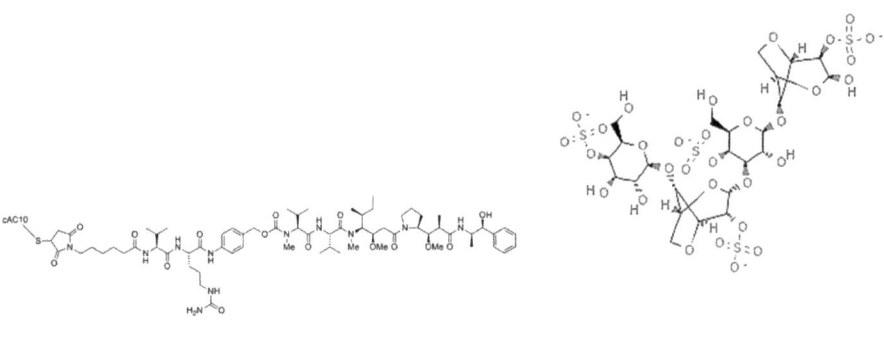

Figure 3. Chemical structures of marine-derived therapeutic compounds approved by the U.S. Food and Drug Administration (FDA).

3. Sustainability and Health

Potential anticancer drugs derived from various marine species are not always present in the environment in sufficient quantities and do not maintain the same functional characteristics over time both in terms of chemical-physical structure and biological potential, thus limiting their characterization. These molecules, before being used as drugs, need to be submitted to rigorous scientific research and to quality control according to precise standards and procedures created ad hoc to ensure their best implementation. One of the aspects that influences their production is represented by the conditions of the marine environment, which has a fundamental impact on development, research and on new strategies applied to marine biotechnology. The sea must be considered not only an environment to be exploited, but also to be safeguarded, since its protection has crucial benefits for human health. Apart from human activities, climate change, the availability of nutrients, the attack of predators also strongly affecting the production of bioactive compounds, for which we are increasingly trying to enhance sustainability, well-being and health, both in environmental protection and in socio-economic terms.

4. (Poly)phenolic Compounds

(Poly)phenolic compounds are one of the main classes of marine-derived secondary metabolites. They can be found in different pelagic organisms and their production varies across genera as well as growing conditions, geographical location, and abiotic/biotic factors. These compounds can be distinguished by the presence of one (phenolic acids) or more (polyphenols) aromatic rings annexed to hydroxyl groups in their structures, which confer very strong antioxidant properties. Their bioactivity is also linked to other enzymatic inhibitory effects as well as to anticancer, antidiabetic, or anti-inflammatory actions, with beneficial results for human health [33–35]. In addition, their role as scavengers of singlet oxygen and free radicals and/or reducing and chelating agents is a very promising area for the study and treatment of cancer, as they display interesting epigenetic molecular mechanisms that modulate gene expression as well as DNA damage and repair. The following subsections focus on the most studied natural phenolic compounds and their derivatives in terms of their epigenetic role in cancer and their use in clinical trials (Table 1 and Supplementary Table S1).

4.1. Psammaplin A

Psammaplins belong to a group of bromotyrosine phenols, whose common ancestor is Psammaplin A (PsA), a natural phenolic product isolated for the first time from the *Psammaplin aplysilla* marine sponge and from an unknown sponge (probably *Thorectopsamma xana*) in 1987 [36]. This marine metabolite was the first natural product containing oxime and disulfide moieties to be isolated from a marine sponge [29,37], and is characterized by a disulfide bridge and a bromotyrosine ring occurring in nature in the form of monomers or dimers. PsA exhibits anticancer activities by modulating different human enzymes, which in turn regulate DNA replication, transcription, differentiation, apoptosis, proliferation, tumor invasion, and migration. PsA also inhibits topoisomerase II, aminopeptidase N, chitinases, farnesyl protein transferase, leucine aminopeptidase, and other enzymes [36,38–41]. PsA is reported to act as an antiproliferative agent in various human cancer cell lines, such as endometrial, breast, and triple negative metastatic breast cancer, as well as in in vivo models [15,42,43] by exerting potentially inhibitory effects on HDACs and DNMTs. PsA was also shown to sensitize human lung and glioblastoma cancer cells to radiation in vitro; PsA pretreatment in these cells increased the sub-G1 phase of the cell cycle, induced an increased expression of cleaved caspase-3, and led to a drastic depletion of DNMT1 and DNMT3A, suggesting inhibition of the DNA damage repair process elicited by the DNA damage marker γH2AX [44]. The mechanism of action underlying the HDAC inhibitory effect of PsA involves a change in the redox state of the disulfide bond. Replacement of the sulfur atom leads to the formation of a mercaptan, which in turn chelates the Zn^+ ion present in the characteristic active site of the HDAC enzyme, modifying its conformational state and thus preventing its accessibility to the natural substrate [45]. This new conformational state determines an increase in acetylation levels of histone H3, a well-known epigenetic marker of chromatin structure and function, suggesting selectivity for HDACs.

4.2. Indole-Derived Psammaplin a Analogues

Because of the limits relating to the extraction and instability of PsA, several indole-derived analogues have been designed and many studies undertaken to improve the inhibitory effect of this promising natural drug. A computational-based study was carried out to discover and biologically test novel potent and selective HDAC inhibitors (HDACi) from thioester-derivatives and analogues of PsA [46]. Although chemically reduced PsAs and thiol-derived analogues both showed a good inhibitory effect at the nanomolar level in vitro, when they were tested in cancer cell models, their potency was much lower. This biological effect was probably due to the low permeability/stability of thiol in malignant cells. In order to overcome this issue, a novel approach was adopted to "protect" free thiol and enhance its effectiveness in cancer cells. This strategy was developed thanks to the production of novel thioester-active PsA analogues, whose molecular mechanism is mediated by thioester hydrolysis, identified by in vitro assay, and followed by cleavage of the acetyl group by HDAC1 and six enzymes. These newly synthetized thioesters displayed significant cytotoxicity against several cancer cell lines as well as robust enzymatic activity [46]. After confirming the epigenetic role of PsA using in vitro and cell-based assays, a structure–activity relationship (SAR) study was performed by modifying the original scaffold of PsA based on the β-indole-α-oximinoamido protection group and by the replacement of the o-bromophenol unit by an indole ring. These new derivatives were evaluated by several biological assays, displaying cell cycle arrest and p21 induction in acute myeloid leukemia (AML), breast, and prostate cancer cells, as well as histone H3 and alpha tubulin acetylation, showing multiple epigenetic activities [47]. Novel PsA derivatives were synthetized as bisulfide bromotyrosine products, including psammaplins F, G, and H, while two new bromotyrosine derivatives were characterized as psammaplins B, C, D, bisaprasin, I and J, along with the known PsA. [48–51]. PsA, psammaplin G, and bisaprasin displayed both HDAC and DNMT inhibitory activities, while all the others substantially exhibited HDAC inhibition in vitro.

Given the growing interest in new epigenetic modulators in cancer, research has been focusing on the role of PsA and its derivatives as potential epigenetic markers and investigating their biological activity. Many other computational and biological-based assays have been carried out to optimize the selectivity of psammaplin compounds and determine the best trade-off between chemical stability and epigenetic-based biological function.

4.2.1. UVI5008

The molecular characterization and anticancer activities of UVI5008, a novel synthetic derivative of PsA that exerts multiple epigenetic effects in several cancer cell lines via simultaneous targeting of HDACs, DNMTs, and sirtuins (class III HDACs). UVI5008 is a powerful HDACi, displaying histone H3 acetylation and HDAC inhibition. UVI5008 also inhibits DNA methylation in the promoter region of tumor suppressor gene *p16INK4a* and alters the acetylation status of chromatin on tumor necrosis factor-related apoptosis-inducing ligand (TRAIL). The inhibitory activity of UVI5008 was also tested on sirtuin 1 and 2, and was found to impact p53 acetylation levels. UVI5008 affects death and ROS pathways in HDAC-resistant and -mutated cancer cells and tumors, providing a potentially valid alternative to combination cancer therapy (patent WO2008125988A1) [52].

4.2.2. Panobinostat

Cinnamic acids play a crucial role in the formation of other more complex phenolic compounds. Panobinostat, (LBH-589; Farydak®, Novartis Pharmaceuticals Corporation, East Hanover, NJ, USA), a synthetic analogue of PsA, is one of the most potent pan HDACi and in 2015 received FDA approval for therapeutic application in patients with multiple myeloma (MM). To date, panobinostat has been investigated in numerous completed clinical trials for the treatment of solid and hematological cancers, alone or in combination (NCT01242774, NCT01802879, NCT01336842, NCT01460940, NCT01065467) and about ten clinical studies are currently recruiting (NCT04326764, NCT04341311, NCT02717455, NCT04150289, NCT02386800, NCT02506959, NCT02890069, NCT04315064, NCT01543763, NCT04264143, NCT03143036, NCT03878524). Many reports also confirm the antiangiogenic role of this natural molecule in hepatocellular carcinoma both in vitro and in vivo through the epigenetically regulated connective tissue growth factor [53]. In vitro findings demonstrated that panobinostat inhibits tumor growth in an orthotopic xenograft model of ovarian cancer and that its effect is characterized by acetylation of histone H2B and upregulation of pH2AX, suggesting that these mechanisms are mediated by HDAC inhibition [54]. Panobinostat treatment also showed effective HDAC inhibition in breast, prostate, colon, and pancreatic cancer cell lines, while its effects on normal cells were marginal [55,56], suggesting its cancer-specific selectivity.

4.2.3. NVP-LAQ824

NVP-LAQ824 (dacinostat), another PsA analogue, is a derivative of 4-aminomethylcinnamic hydroxamic acid, which has entered phase I clinical trials [57,58] for the treatment of solid tumors and leukemia. NVP-LAQ824 inhibits HDAC activities and exerts anticancer effects at nanomolar concentrations through a mechanism of action involving the disruption of the charge-relay network via zinc chelation. Dacinostat may interfere with epidermal growth factor-mediated signaling in breast cancer via two independent epigenetic mechanisms involving a decrease in human epidermal growth factor receptor 2 (HER2) mRNA levels and by proteasomal degradation via an increase in the chaperone protein Hsp90. This effect is due to a further increase in acetylation levels induced by a dacinostat-mediated inhibitory mechanism [59]. NVP-LAQ824 was also proposed as a novel HDACi due to its ability to activate p21 at promoter and protein expression level, inhibit cyclin-dependent kinase 2 kinase activity, reduce retinoblastoma phosphorylation, and cause cell cycle arrest selectively in different cancer cell lines and in vivo models [60]. NVP-LAQ824 can also epigenetically modulate macrophage immune response through a mechanism involving recruitment of the transcriptional repressors HDAC11 and PU.1 to the *IL-10* gene promoter. This biological effect results in *IL-10* inhibition and improved responsiveness of CD4+ T cells [61].

4.2.4. Trichostatin A

Trichostatin A (TSA) is an hydroxamic acid originally isolated from the bacterium *Streptomyces platensis*, present in soil, which exerts antifungal, antibacterial, and antineoplastic activities as well as a broad spectrum of reversible HDAC inhibitory functions. Clinical trials investigating TSA in cancer are currently recruiting (NCT03838926, NCT03784417). In a recent study, malignant melanoma cells were treated with TSA and subjected to whole-transcriptome profiling. Data analysis showed that TSA was able to drastically change the transcriptome and several up- and downregulated transcripts were identified within BRAF-mutated melanoma cells. Specifically, TSA was able to downregulate MAPK/MEK/BRAF axis without affecting HDAC and BRAF pathways [62]. Sirtuin 6 is a class III HDAC enzyme involved in various epigenetic-like activities such as gene silencing regulation and DNA repair mechanisms, as well as blood glucose level regulation and stress resistance. Dysregulation of sirtuin 6 has a strong impact in various diseases including dysmetabolism, neurodegeneration, diabetes, and cancer. Since the tumor suppressor protein p53 upregulates sirtuin 6 via a deacetylation mechanism, histone H3 and p53 acetylation (via suppression of sirtuin 6) by TSA has a robust action on cancer cells as the posttranslational modification mediated by acetylation restores the regulation of p53 to normal physiological conditions [63]. TSA analogues such as trichostatic acid, JBIR-109, JBIR-110, and JBIR-111 derive from cultures of the marine sponge-derived *Streptomyces* sp. strain RM72 [64]. The JBIR-17 analogue was instead isolated from *Streptomyces* sp.

26634, in turn isolated from a leaf of the *Kerria japonica* shrub collected in Iwata, Japan [65]. These derivatives display similar biological effects and may be used as lead compounds for the generation of more active drugs.

4.2.5. Vorinostat

Vorinostat (SAHA, ZOLINZA®, Merck & Co., Inc., Kenilworth, NJ, USA) was the first HDACi approved by the FDA for the treatment of cutaneous T-cell lymphoma (CTCL) in 2006. Vorinostat is a synthetic derivative of the first natural hydroxamate HDACi identified, TSA, described in the previous subsection [66]. Vorinostat is a pan HDAC inhibitor and the most studied synthetic derivative compound from a natural source. Currently, about 40 clinical trials are in the recruitment phase (the most recent are NCT04308330, NCT04339751, NCT03803605, NCT03056495, NCT02638090, NCT04357873, NCT03167437, NCT03843528, NCT03842696) for a wide variety of diseases. Furthermore, a broad spectrum of datasets present in literature describe and demonstrate the multiple epigenetic roles of vorinostat in cancer and other disorders, as most recently reported in [67–74].

Table 1. Natural phenolic compounds and their derivatives, and their epigenetic role in cancer.

Compound	Structural Formula	Chemical Class	Source	Species	Epigenetic Mechanism	Ref
Psammaplin A		Phenolic compound	Sponge	*Psammaplin aplysilla, Thorectopsammaxana*	DNMT inhibition (in vitro)	[36,44,47,50]
					HDAC inhibition (in vitro)	[37,42,43,46,47,57–59,61,64,66]
					Topoisomerase II inhibition (in vitro)	[39]
					Inhibition of DNA regulation (in vitro)	[36]
					Aminopeptidase N inhibition (in vitro)	[40]
					SIRT1 induction (in vitro)	[47]
					HDAC inhibition (in vitro)	[46]
					Increased H3 acetylation (in vitro)	
Psammaplin F		Phenolic compound	Sponge	*Pseudoceratina purpurea*	HDAC inhibition (in vitro)	[50]

Table 1. Cont.

Compound	Structural Formula	Chemical Class	Source	Species	Epigenetic Mechanism	Ref
Psammaplin G		Phenolic compound	Sponge	*Pseudoceratina purpurea*	DNMT inhibition (in vitro)	[50]
Bisaprasin		Phenolic compound	Sponge	*Pseudoceratina purpurea*	DNMT inhibition (in vitro)	[50]
UVI5008		Phenolic compound		*Psammaplin derivative*	DNMT3a inhibition (in vitro)	[52]

Table 1. Cont.

Compound	Structural Formula	Chemical Class	Source	Species	Epigenetic Mechanism	Ref
					H3 hyperacetylation (ex vivo)	
					HDAC inhibition (in vitro)	
					HDAC1–4 inhibition (in vitro)	
					SIRT inhibition (in vitro)	
NVP-LAQ824 (dacinostat)		Hydroxamic acid		Psammaplin derivative	HDAC inhibition (in vitro)	[57,59,60]
					HDAC inhibition (in vivo)	[57,58]
					Increased H3 acetylation (in vitro)	[59–61]
					Increased H4 acetylation (in vitro)	[60,61]

Table 1. Cont.

Compound	Structural Formula	Chemical Class	Source	Species	Epigenetic Mechanism	Ref
Trichostatin A		Hydroxamic acid	Bacterium	*Streptomyces platensis*	HDAC inhibition (in vitro)	[62,66]
					MAPK/MEK/BRAF downregulation (in vitro)	[62]
					Increased H3 acetylation (in vitro)	[63]
JBIR-109		Trichostatin analogue	Sponge	*Streptomyces* sp. strain RM72	HDAC inhibition (in vitro)	[64]

Table 1. Cont.

Compound	Structural Formula	Chemical Class	Source	Species	Epigenetic Mechanism	Ref
JBIR-110		Trichostatin analogue	Sponge	*Streptomyces* sp. strain RM72	HDAC inhibition (in vitro)	[64]
JBIR-111		Trichostatin analogue	Sponge	*Streptomyces* sp. strain RM72	HDAC inhibition (in vitro)	[64]
JBIR-17		Phenolic compound	Bacterium	*Kerria japonica*	HDAC inhibition (in vitro)	[65]

Table 1. Cont.

Compound	Structural Formula	Chemical Class	Source	Species	Epigenetic Mechanism	Ref
Panobinostat		Phenolic compound	Sponge	*Psammaplin aplysilla*	Pan-HDAC inhibition (in vitro)	[53,54]
					HDAC inhibition (in vitro)	[55]
Vorinostat		Hydroxamic acid		Trichostatin A derivative	Pan HDAC inhibition (in vitro)	[67]
					HDAC inhibition (in vitro)	[66,69,70,73]
					HDAC inhibition (in vivo)	[67,68]
					mTOR inhibition (in vivo)	[68]
					PLD-1 upregulation (in vitro)	[70]

5. Cyclic Peptides

Marine-derived secondary metabolites are a huge source of multi-structured peptides possessing unique features able to regulate epigenetic mechanisms in cancer. The majority of these compounds are of natural origin and their backbone, characterized by a ring structure, has been used for the novel synthesis of more active and specific therapeutic drugs. This section mainly discusses depsipeptides and cyclic tetrapeptides (CTPs) as epigenetic-like anticancer agents. Depsipeptides are non-ribosomal peptides in which one or more amine bonds are replaced by the corresponding ester. These derivatives often contain non-protein amino acids and are found in the marine environment. Their synthesis is very straightforward and may lead to the development of several structural combinations useful for identifying the most effective anticancer agents. For instance, modifying amine groups to esters leads to an increase in lipophilicity, thus increasing their cell permeability [75]. Unlike depsipeptides, CTPs are very difficult to synthetize due to their highly complex structure characterized by four amino acids linked by eupeptide bonds. Specifically, CPTs contain L-, D-, and cyclic amino acids, which reduce the cyclic tension associated with CTPs. Many biochemical approaches coupled with extensive studies of three-dimensional structures by X-ray crystallography and NMR have been developed [76] to produce novel and more bioactive molecular structures. The following subsections describe the epigenetic role exhibited by marine-derived cyclic peptides displaying strong anticancer and anticancer-associated biological activities, which may have important implications for human health (Table 2 and Supplementary Table S2).

5.1. Romidepsin

Romidepsin ((Istodax®, Celgene Corp, Summit, NJ, USA) is a depsipeptide derived from the marine bacterium *Chromobacterium violaceum* and was the first epigenetic-like peptide approved by the FDA for the treatment of CTCL and other peripheral T-cell lymphomas in 2009 and 2011, respectively [77]. Romidepsin is mainly active against class I HDACs via a mechanism involving the release of a thiol by the disulfide bond of the peptide. The resulting mercaptan interacts with zinc at the HDAC binding site, thus inhibiting its activity. Romidepsin is currently the subject of about ten recruiting studies on cancer NCT02512497, NCT01947140, NCT02232516, NCT02616965, NCT03742921, NCT03161223, NCT02783625, NCT04257448, NCT03703375, NCT03593018, NCT02551718). About fifty trials investigating the role of romidepsin in cancer have been completed (the most recent are NCT02296398, NCT01913119, NCT01537744, NCT01324310, NCT01822886, NCT01353664). Other depsipeptide molecules include spiruchostatins [78,79], burkholdacs [80,81], and thailandepsin B [82,83], which are the product of the bacterium *Burkholderia thailandensis*, while FR901375 [84] and largazole [85] are derived from *Pseudomonas chlororaphis* and the cyanobacterium *Symploca* sp., respectively.

5.2. Plitidepsin

Also known as dehydrodidemnin B, plitidepsin (Aplidin®, PharmaMar, S.A., Colmenar Viejo, Spain) belongs to the class of didemnins isolated from the tunicate *Aplidium albicans* of the genus *Trididemnum* and is a natural HDACi with a broad spectrum of anticancer effects [86,87]. To date, six studies investigating the anticancer effects of plitidepsin have been completed (NCT01102426, NCT00884286, NCT01149681, NCT02100657, NCT00788099, NCT00229203), five have been terminated (NCT03117361, NCT00780143, NCT03070964, NCT00780975, NCT01876043), and only one is active for patients with COVID-19 (NCT04382066). Plitidepsin displays a strong inhibitory effect on cell growth and apoptosis in MM patients and cell lines, including those resistant to conventional therapies. This bioproduct also potently inhibits osteoclast differentiation and bone resorptive activity both in vivo and in vitro [88]. Among hundreds of plitidepsin analogues, PM01215 and PM02781 (patent WO 2002002596) were identified for their antiangiogenic effect in human primary cells [89].

5.3. Largazole

Largazole is a macrocyclic depsipeptide deriving from the marine cyanobacterium *Symploca* sp. [90]. This molecule is considered a superior hybrid thanks to its structural characteristics: it contains a thiazole unit linked to a 4-methylthiazoline, a nonmodified L-valine amino acid, and a thioester responsible for its mechanism of action. Largazole acts as an HDACi and is particularly active in colon cancer cell lines, as documented by a screening of 60 cell lines from the National Cancer Institute. In vivo and in vitro studies showed its apoptotic and antiproliferative activities as well as histone H3 hyperacetylation. Many similarities in terms of gene regulation were also found with two other potent HDACi, vorinostat and FK228, by gene transcriptomic profiling [85,91].

5.4. Azumamides

Azumamides are a group of CTPs isolated from the Japanese marine sponge *Mycale izuensis*, with five isoforms (A, B, C, D, E). Azumamides A–E were the first cyclic peptides with HDAC inhibitory activity isolated from marine organisms, and are characterized by four non-ribosomal amino acid residues, three of which are D-series amino acids while only one is a beta amino acid [92]. Azumamides A–E were identified for the first time as potent HDACi in a chronic myeloid leukemia cell line [93] following in vitro evaluation of HDAC activity. Specifically, increasing concentrations of azumamide A induced histone H3 acetylation while producing cytotoxic effects in colon cancer and chronic leukemia cells. Azumamide variants B, C, and E produced an HDAC inhibitory effect in human carcinoma cell lines with IC50 values in the micromolar range. Derivative E resulted the most active compound with inhibitory activities due to its different chemical structure represented by a carboxylic acid, which has a higher affinity for thee HDAC active site containing zinc ion, unlike the amide group present in the other azumamides A, B, and D [94]. From a mechanistic perspective, azumamide E was the only isoform found able to induce overexpression of p21, a well-known marker regulating cell cycle progression, in murine induced pluripotent stem cells [95].

5.5. Trapoxins

Trapoxin (TPX) A is a fungal-derived HDACi with a homodetic cyclic tetrapeptidic structure isolated from the species *Helicoma ambiens*. This molecule is an epoxyketone and exerts irreversible inhibitory effects on class I HDACs due to the analogous structure of its ketone carbonyl group and the carbonyl of the substrate acetyl-L-lysine of HDACs. A study reporting the creation of a novel X-ray structure characterized by trapoxin A bound to HDAC8 demonstrated that trapoxin A is a non-covalent HDAC8 inhibitor thanks to an α,β-epoxyketone side chain, which by chemical transition state is able to bind the HDAC active site containing zinc [96]. Cyclic hydroxamic acid-containing peptide (CHAP) 1 is a hybrid compound deriving from trapoxin A and TSA, in which the epoxyketone group is substituted by the hydroxamic acid instead of the epoxyketone and can reversibly inhibit HDACs at low nanomolar concentrations. Although several CHAP derivatives have been produced, only one showed antitumor activity in BDF1 mice bearing B16/BL6 tumor cells, suggesting the possibility of an improved synthesis of new hybrids [97].

Table 2. Cyclic peptides and alkaloids with their epigenetic anticancer role.

Compound	Structural Formula	Chemical Class	Source	Species	Epigenetic Mechanism	Ref
Romidepsin		Depsipeptide	Bacterium	*Chromobacterium violaceum*	HDAC inhibition (in vitro)	[80,82–84]
Plitidepsin		Cyclic tetrapeptide	Tunicate	*Aplidium albicans*	Caspase-3 upregulation (in vitro)	[87]
					Dephosphorylation of ERK1/2 and 5 (in vitro)	[88]
PM01215			Aplidin analogues		p16INK4A induction (in vitro)	[89]
					VEGF downregulation (in vitro)	

Table 2. Cont.

Compound	Structural Formula	Chemical Class	Source	Species	Epigenetic Mechanism	Ref
PM02781			Aplidin analogues		p16INK4A induction (in vitro)	[89]
Largazole		Macrocyclic depsipeptide	Cyanobacterium	*Symplocasp*	HDAC inhibition (in vitro)	[85,91]
					HDAC inhibition (in vivo)	[85]
Azumamides		Cyclic tetrapeptide	Sponge	*Mycale izuensis*	HDAC inhibition (in vitro)	[92,93,95]

Table 2. Cont.

Compound	Structural Formula	Chemical Class	Source	Species	Epigenetic Mechanism	Ref
Trapoxins		Cyclic tetrapeptide	Fungus	*Helicoma ambiens*	Increased H3 acetylation (in vitro)	[94]
					Class I HDAC inhibition (in vitro)	[96]
Apicidin		Cyclic tetrapeptide	Fungus	*Fusarium pallidoroseum*	HDAC inhibition (in vitro)	[97]
					HDAC8 inhibition (in vivo)	[98]
					p21 upregulation (in vitro)	[99]
					HDAC inhibition (in vitro)	[99,100]
					DNMT inhibition (in vitro)	[42]
					HDACs2/3 inhibition (in vitro)	[42]

Table 2. *Cont.*

Compound	Structural Formula	Chemical Class	Source	Species	Epigenetic Mechanism	Ref
Microsporins A and B		Cyclic peptide	Fungus	*Microsporum* cf. *gypseum*	HDAC inhibition (in vitro)	[101]
Isofistularin-3		Alkaloid	Sponge	*Aplysina aerophoba*	HDAC8 inhibition (in vitro) DNMT1 inhibition (in vitro)	[33]
Cyclostellettamines		Alkaloid	Sponge	*Xestospongia*	HDAC inhibition (in vitro)	[102,103]

5.6. Apicidin

Apicidin is a fungal metabolite derived from the species *Fusarium pallidoroseum*, in the *Sordariomycetes* class. It is an HDAC2 and 3 inhibitor and acts as a trapoxin A analogue, but lacks the epoxyketone functional group. Several studies described the anticancer activities of apicidin in vitro and in vivo [42,98,99]. A recent report investigated the characterization of HDAC3 in Notch signaling by comparing data obtained following apicidin treatment and HDAC3 loss of function in APRE T cell models. Gene expression data from RNA sequencing revealed a cluster of 65 upregulated genes and another of 368 downregulated genes in both HDAC knockdown and apicidin-treated cells. Many of the identified downregulated genes affected Notch signaling, and in particular apicidin treatment led to an increase in epigenetic markers such as acetylation levels of histone H3 lysine 27 (H3K27), histone H3 lysine 18 (H3K18), and histone H3 lysine 9 (H3K9), while a decrease in H3K27 acetylation was detected at the recombination signal binding protein for immunoglobulin kappa J region binding sites associated with Notch target genes. Apicidin treatment affected NOTCH1 intracellular domain stability via a mechanism driven by proteasomal degradation mediated by ubiquitination [100]. Microsporins A and B are also marine-derived metabolites from the fungus *Microsporum* cf. *gypseum* that display HDACi action. Their cytotoxic-related activities were reported in colon adenocarcinoma cells and a precursor to the unusual amino acid residue of the anticancer agent microsporin B was subsequently synthetized as (S)-2-Boc-Amino-8-(R)-(tert-butyldimethylsilanyloxy) decanoic acid [101].

6. Alkaloids

Alkaloids are natural compounds characterized by a nitrogen-heterocyclic structure. Specifically, marine alkaloids have an amine nitrogen group and a carbon ring and mainly derive from marine organisms such as sponges, algae (green, brown, and red), coelenterates, and tunicates. These metabolites display several properties, acting as antitumor, antiviral, antimalarial, antifungal, and anti-osteoporosis agents. Marine alkaloids may be used as chemotherapeutics or as lead compounds for structural modification (Table 2).

6.1. Brominated Alkaloids: Isofistularin-3

Brominated alkaloids (BAs) include the promising natural molecule isofistularin-3 (Iso-3), whose source is the sponge Aplysina aerophoba. Structurally, this compound shows similarities with PsA, a well-known bromotyrosine derivative. Iso-3 was screened for its DNMT1 inhibitory activities in vitro together with a library of compounds. The conformational structure of this compound was also analyzed by molecular docking prediction, revealing an inhibition interaction between DNMT1 and DNA via a conserved CXXC motif affecting binding activity via positively charged residues. BAs lack a thiol linker moiety, explaining the absence of HDAC inhibitory activity. Iso-3 was shown to have anticancer potential in lymphoma cells, leading to cell cycle arrest, morphological changes, and authophagy as well as caspase-dependent and -independent cell death [33].

6.2. Bispyridinium Alkaloids: Cyclostellettamines

Marine-derived alkaloids include a group of compounds with a macrocyclic ring of the precursor bispyridinium alkaloid called cyclostellettamines. Cyclostellettamines A and G together with dehydrocyclostellettamine D and E, shown to act as HDAC inhibitors in the myelogenous leukemia K562 cell line, were isolated from a marine sponge of the genus Xestospongia [102]. The inhibitory effect of these compounds was very weak, with cytotoxic activities observed in human cervix carcinoma, mouse leukemia, and rat fibroblasts, suggesting that multifunctional targets of these molecules can modulate their cytotoxic effects. A synthetic route for cyclostellectamines A–L and dehdrocyclostellettamines D and E was developed using bispyridinium dienes precursors and subsequent catalytic hydrogenation. The compounds obtained and their precursors were tested in vitro in an AML cell line for HDAC activity, cell cycle modulation, acetylation levels of histone H3 and tubulin, differentiation, and apoptosis. The precursors were found to have more potent activities than the natural compounds [103].

7. Conclusions

Anticancer therapy-associated drawbacks include resistance to drug treatments and the occurrence of relapses, whereby, finding and characterizing new drugs is one of the main objectives. The development of new drugs with anticancer activity follows a multidisciplinary approach that generally begins with the identification and retrieval of new bioactive molecules from natural sources, which in turn undergo preliminary evaluations assessing biological activity, toxicological tests, and chemical/biotechnological synthesis [23]. The difficulty in finding natural substances of marine origin and collecting sufficient quantities for clinical and preclinical experimentation often hinders the possibility of isolating natural biomolecules, preventing the development of promising compounds. Although the epigenetic role of natural compounds has been discussed in previous studies, the aspects related to the discovery of new marine-derived anticancer bio-compounds highlighting the variability that characterizes the organisms themselves and their surrounding environment that, have not been extensively discussed previously. The chemical-physical-biological characteristics of natural marine compounds are unique and cannot be found in the terrestrial environment, but the properties of already characterized molecules can be exploited for a new chemical synthesis and molecular modeling of new products to refine their anticancer activity. Natural marine bio-compounds are produced in co-evolution with biological systems and can be specific mediators of epigenetic processes in cancer, in turn influencing the abundance and distribution of species in nature and the functioning of ecosystems. A very important aspect also involves the concept of environmental sustainability, linked to the strong need to reduce the impact of the ecosystem on natural resources and the need to safeguard the marine environment to maintain and preserve biodiversity and prevent as much as possible the decrease of ecosystem functions. Marine biotechnologies are increasingly specializing in the development of new methods based on the evaluation of the sustainability of organisms sampling for their subsequent use associated with new selection criteria and the creation of marine biobanks.

Marine organisms produce secondary metabolites whose chemical-physical and biological characteristics are extremely variable due to biotic and abiotic factors, adding a further level of complexity to research and development efforts in this field. Most compounds of marine origin can be synthesized and more than 10 are currently at an advanced clinical stage [104]. Furthermore, new and advanced technologies allow the biotechnological production of these molecules either through cloning techniques or gene cluster manipulation, overcoming a number of obstacles including those linked to environmental risks associated with the potential loss of genetic resources caused by overharvesting of producer organisms. Major interest is currently focusing on the identification and biosynthetic characterization of natural marine compounds, particularly those derived from the secondary metabolism, potentially available as active principles (lead compounds) or biochemically comparable (biosynthetic analogues) to active compounds, for the development of new epigenetic drugs. Many marine compounds with anticancer activity capable of modulating microRNA and epigenetic mechanisms such as DNA methylation, acetylation, and histone methylation, have a considerable impact on the regulation of gene expression [105]. Marine organisms are themselves subject to intrinsic epigenetic changes induced by the surrounding environment, causing them to produce biomolecules with unique structural characteristics that can act as an imprint to produce a novel synthesis. An example of a response to ecological changes is represented by dimethylsulfoniopropionate (DMSP), a metabolite that can be degraded by phytoplankton or bacteria to produce dimethylsulfide (DMS). Inducing the bloom of the Gulf of Mexico phytoplankton, bacterioplankton cells can demethylate this metabolite via the dmdA gene pointing out several dmdA subclases identified in response to ecological alteration [106]. Epigenetic mechanisms such as DNA methylation and histone modifications may also affect coral adaptation to climate change [107] spreading to subsequent generations, but these mechanisms still need to be further studied [108]. The chromosomal characterization of different species of sponges has been carried out on the basis of their phylogenetic relationships, identifying similar karyotypes, harboring a diploid chromosome number. A high variability in the extent of the genome has been defined also in species belonging to the same class, reflecting distinct genomic organization [109]. Further studies will allow to understand how epigenetic mechanisms, which are sometimes stochastic events and often are responsible for locus-specific gene expression via chromatin modifications, can be correlated with organism ploidy. As cancer treatments are increasingly based on personalized medicine due to the complexity of the disease and the multitude of hallmarks involved, including epigenetic alterations, developing new bioactive molecules derived from marine sources will provide a vast repertoire of substances with pharmacological activity that can be used alone or in combination with other epigenetic drugs, chemotherapy, or radiotherapy.

Supplementary Materials: The following are available online at https://www.mdpi.com/1660-3397/19/1/15/s1. Table S1: Recent registered clinical trials on phenolic compounds with epigenetic mechanisms in different cancers alone and in co-treatment. Table S2: Recent registered clinical trials on cyclic peptides with epigenetic mechanisms in different cancers alone and in co-treatment.

Author Contributions: M.C. conceived the article and wrote the manuscript. E.F. participated in data collection and wrote the manuscript. L.A. and A.N. reviewed and revised the final draft. All authors have read and agreed to the published version of the manuscript.

Funding: This work was funded by Vanvitelli per la Ricerca "AdipCare" (ID 263), Campania Regional Government Technology Platform Lotta alle Patologie Oncologiche: iCURE (B21C17000030007), Campania Regional Government FASE2: IDEAL (B63D18000560007), MIUR, Proof of Concept POC01_00043, Programma V: ALERE 2020—Progetto competitivo "NETWINS" -D.R. no. 138 of 17/02/2020.

Institutional Review Board Statement: Not applicable.

Informed Consent Statement: Not applicable.

Acknowledgments: We thank C. Fisher for English language editing.

Conflicts of Interest: The authors declare no conflict of interest.

References

1. Poli, A.; Finore, I.; Romano, I.; Gioiello, A.; Lama, L.; Nicolaus, B. Microbial Diversity in Extreme Marine Habitats and Their Biomolecules. *Microorganisms* **2017**, *5*, 25. [CrossRef] [PubMed]
2. Firn, R.D.; Jones, C.G. The evolution of secondary metabolism-a unifying model. *Mol. Microbiol.* **2000**, *37*, 989–994. [CrossRef] [PubMed]
3. Giordano, D.; Coppola, D.; Russo, R.; Denaro, R.; Giuliano, L.; Lauro, F.M.; di Prisco, G.; Verde, C. Marine Microbial Secondary Metabolites: Pathways, Evolution and Physiological Roles. *Adv. Microb. Physiol.* **2015**, *66*, 357–428. [PubMed]
4. Carneiro, V.C.; Lyko, F. Rapid Epigenetic Adaptation in Animals and Its Role in Invasiveness. *Integr. Comp. Biol.* **2020**, *60*, 267–274. [CrossRef]
5. Mirbahai, L.; Chipman, J.K. Epigenetic memory of environmental organisms: A reflection of lifetime stressor exposures. *Mutat. Res. Genet. Toxicol. Environ. Mutagen.* **2014**, *764–765*, 10–17. [CrossRef]
6. Jeremias, G.; Barbosa, J.; Marques, S.M.; Asselman, J.; Goncalves, F.J.M.; Pereira, J.L. Synthesizing the role of epigenetics in the response and adaptation of species to climate change in freshwater ecosystems. *Mol. Ecol.* **2018**, *27*, 2790–2806. [CrossRef]
7. Seca, A.M.L.; Pinto, D. Plant Secondary Metabolites as Anticancer Agents: Successes in Clinical Trials and Therapeutic Application. *Int. J. Mol. Sci.* **2018**, *19*, 263. [CrossRef]
8. Kiuru, P.; D'Auria, M.V.; Muller, C.D.; Tammela, P.; Vuorela, H.; Yli-Kauhaluoma, J. Exploring marine resources for bioactive compounds. *Planta Med.* **2014**, *80*, 1234–1246. [CrossRef]
9. Lindequist, U. Marine-Derived Pharmaceuticals-Challenges and Opportunities. *Biomol. Ther.* **2016**, *24*, 561–571. [CrossRef]
10. Sun, W.; Wu, W.; Liu, X.; Zaleta-Pinet, D.A.; Clark, B.R. Bioactive Compounds Isolated from Marine-Derived Microbes in China: 2009–2018. *Mar. Drugs* **2019**, *17*, 339. [CrossRef]
11. Weinhold, B. Epigenetics: The science of change. *Environ. Health Perspect.* **2006**, *114*, A160–A167. [CrossRef] [PubMed]
12. Baylin, S.B.; Jones, P.A. Epigenetic Determinants of Cancer. *Cold Spring Harb. Perspect. Biol.* **2016**, *8*, a019505. [CrossRef] [PubMed]
13. D'Urso, A.; Brickner, J.H. Mechanisms of epigenetic memory. *Trends Genet.* **2014**, *30*, 230–236. [CrossRef] [PubMed]

14. Thomas, M.L.; Marcato, P. Epigenetic Modifications as Biomarkers of Tumor Development, Therapy Response, and Recurrence across the Cancer Care Continuum. *Cancers* **2018**, *10*, 101. [CrossRef] [PubMed]
15. Yang, A.Y.; Kim, H.; Li, W.; Kong, A.N. Natural compound-derived epigenetic regulators targeting epigenetic readers, writers and erasers. *Curr. Top. Med. Chem.* **2016**, *16*, 697–713. [CrossRef] [PubMed]
16. Torres, I.O.; Fujimori, D.G. Functional coupling between writers, erasers and readers of histone and DNA methylation. *Curr. Opin. Struct. Biol.* **2015**, *35*, 68–75. [CrossRef]
17. Biswas, S.; Rao, C.M. Epigenetic tools (The Writers, The Readers and The Erasers) and their implications in cancer therapy. *Eur. J. Pharmacol.* **2018**, *837*, 8–24. [CrossRef]
18. Atanasov, A.G.; Waltenberger, B.; Pferschy-Wenzig, E.M.; Linder, T.; Wawrosch, C.; Uhrin, P.; Temml, V.; Wang, L.; Schwaiger, S.; Heiss, E.H.; et al. Discovery and resupply of pharmacologically active plant-derived natural products: A review. *Biotechnol. Adv.* **2015**, *33*, 1582–1614. [CrossRef]
19. Bosch, T.C.; Adamska, M.; Augustin, R.; Domazet-Loso, T.; Foret, S.; Fraune, S.; Funayama, N.; Grasis, J.; Hamada, M.; Hatta, M.; et al. How do environmental factors influence life cycles and development? An experimental framework for early-diverging metazoans. *Bioessays* **2014**, *36*, 1185–1194. [CrossRef]
20. Dias, B.G.; Maddox, S.; Klengel, T.; Ressler, K.J. Epigenetic mechanisms underlying learning and the inheritance of learned behaviors. *Trends Neurosci.* **2015**, *38*, 96–107. [CrossRef]
21. Seca, A.M.L.; Pinto, D. Biological Potential and Medical Use of Secondary Metabolites. *Medicines* **2019**, *6*, 66. [CrossRef] [PubMed]
22. Vetrivel, I.; Mahajan, S.; Tyagi, M.; Hoffmann, L.; Sanejouand, Y.H.; Srinivasan, N.; de Brevern, A.G.; Cadet, F.; Offmann, B. Knowledge-based prediction of protein backbone conformation using a structural alphabet. *PLoS ONE* **2017**, *12*, e0186215. [CrossRef] [PubMed]
23. Khalifa, S.A.M.; Elias, N.; Farag, M.A.; Chen, L.; Saeed, A.; Hegazy, M.F.; Moustafa, M.S.; Abd El-Wahed, A.; Al-Mousawi, S.M.; Musharraf, S.G.; et al. Marine Natural Products: A Source of Novel Anticancer Drugs. *Mar. Drugs* **2019**, *17*, 491. [CrossRef] [PubMed]
24. Lin, D.; Xiao, M.; Zhao, J.; Li, Z.; Xing, B.; Li, X.; Kong, M.; Li, L.; Zhang, Q.; Liu, Y.; et al. An Overview of Plant Phenolic Compounds and Their Importance in Human Nutrition and Management of Type 2 Diabetes. *Molecules* **2016**, *21*, 1374. [CrossRef] [PubMed]
25. Baral, B.; Akhgari, A.; Metsa-Ketela, M. Activation of microbial secondary metabolic pathways: Avenues and challenges. *Synth. Syst. Biotechnol.* **2018**, *3*, 163–178. [CrossRef] [PubMed]
26. Tomizawa, D.; Tanaka, S.; Hasegawa, D.; Iwamoto, S.; Hiramatsu, H.; Kiyokawa, N.; Miyachi, H.; Horibe, K.; Saito, A.M.; Taga, T.; et al. Evaluation of high-dose cytarabine in induction therapy for children with de novo acute myeloid leukemia: A study protocol of the Japan Children's Cancer Group Multi-Center Seamless Phase II-III Randomized Trial (JPLSG AML-12). *Jpn. J. Clin. Oncol.* **2018**, *48*, 587–593. [CrossRef]
27. Tamborini, L.; Previtali, C.; Annunziata, F.; Bavaro, T.; Terreni, M.; Calleri, E.; Rinaldi, F.; Pinto, A.; Speranza, G.; Ubiali, D.; et al. An Enzymatic Flow-Based Preparative Route to Vidarabine. *Molecules* **2020**, *25*, 1223. [CrossRef]
28. McDowell, G.C., 2nd; Pope, J.E. Intrathecal Ziconotide: Dosing and Administration Strategies in Patients with Refractory Chronic Pain. *Neuromodulation* **2016**, *19*, 522–532. [CrossRef]
29. Czyz, K.; Sokola-Wysoczanska, E.; Bodkowski, R.; Cholewinska, P.; Wyrostek, A. Dietary Omega-3 Source Effect on the Fatty Acid Profile of Intramuscular and Perimuscular Fat-Preliminary Study on a Rat Model. *Nutrients* **2020**, *12*, 3382. [CrossRef]
30. Nakano, K.; Hayakawa, K.; Funauchi, Y.; Tanizawa, T.; Ae, K.; Matsumoto, S.; Tomomatsu, J.; Ono, M.; Taira, S.; Nishizawa, M.; et al. Differences in the efficacy and safety of eribulin in patients with soft tissue sarcoma by histological subtype and treatment line. *Mol. Clin. Oncol.* **2020**, *14*, 13. [CrossRef]
31. Oberic, L.; Delzor, F.; Protin, C.; Perriat, S.; Laurent, C.; Grand, A.; Canonge, J.M.; Borel, C.; Gauthier, M.; Ysebaert, L.; et al. Brentuximab vedotin in real life, a seven year experience in patients with refractory/relapsed CD30+ T cell lymphoma. *J. Oncol. Pharm. Pract.* **2020**, 1078155220968615. [CrossRef] [PubMed]
32. Eccles, R.; Winther, B.; Johnston, S.L.; Robinson, P.; Trampisch, M.; Koelsch, S. Efficacy and safety of iota-carrageenan nasal spray versus placebo in early treatment of the common cold in adults: The ICICC trial. *Respir. Res.* **2015**, *16*, 121. [CrossRef] [PubMed]
33. Florean, C.; Schnekenburger, M.; Lee, J.Y.; Kim, K.R.; Mazumder, A.; Song, S.; Kim, J.M.; Grandjenette, C.; Kim, J.G.; Yoon, A.Y.; et al. Discovery and characterization of Isofistularin-3, a marine brominated alkaloid, as a new DNA demethylating agent inducing cell cycle arrest and sensitization to TRAIL in cancer cells. *Oncotarget* **2016**, *7*, 24027–24049. [CrossRef] [PubMed]
34. Del Rio, D.; Rodriguez-Mateos, A.; Spencer, J.P.; Tognolini, M.; Borges, G.; Crozier, A. Dietary (poly)phenolics in human health: Structures, bioavailability, and evidence of protective effects against chronic diseases. *Antioxid. Redox Signal.* **2013**, *18*, 1818–1892. [CrossRef] [PubMed]
35. Ferreira, I.; Martins, N.; Barros, L. Phenolic Compounds and Its Bioavailability: In Vitro Bioactive Compounds or Health Promoters? *Adv. Food Nutr. Res.* **2017**, *82*, 1–44. [PubMed]
36. Godert, A.M.; Angelino, N.; Woloszynska-Read, A.; Morey, S.R.; James, S.R.; Karpf, A.R.; Sufrin, J.R. An improved synthesis of psammaplin A. *Bioorg. Med. Chem. Lett.* **2006**, *16*, 3330–3333. [CrossRef]
37. Jing, Q.; Hu, X.; Ma, Y.; Mu, J.; Liu, W.; Xu, F.; Li, Z.; Bai, J.; Hua, H.; Li, D. Marine-Derived Natural Lead Compound Disulfide-Linked Dimer Psammaplin A: Biological Activity and Structural Modification. *Mar. Drugs* **2019**, *17*, 384. [CrossRef]

38. Kim, D.; Lee, I.S.; Jung, J.H.; Yang, S.I. Psammaplin A, a natural bromotyrosine derivative from a sponge, possesses the antibacterial activity against methicillin-resistant *Staphylococcus aureus* and the DNA gyrase-inhibitory activity. *Arch. Pharm. Res.* **1999**, *22*, 25–29. [CrossRef]
39. Jiang, Y.; Ahn, E.Y.; Ryu, S.H.; Kim, D.K.; Park, J.S.; Yoon, H.J.; You, S.; Lee, B.J.; Lee, D.S.; Jung, J.H. Cytotoxicity of psammaplin A from a two-sponge association may correlate with the inhibition of DNA replication. *BMC Cancer* **2004**, *4*, 70. [CrossRef]
40. Shim, J.S.; Lee, H.S.; Shin, J.; Kwon, H.J. Psammaplin A, a marine natural product, inhibits aminopeptidase N and suppresses angiogenesis in vitro. *Cancer Lett.* **2004**, *203*, 163–169. [CrossRef]
41. Salam, K.A.; Furuta, A.; Noda, N.; Tsuneda, S.; Sekiguchi, Y.; Yamashita, A.; Moriishi, K.; Nakakoshi, M.; Tsubuki, M.; Tani, H.; et al. Psammaplin A inhibits hepatitis C virus NS3 helicase. *J. Nat. Med.* **2013**, *67*, 765–772. [CrossRef] [PubMed]
42. You, J.S.; Kang, J.K.; Lee, E.K.; Lee, J.C.; Lee, S.H.; Jeon, Y.J.; Koh, D.H.; Ahn, S.H.; Seo, D.W.; Lee, H.Y.; et al. Histone deacetylase inhibitor apicidin downregulates DNA methyltransferase 1 expression and induces repressive histone modifications via recruitment of corepressor complex to promoter region in human cervix cancer cells. *Oncogene* **2008**, *27*, 1376–1386. [CrossRef] [PubMed]
43. Zhou, Y.D.; Li, J.; Du, L.; Mahdi, F.; Le, T.P.; Chen, W.L.; Swanson, S.M.; Watabe, K.; Nagle, D.G. Biochemical and Anti-Triple Negative Metastatic Breast Tumor Cell Properties of Psammaplins. *Mar. Drugs* **2018**, *16*, 442. [CrossRef]
44. Kim, H.J.; Kim, J.H.; Chie, E.K.; Young, P.D.; Kim, I.A.; Kim, I.H. DNMT (DNA methyltransferase) inhibitors radiosensitize human cancer cells by suppressing DNA repair activity. *Radiat. Oncol.* **2012**, *7*, 39. [CrossRef] [PubMed]
45. Ahn, M.Y.; Jung, J.H.; Na, Y.J.; Kim, H.S. A natural histone deacetylase inhibitor, Psammaplin A, induces cell cycle arrest and apoptosis in human endometrial cancer cells. *Gynecol. Oncol.* **2008**, *108*, 27–33. [CrossRef]
46. Baud, M.G.; Leiser, T.; Petrucci, V.; Gunaratnam, M.; Neidle, S.; Meyer-Almes, F.J.; Fuchter, M.J. Thioester derivatives of the natural product psammaplin A as potent histone deacetylase inhibitors. *Beilstein J. Org. Chem.* **2013**, *9*, 81–88. [CrossRef]
47. Pereira, R.; Benedetti, R.; Pérez-Rodríguez, S.; Nebbioso, A.; García-Rodríguez, J.; Carafa, V.; Stuhldreier, M.; Conte, M.; Rodríguez-Barrios, F.; Stunnenberg, H.G.; et al. Indole-derived psammaplin A analogues as epigenetic modulators with multiple inhibitory activities. *J. Med. Chem.* **2012**, *55*, 9467–9491. [CrossRef]
48. Mujumdar, P.; Teruya, K.; Tonissen, K.F.; Vullo, D.; Supuran, C.T.; Peat, T.S.; Poulsen, S.A. An Unusual Natural Product Primary Sulfonamide: Synthesis, Carbonic Anhydrase Inhibition, and Protein X-ray Structures of Psammaplin C. *J. Med. Chem.* **2016**, *59*, 5462–5470. [CrossRef]
49. Yang, Q.; Liu, D.; Sun, D.; Yang, S.; Hu, G.; Wu, Z.; Zhao, L. Synthesis of the marine bromotyrosine psammaplin F and crystal structure of a psammaplin A analogue. *Molecules* **2010**, *15*, 8784–8795. [CrossRef]
50. Piña, I.C.; Gautschi, J.T.; Wang, G.Y.; Sanders, M.L.; Schmitz, F.J.; France, D.; Cornell-Kennon, S.; Sambucetti, L.C.; Remiszewski, S.W.; Perez, L.B.; et al. Psammaplins from the sponge *Pseudoceratina purpurea*: Inhibition of both histone deacetylase and DNA methyltransferase. *J. Org. Chem.* **2003**, *68*, 3866–3873. [CrossRef]
51. Park, Y.; Liu, Y.; Hong, J.; Lee, C.O.; Cho, H.; Kim, D.K.; Im, K.S.; Jung, J.H. New bromotyrosine derivatives from an association of two sponges, *Jaspis wondoensis* and *Poecillastra wondoensis*. *J. Nat. Prod.* **2003**, *66*, 1495–1498. [CrossRef] [PubMed]
52. Nebbioso, A.; Pereira, R.; Khanwalkar, H.; Matarese, F.; García-Rodríguez, J.; Miceli, M.; Logie, C.; Kedinger, V.; Ferrara, F.; Stunnenberg, H.G.; et al. Death receptor pathway activation and increase of ROS production by the triple epigenetic inhibitor UVI5008. *Mol. Cancer Ther.* **2011**, *10*, 2394–2404. [CrossRef] [PubMed]
53. Gahr, S.; Mayr, C.; Kiesslich, T.; Illig, R.; Neureiter, D.; Alinger, B.; Ganslmayer, M.; Wissniowski, T.; Fazio, P.D.; Montalbano, R.; et al. The pan-deacetylase inhibitor panobinostat affects angiogenesis in hepatocellular carcinoma models via modulation of CTGF expression. *Int. J. Oncol.* **2015**, *47*, 963–970. [CrossRef] [PubMed]
54. Helland, O.; Popa, M.; Bischof, K.; Gjertsen, B.T.; McCormack, E.; Bjorge, L. The HDACi Panobinostat Shows Growth Inhibition Both In Vitro and in a Bioluminescent Orthotopic Surgical Xenograft Model of Ovarian Cancer. *PLoS ONE* **2016**, *11*, e0158208. [CrossRef] [PubMed]
55. Atadja, P. Development of the pan-DAC inhibitor panobinostat (LBH589): Successes and challenges. *Cancer Lett.* **2009**, *280*, 233–241. [CrossRef] [PubMed]
56. Johnstone, R.W. Histone-deacetylase inhibitors: Novel drugs for the treatment of cancer. *Nat. Rev. Drug Discov.* **2002**, *1*, 287–299. [CrossRef]
57. Remiszewski, S.W. The discovery of NVP-LAQ824: From concept to clinic. *Curr. Med. Chem.* **2003**, *10*, 2393–2402. [CrossRef]
58. Cuneo, K.C.; Fu, A.; Osusky, K.; Huamani, J.; Hallahan, D.E.; Geng, L. Histone deacetylase inhibitor NVP-LAQ824 sensitizes human nonsmall cell lung cancer to the cytotoxic effects of ionizing radiation. *Anticancer Drugs* **2007**, *18*, 793–800. [CrossRef]
59. Fuino, L.; Bali, P.; Wittmann, S.; Donapaty, S.; Guo, F.; Yamaguchi, H.; Wang, H.G.; Atadja, P.; Bhalla, K. Histone deacetylase inhibitor LAQ824 down-regulates Her-2 and sensitizes human breast cancer cells to trastuzumab, taxotere, gemcitabine, and epothilone B. *Mol. Cancer Ther.* **2003**, *2*, 971–984.
60. Atadja, P.; Gao, L.; Kwon, P.; Trogani, N.; Walker, H.; Hsu, M.; Yeleswarapu, L.; Chandramouli, N.; Perez, L.; Versace, R.; et al. Selective growth inhibition of tumor cells by a novel histone deacetylase inhibitor, NVP-LAQ824. *Cancer Res.* **2004**, *64*, 689–695. [CrossRef]
61. Wang, H.; Cheng, F.; Woan, K.; Sahakian, E.; Merino, O.; Rock-Klotz, J.; Vicente-Suarez, I.; Pinilla-Ibarz, J.; Wright, K.L.; Seto, E.; et al. Histone deacetylase inhibitor LAQ824 augments inflammatory responses in macrophages through transcriptional regulation of IL-10. *J. Immunol.* **2011**, *186*, 3986–3996. [CrossRef] [PubMed]

62. Mazzio, E.A.; Soliman, K.F.A. Whole-transcriptomic Profile of SK-MEL-3 Melanoma Cells Treated with the Histone Deacetylase Inhibitor: Trichostatin, A. *Cancer Genom. Proteom.* **2018**, *15*, 349–364. [CrossRef] [PubMed]
63. Wood, M.; Rymarchyk, S.; Zheng, S.; Cen, Y. Trichostatin A inhibits deacetylation of histone H3 and p53 by SIRT6. *Arch. Biochem. Biophys.* **2018**, *638*, 8–17. [CrossRef] [PubMed]
64. Hosoya, T.; Hirokawa, T.; Takagi, M.; Shin-ya, K. Trichostatin analogues JBIR-109, JBIR-110, and JBIR-111 from the marine sponge-derived *Streptomyces* sp. RM72. *J. Nat. Prod.* **2012**, *75*, 285–289. [CrossRef]
65. Ueda, J.Y.; Hwang, J.H.; Maeda, S.; Kato, T.; Ochiai, K.; Isshiki, K.; Yoshida, M.; Takagi, M.; Shin-ya, K. JBIR-17, a novel trichostatin analog from Streptomyces sp. 26634. *J. Antibiot.* **2009**, *62*, 283–285. [CrossRef]
66. Codd, R.; Braich, N.; Liu, J.; Soe, C.Z.; Pakchung, A.A. Zn(II)-dependent histone deacetylase inhibitors: Suberoylanilide hydroxamic acid and trichostatin A. *Int. J. Biochem. Cell Biol.* **2009**, *41*, 736–739. [CrossRef]
67. Makena, M.R.; Nguyen, T.H.; Koneru, B.; Hindle, A.; Chen, W.H.; Verlekar, D.U.; Kang, M.H.; Reynolds, C.P. Vorinostat and fenretinide synergize in preclinical models of T-cell lymphoid malignancies. *Anticancer Drugs* **2020**, *32*, 34–43. [CrossRef]
68. Janku, F.; Park, H.; Call, S.G.; Madwani, K.; Oki, Y.; Subbiah, V.; Hong, D.S.; Naing, A.; Velez-Bravo, V.M.; Barnes, T.G.; et al. Safety and Efficacy of Vorinostat Plus Sirolimus or Everolimus in Patients with Relapsed Refractory Hodgkin Lymphoma. *Clin. Cancer Res.* **2020**, *26*, 5579–5587. [CrossRef]
69. Abdel-Ghany, S.; Raslan, S.; Tombuloglu, H.; Shamseddin, A.; Cevik, E.; Said, O.A.; Madyan, E.F.; Senel, M.; Bozkurt, A.; Rehman, S.; et al. Vorinostat-loaded titanium oxide nanoparticles (anatase) induce G2/M cell cycle arrest in breast cancer cells via PALB2 upregulation. *3 Biotech.* **2020**, *10*, 407. [CrossRef]
70. Kang, D.W.; Hwang, W.C.; Noh, Y.N.; Kang, Y.; Jang, Y.; Kim, J.A.; Min, D.S. Phospholipase D1 is upregulated by vorinostat and confers resistance to vorinostat in glioblastoma. *J. Cell Physiol.* **2020**, *236*, 549–560. [CrossRef]
71. Skelton, W.P., 4th; Turba, E.; Sokol, L. Durable Complete Response to AMG 655 (Conatumumab) and Vorinostat in a Patient with Relapsed Classical Hodgkin Lymphoma: Extraordinary Response from a Phase 1b Clinical Protocol. *Clin. Lymphoma Myeloma Leuk.* **2020**, *20*, e944–e946. [CrossRef] [PubMed]
72. Kaufman, J.L.; Mina, R.; Shah, J.J.; Laubach, J.P.; Nooka, A.K.; Lewis, C.; Gleason, C.; Sharp, C.; Harvey, R.D.; Heffner, L.T.; et al. Phase 1 Trial Evaluating Vorinostat Plus Bortezomib, Lenalidomide, and Dexamethasone in Patients with Newly Diagnosed Multiple Myeloma. *Clin. Lymphoma Myeloma Leuk.* **2020**, *20*, 797–803. [CrossRef] [PubMed]
73. Fujimoto, K.; Shinojima, N.; Hayashi, M.; Nakano, T.; Ichimura, K.; Mukasa, A. Histone deacetylase inhibition enhances the therapeutic effects of methotrexate on primary central nervous system lymphoma. *Neurooncol. Adv.* **2020**, *2*, vdaa084. [PubMed]
74. Terranova-Barberio, M.; Pawlowska, N.; Dhawan, M.; Moasser, M.; Chien, A.J.; Melisko, M.E.; Rugo, H.; Rahimi, R.; Deal, T.; Daud, A.; et al. Exhausted T cell signature predicts immunotherapy response in ER-positive breast cancer. *Nat. Commun.* **2020**, *11*, 3584. [CrossRef] [PubMed]
75. Naylor, M.R.; Ly, A.M.; Handford, M.J.; Ramos, D.P.; Pye, C.R.; Furukawa, A.; Klein, V.G.; Noland, R.P.; Edmondson, Q.; Turmon, A.C.; et al. Lipophilic Permeability Efficiency Reconciles the Opposing Roles of Lipophilicity in Membrane Permeability and Aqueous Solubility. *J. Med. Chem.* **2018**, *61*, 11169–11182. [CrossRef]
76. Sarojini, V.; Cameron, A.J.; Varnava, K.G.; Denny, W.A.; Sanjayan, G. Cyclic Tetrapeptides from Nature and Design: A Review of Synthetic Methodologies, Structure, and Function. *Chem. Rev.* **2019**, *119*, 10318–10359. [CrossRef]
77. Bates, S.E. Epigenetic Therapies for Cancer. *N. Engl. J. Med.* **2020**, *383*, 650–663. [CrossRef]
78. Narita, K.; Kikuchi, T.; Watanabe, K.; Takizawa, T.; Oguchi, T.; Kudo, K.; Matsuhara, K.; Abe, H.; Yamori, T.; Yoshida, M.; et al. Total synthesis of the bicyclic depsipeptide HDAC inhibitors spiruchostatins A and B, 5"-epi-spiruchostatin B, FK228 (FR901228) and preliminary evaluation of their biological activity. *Chemistry* **2009**, *15*, 11174–11186. [CrossRef]
79. Narita, K.; Fukui, Y.; Sano, Y.; Yamori, T.; Ito, A.; Yoshida, M.; Katoh, T. Total synthesis of bicyclic depsipeptides spiruchostatins C and D and investigation of their histone deacetylase inhibitory and antiproliferative activities. *Eur. J. Med. Chem.* **2013**, *60*, 295–304. [CrossRef]
80. Fukui, Y.; Narita, K.; Dan, S.; Yamori, T.; Ito, A.; Yoshida, M.; Katoh, T. Total synthesis of burkholdacs A and B and 5,6,20-tri-epi-burkholdac A: HDAC inhibition and antiproliferative activity. *Eur. J. Med. Chem.* **2014**, *76*, 301–313. [CrossRef]
81. Biggins, J.B.; Gleber, C.D.; Brady, S.F. Acyldepsipeptide HDAC inhibitor production induced in *Burkholderia thailandensis*. *Org. Lett.* **2011**, *13*, 1536–1539. [CrossRef] [PubMed]
82. Narita, K.; Katoh, T. Total Synthesis of Thailandepsin B, a Potent HDAC Inhibitor Isolated from a Microorganism. *Chem. Pharm. Bull.* **2016**, *64*, 913–917. [CrossRef] [PubMed]
83. Brosowsky, J.; Lutterbeck, M.; Liebich, A.; Keller, M.; Herp, D.; Vogelmann, A.; Jung, M.; Breit, B. Syntheses of Thailandepsin B Pseudo-Natural Products: Access to New Highly Potent HDAC Inhibitors via Late-Stage Modification. *Chemistry* **2020**, *26*, 16241–16245. [CrossRef] [PubMed]
84. Chen, Y.; Gambs, C.; Abe, Y.; Wentworth, P., Jr.; Janda, K.D. Total synthesis of the depsipeptide FR-901375. *J. Org. Chem.* **2003**, *68*, 8902–8905. [CrossRef]
85. Hong, J.; Luesch, H. Largazole: From discovery to broad-spectrum therapy. *Nat. Prod. Rep.* **2012**, *29*, 449–456. [CrossRef]
86. Yao, L. Aplidin PharmaMar. *IDrugs* **2003**, *6*, 246–250.
87. Alonso-Álvarez, S.; Pardal, E.; Sánchez-Nieto, D.; Navarro, M.; Caballero, M.D.; Mateos, M.V.; Martín, A. Plitidepsin: Design, development, and potential place in therapy. *Drug Des. Dev. Ther.* **2017**, *11*, 253–264. [CrossRef]

88. Delgado-Calle, J.; Kurihara, N.; Atkinson, E.G.; Nelson, J.; Miyagawa, K.; Galmarini, C.M.; Roodman, G.D.; Bellido, T. Aplidin (plitidepsin) is a novel anti-myeloma agent with potent anti-resorptive activity mediated by direct effects on osteoclasts. *Oncotarget* **2019**, *10*, 2709–2721. [CrossRef]
89. Borjan, B.; Steiner, N.; Karbon, S.; Kern, J.; Francesch, A.; Hermann, M.; Willenbacher, W.; Gunsilius, E.; Untergasser, G. The Aplidin analogs PM01215 and PM02781 inhibit angiogenesis in vitro and in vivo. *BMC Cancer* **2015**, *15*, 738. [CrossRef]
90. Taori, K.; Paul, V.J.; Luesch, H. Structure and activity of largazole, a potent antiproliferative agent from the Floridian marine cyanobacterium *Symploca* sp. *J. Am. Chem. Soc.* **2008**, *130*, 1806–1807. [CrossRef]
91. Liu, Y.; Salvador, L.A.; Byeon, S.; Ying, Y.; Kwan, J.C.; Law, B.K.; Hong, J.; Luesch, H. Anticolon cancer activity of largazole, a marine-derived tunable histone deacetylase inhibitor. *J. Pharmacol. Exp. Ther.* **2010**, *335*, 351–361. [CrossRef] [PubMed]
92. Schnekenburger, M.; Dicato, M.; Diederich, M. Epigenetic modulators from "The Big Blue": A treasure to fight against cancer. *Cancer Lett.* **2014**, *351*, 182–197. [CrossRef] [PubMed]
93. Izzo, I.; Maulucci, N.; Bifulco, G.; De Riccardis, F. Total synthesis of azumamides A and E. *Angew. Chem. Int. Ed. Engl.* **2006**, *45*, 7557–7560. [CrossRef] [PubMed]
94. Seidel, C.; Florean, C.; Schnekenburger, M.; Dicato, M.; Diederich, M. Chromatin-modifying agents in anti-cancer therapy. *Biochimie* **2012**, *94*, 2264–2279. [CrossRef]
95. Nakao, Y.; Narazaki, G.; Hoshino, T.; Maeda, S.; Yoshida, M.; Maejima, H.; Yamashita, J.K. Evaluation of antiangiogenic activity of azumamides by the in vitro vascular organization model using mouse induced pluripotent stem (iPS) cells. *Bioorg. Med. Chem. Lett.* **2008**, *18*, 2982–2984. [CrossRef]
96. Porter, N.J.; Christianson, D.W. Binding of the Microbial Cyclic Tetrapeptide Trapoxin A to the Class I Histone Deacetylase HDAC8. *ACS Chem. Biol.* **2017**, *12*, 2281–2286. [CrossRef]
97. Yoshida, M.; Furumai, R.; Nishiyama, M.; Komatsu, Y.; Nishino, N.; Horinouchi, S. Histone deacetylase as a new target for cancer chemotherapy. *Cancer Chemother. Pharmacol.* **2001**, *48* (Suppl. S1), S20–S26. [CrossRef]
98. Ahn, M.Y. HDAC inhibitor apicidin suppresses murine oral squamous cell carcinoma cell growth in vitro and in vivo via inhibiting HDAC8 expression. *Oncol. Lett.* **2018**, *16*, 6552–6560. [CrossRef]
99. Ahn, M.Y.; Lee, J.; Na, Y.J.; Choi, W.S.; Lee, B.M.; Kang, K.W.; Kim, H.S. Mechanism of apicidin-induced cell cycle arrest and apoptosis in Ishikawa human endometrial cancer cells. *Chem. Biol. Interact.* **2009**, *179*, 169–177. [CrossRef]
100. Hwang, W.C.; Kang, D.W.; Kang, Y.; Jang, Y.; Kim, J.A.; Min, D.S. Inhibition of phospholipase D2 augments histone deacetylase inhibitor-induced cell death in breast cancer cells. *Biol. Res.* **2020**, *53*, 34. [CrossRef]
101. Gu, W.; Silverman, R.B. Synthesis of (S)-2-Boc-Amino-8-(R)-(tert-butyldimethylsilanyloxy) decanoic acid, a Precursor to the Unusual Amino Acid Residue of the Anticancer Agent Microsporin, B. *Tetrahedron Lett.* **2011**, *52*, 5438–5440. [CrossRef] [PubMed]
102. Oku, N.; Nagai, K.; Shindoh, N.; Terada, Y.; van Soest, R.W.; Matsunaga, S.; Fusetani, N. Three new cyclostellettamines, which inhibit histone deacetylase, from a marine sponge of the genus Xestospongia. *Bioorg. Med. Chem. Lett.* **2004**, *14*, 2617–2620. [CrossRef] [PubMed]
103. Pérez-Balado, C.; Nebbioso, A.; Rodríguez-Graña, P.; Minichiello, A.; Miceli, M.; Altucci, L.; de Lera, A.R. Bispyridinium dienes: Histone deacetylase inhibitors with selective activities. *J. Med. Chem.* **2007**, *50*, 2497–2505. [CrossRef] [PubMed]
104. Newman, D.J.; Cragg, G.M. Marine natural products and related compounds in clinical and advanced preclinical trials. *J. Nat. Prod.* **2004**, *67*, 1216–1238. [CrossRef]
105. Ratovitski, E.A. Anticancer Natural Compounds as Epigenetic Modulators of Gene Expression. *Curr. Genom.* **2017**, *18*, 175–205. [CrossRef]
106. Howard, E.C.; Sun, S.; Reisch, C.R.; del Valle, D.A.; Bürgmann, H.; Kiene, R.P.; Moran, M.A. Changes in dimethylsulfoniopropionate demethylase gene assemblages in response to an induced phytoplankton bloom. *Appl. Environ. Microbiol.* **2011**, *77*, 524–531. [CrossRef]
107. Bourne, D.G.; Morrow, K.M.; Webster, N.S. Insights into the Coral Microbiome: Underpinning the Health and Resilience of Reef Ecosystems. *Annu. Rev. Microbiol.* **2016**, *70*, 317–340. [CrossRef]
108. Quina, A.S.; Buschbeck, M.; Di Croce, L. Chromatin structure and epigenetics. *Biochem. Pharmacol.* **2006**, *72*, 1563–1569. [CrossRef]
109. Ishijima, J.; Iwabe, N.; Masuda, Y.; Watanabe, Y.; Matsuda, Y. Sponge cytogenetics-mitotic chromosomes of ten species of freshwater sponge. *Zool. Sci.* **2008**, *25*, 480–486. [CrossRef]

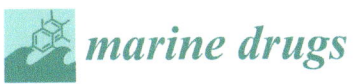

Article

Anti-Leukemic Properties of Aplysinopsin Derivative EE-84 Alone and Combined to BH3 Mimetic A-1210477

Sungmi Song [1,†], Sua Kim [1,†], Eslam R. El-Sawy [2,3], Claudia Cerella [1,4], Barbora Orlikova-Boyer [1,4], Gilbert Kirsch [3], Christo Christov [5], Mario Dicato [4] and Marc Diederich [1,*]

1. Department of Pharmacy, College of Pharmacy, Seoul National University, 1 Gwanak-ro, Gwanak-gu, Seoul 08626, Korea; sson35@snu.ac.kr (S.S.); suakim@snu.ac.kr (S.K.); claudia.cerella@lbmcc.lu (C.C.); barbora.orlikova@lbmcc.lu (B.O.-B.)
2. Chemistry Department of Natural Compounds, National Research Centre, Dokki, 12622 Giza, Egypt; eslamelsawy@gmail.com
3. UMR CNRS 7565 SRSMC, Université du Lorraine, 57070 Metz, France; gilbert.kirsch@univ-lorraine.fr
4. Laboratoire de Biologie Moléculaire et Cellulaire du Cancer, Hôpital Kirchberg, 9, Rue Edward Steichen, 2540 Luxembourg, Luxembourg; dicato.mario@chl.lu
5. Service d'Histologie, Faculté de Médicine, Université de Lorraine, INSERM U1256 NGERE, 54000 Nancy, France; christo.christov@univ-lorraine.fr
* Correspondence: marcdiederich@snu.ac.kr; Tel.: +82-2-880-8919
† These authors equally contributed to this work.

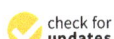

Citation: Song, S.; Kim, S.; El-Sawy, E.R.; Cerella, C.; Orlikova-Boyer, B.; Kirsch, G.; Christov, C.; Dicato, M.; Diederich, M. Anti-Leukemic Properties of Aplysinopsin Derivative EE-84 Alone and Combined to BH3 Mimetic A-1210477. *Mar. Drugs* 2021, 19, 285. https://doi.org/10.3390/md19060285

Academic Editor: Orazio Taglialatela-Scafati

Received: 1 March 2021
Accepted: 13 May 2021
Published: 21 May 2021

Publisher's Note: MDPI stays neutral with regard to jurisdictional claims in published maps and institutional affiliations.

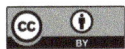

Copyright: © 2021 by the authors. Licensee MDPI, Basel, Switzerland. This article is an open access article distributed under the terms and conditions of the Creative Commons Attribution (CC BY) license (https://creativecommons.org/licenses/by/4.0/).

Abstract: Aplysinopsins are a class of marine indole alkaloids that exhibit a wide range of biological activities. Although both the indole and N-benzyl moieties of aplysinopsins are known to possess antiproliferative activity against cancer cells, their mechanism of action remains unclear. Through in vitro and in vivo proliferation and viability screening of newly synthesized aplysinopsin analogs on myelogenous leukemia cell lines and zebrafish toxicity tests, as well as analysis of differential toxicity in noncancerous RPMI 1788 cells and PBMCs, we identified EE-84 as a promising novel drug candidate against chronic myeloid leukemia. This indole derivative demonstrated drug-likeness in agreement with Lipinski's rule of five. Furthermore, EE-84 induced a senescent-like phenotype in K562 cells in line with its cytostatic effect. EE-84-treated K562 cells underwent morphological changes in line with mitochondrial dysfunction concomitant with autophagy and ER stress induction. Finally, we demonstrated the synergistic cytotoxic effect of EE-84 with a BH3 mimetic, the Mcl-1 inhibitor A-1210477, against imatinib-sensitive and resistant K562 cells, highlighting the inhibition of antiapoptotic Bcl-2 proteins as a promising novel senolytic approach against chronic myeloid leukemia.

Keywords: aplysinopsin analogs; indole alkaloids; marine source; chronic myeloid leukemia; BH3 mimetics

1. Introduction

Chronic myeloid leukemia (CML) is characterized by the oncogenic *BCR-ABL1* fusion gene expression, which codes for a leukemogenic tyrosine kinase [1]. The first-line therapy for CML is imatinib, a tyrosine kinase inhibitor (TKI) that selectively inhibits the activity of the BCR-ABL fusion protein. Since the discovery of imatinib, the overall survival rate of patients with CML has drastically increased, with patients showing durable responses after imatinib treatment [2]. Leukemia cells, however, develop resistance mechanisms to escape chemotherapy; therefore, despite the high remission rate, a significant number of patients develop resistance or become intolerant to imatinib treatment. Furthermore, 33% of patients who receive imatinib treatment do not achieve a complete cytogenetic response (CCyR) [3]. Thus, alternative strategies for the management of CML are needed to combat chemoresistance, for which compounds of natural origin have shown promise as potential therapeutic agents by their capacity to induce cellular stress mechanisms sensitizing leukemia cells against cytotoxic treatments.

The endoplasmic reticulum (ER) is responsible for protein translocation, proper folding, and protein post-translational modifications [4]. Altered cell metabolism and inflammation may disrupt this balance and result in ER stress that can trigger the unfolded protein response (UPR) [5]. The UPR represents a series of adaptive cellular mechanisms designed to restore protein homeostasis [2], and ER stress activates apoptotic cell death under severe or chronic stress conditions [6]. Autophagy is also a stress-induced cell survival program that involves a catabolic process to degrade large protein aggregates and damaged organelles in autophagosomes [7]. Although autophagy and ER stress function independently, increasing evidence supports that these processes can be coactivated [8].

Aplysinopsin and its derivatives possess rich structural diversity and have been reported to exhibit a wide range of medicinal and biological activities. For example, they act as neuromodulators [9] and possess antineoplastic [9], antiplasmodial [10], and antimicrobial activities [11]. Interestingly, aplysinopsins display cytotoxicity against a range of cancer cell lines [12]. However, their anticancer potential in leukemic cell lines and the corresponding molecular mechanisms remain to be further investigated.

Here we evaluated the anti-leukemic activity of aplysinopsin (EE-115) and analogs EE-31, EE-80, EE-84, and EE-92 (Scheme 1) against chronic myeloid leukemia cell lines. EE-84 exhibited drug-like properties in line with Lipinski's rule of five and showed a stronger cytostatic and cytotoxic effect on leukemia cells than healthy cell models. Furthermore, its safety profile was validated in vivo by using developing zebrafish larvae. Mechanistically, EE-84 induced a senescent-like phenotype in line with its cytostatic activity, triggered autophagy, ER stress, metabolic alterations, and mitochondrial dysfunction. In addition, EE-84 sensitized imatinib-sensitive and -resistant K562 cells against the Mcl-1 inhibitor A-12101477 to induce caspase-dependent apoptosis. Altogether, this study warrants further investigation of the aplysinopsin analog EE-84 as a preclinical drug candidate against chronic myeloid leukemia.

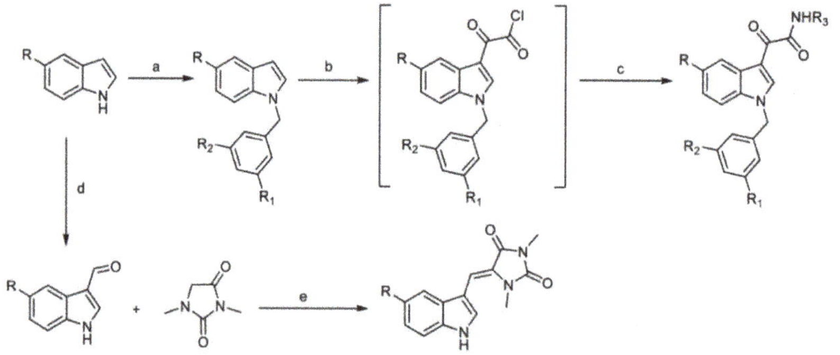

Scheme 1. Synthetic pathway for the preparation of aplysinopsin EE-115 and its analogs EE-31, EE-80, EE-84, and EE-92. Reagents and conditions: (**a**) benzyl chlorides, NaH, DMF; (**b**) oxalyl chloride, dry ethyl ether, heating; (**c**) the reactant amines 2-cyanoacetohydrazide and 1-(2-amino-5-methyl-4,5,6,7-tetrahydrobenzo[b]thiophen-3-yl)ethan-1-one, dry THF, TEA, stirring, 3 h; (**d**) POCl$_3$ DMF, 0 °C, NaOH; (**e**) piperidine, reflux, 4 h.

2. Results

2.1. Aplysinopsin Analogs Display Cytostatic Activities in Myeloid Leukemia Cells

Aplysinopsin (EE-115) and its analogs EE-31, EE-80, EE-84, and EE-92 (Figure 1) were tested for their anti-leukemic effects on the myeloid leukemia cell line K562, using the trypan blue exclusion test (Tables 1 and 2 and Figure S1). NMR spectrum data of ^{1}H of the compounds EE-31, EE-80, EE-84, EE-92, and EE-115 (Figure S2) and ^{13}C NMR spectrum data of the compounds EE-31, EE-80, EE-84, and EE-92 (Figure S3) were provided.

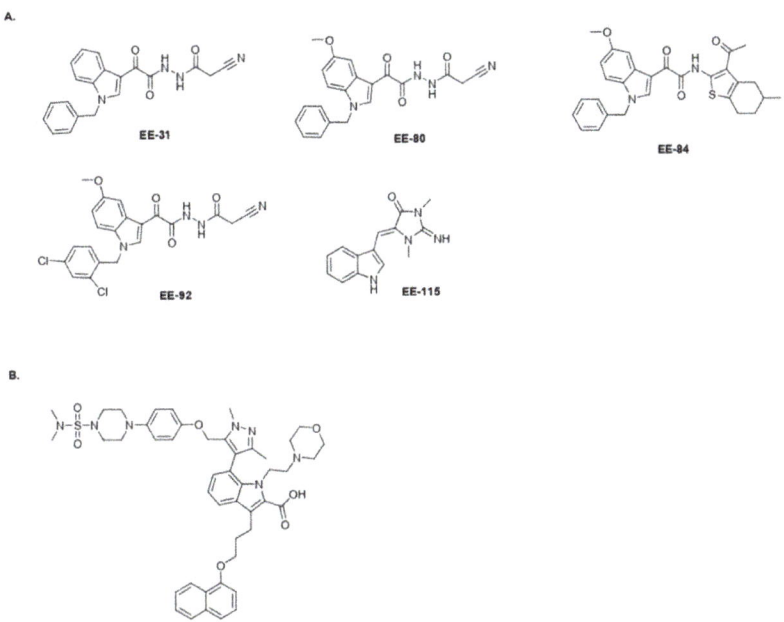

Figure 1. Chemical structures. (**A**) Aplysinopsin (EE-115) and analogs (EE-31, EE-80, EE-84, EE-92). (**B**) A-1210477.

Table 1. GI_{50} of EE-84 in CML cell lines. GI_{50} (µM) values were calculated after indicated times of treatment.

Compound	Cell Line	GI_{50} (µM)		
		24 h	48 h	72 h
EE-84	KBM5	>50	33.95 ± 1.89	28.14 ± 1.68
	MEG01	>50	48.40 ± 5.02	28.89 ± 1.52
	K562IR	>100	95.63 ± 16.56	55.09 ± 3.28
	KBM5IR	>100	32.77 ± 2.25	29.15 ± 2.05

GI_{50} values were calculated after trypan blue staining and represent the mean ± S.D. of three independent experiments. GI_{50} indicates the concentration required to cause 50% overall growth inhibition.

Compounds EE-31, EE-80, EE-92, and EE-115 only weakly affected the overall growth (Figure S1A) and viability (Figure S1B) of K562 cells at concentrations up to 50 µM. Interestingly, EE-84 inhibited the growth of K562 with a GI_{50} of 32.22 ± 3.91 µM and 19.07 ± 0.80 µM after 48 and 72 h, respectively (Figure S1A).

Based on the GI_{50} results in the K562 cell line, we selected EE-84 for further investigations compared to EE-115, the parental compound. To generalize the antiproliferative effect of EE-84 in CML, GI_{50} values of EE-84 were calculated on imatinib-sensitive (KBM5, MEG01) and -resistant (IR) (K562IR and KBM5IR) CML cells (Table 1). We next validated the cytostatic profiles of EE-84 by Methocult colony formation assays (CFA) to assess the compounds' effects on the clonogenic potential in a 3D culture environment (Figure 2A–E). EE-84 reduced the total surface area and average size of K562 colonies after a 48-h pretreatment (Figure 2A). Similar results were observed for other CML cell lines (Figure 2A–E).

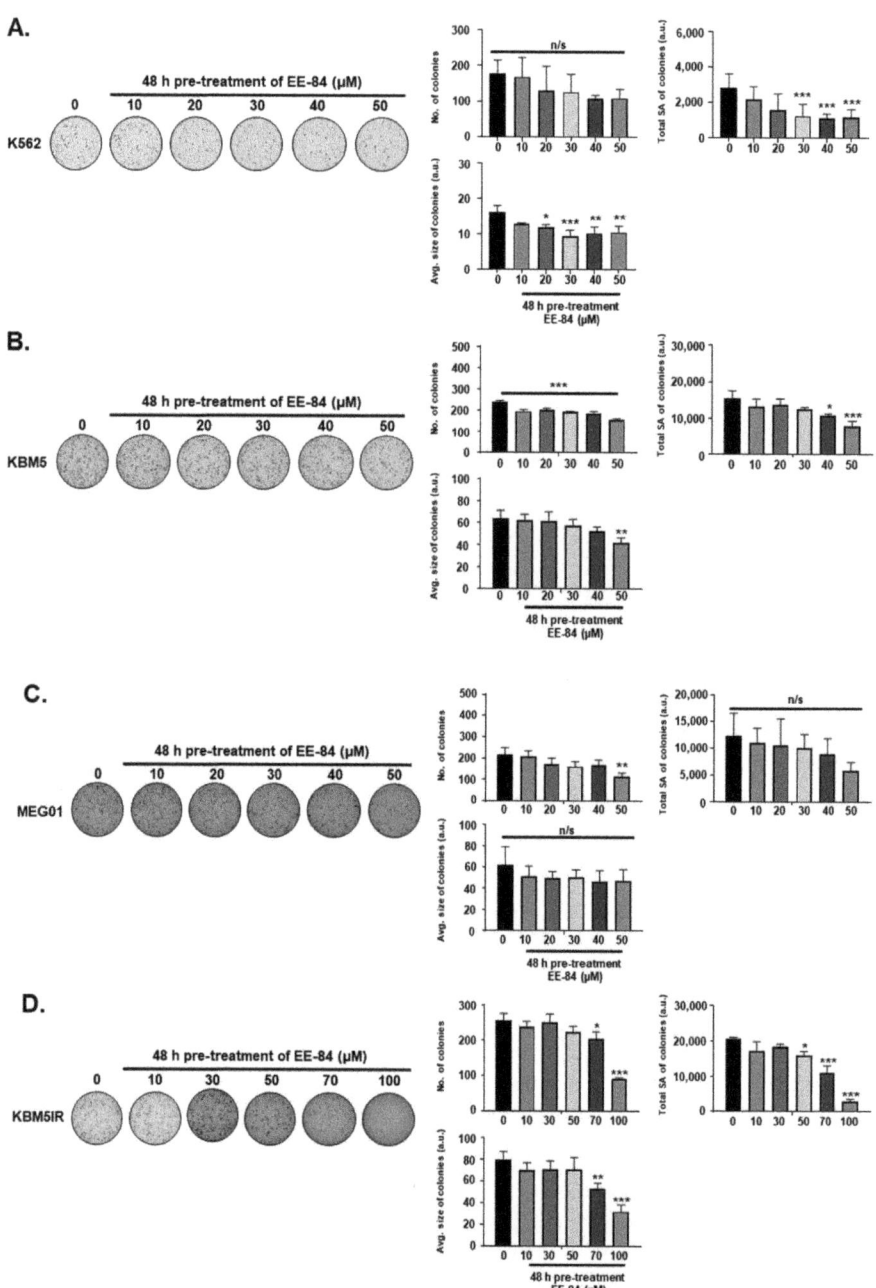

Figure 2. *Cont.*

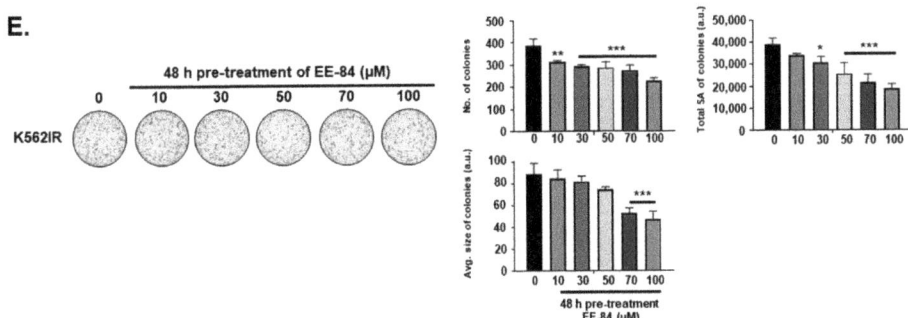

Figure 2. Differential anti-leukemic effects observed by CFA after aplysinopsin treatments (**A–E**). Representative pictures from three independent experiments of clonogenic assays after 48 h pretreatment of EE-84 (**A**) K562, (**B**) KBM5, (**C**) MEG01, (**D**) KBM5IR, (**E**) K562IR cells are shown on the left. Corresponding quantifications (number of colonies, the total surface area of colonies, and average size of colonies) are indicated on the right. Statistical analysis was performed by one-way ANOVA, followed by Sidak's multiple comparisons test. Differences were considered significant when * $p < 0.05$, ** $p < 0.01$, *** $p < 0.001$ compared to control. n/s: not significant.

Considering the moderate cytotoxic effect of 50 µM EE-84 and EE-115 at 72 h in K562 cells (Figure S1), we quantified cell death induction using Hoechst/PI staining by fluorescent microscopy (Figure 3A). EE-84 reduced K562 cell viability leading to $11.0 \pm 4.23\%$ of propidium iodide (PI)-positive cells without nuclear fragmentation. A similar percentage of cell death was shown after quantification of Annexin V APC/PI by FACS (Figure 3B). EE-84 induced approximately 16.5% cell death (Table 2) at the highest concentration of 50 µM. Imatinib (1 µM) was used as a control. Cell cycle analysis showed an accumulation of cells in the sub-G1 phase of $8.34 \pm 1.51\%$ after 48 h and $13.03 \pm 1.19\%$ after 72 h with EE-84 (50 µM), concomitant with a reduction of the G1 population from $58.40 \pm 2.81\%$ at 48 h to $52.03 \pm 2.99\%$ at 72 h (Figure 3C and Table 3). Celecoxib (40 µM) was used as a control.

Table 2. Percentage of cell death after treatment of K562 cells with increasing concentrations of EE-84. (Data from Figure 3B).

	EE-84 (µM)						Ima (µM)
	0	10	20	30	40	50	1
AnnV+/PI− (%)	5.12 ± 1.19	7.05 ± 1.46	5.60 ± 1.98	6.65 ± 2.29	7.71 ± 2.10	8.22 ± 3.12	51.77 ± 2.29
AnnV+/PI+ (%)	2.68 ± 0.77	2.50 ± 0.62	4.40 ± 0.94	7.51 ± 2.70	8.97 ± 1.03	8.25 ± 1.95	31.27 ± 5.24
Combined cell death (%)	7.80 ± 1.73	9.55 ± 3.22	10.00 ± 0.85	14.16 ± 0.61	16.68 ± 0.89	16.46 ± 0.02	83.03 ± 14.50

Results are the mean ± S.D. of three independent experiments.

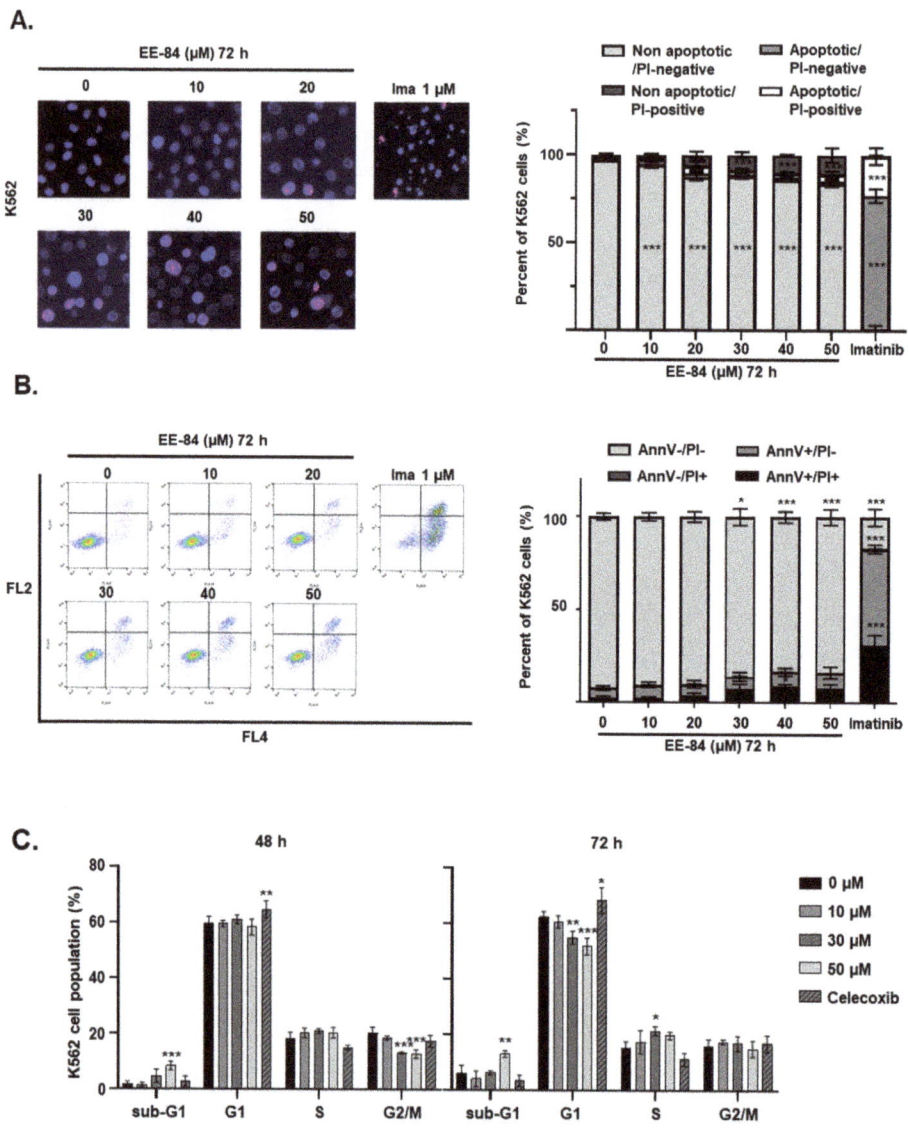

Figure 3. Percentage of cell death after increasing concentrations of EE-84 treatment in K562 cells. (**A**) Representative microscopy images of Hoechst 33342/PI double-stained nuclei of K562 cells exposed to different concentrations of aplysinopsin derivatives at indicated times are shown. The percentage of apoptotic cells was calculated from three independent experiments. (**B**) Results obtained after Annexin V APC/PI staining and quantification by FACS. Ima: imatinib (1 μM). (**C**) For cell cycle analysis, K562 cells were treated with 10, 30, and 50 μM EE-84 for 48 and 72 h. Cell cycle phase distribution was determined by FACS. All data were expressed as mean ± SD of three independent experiments. Statistical analysis was performed by two-way ANOVA, followed by Dunnett's multiple comparisons test (Microscopy, Cell cycle); by Sidak's multiple comparisons test (Annexin V/PI); * $p < 0.05$, ** $p < 0.01$, *** $p < 0.001$ compared to controls.

Table 3. Cell cycle phase distribution after treatment of K562 cells with increasing concentrations of EE-84. (Data from Figure 3C).

48 h Treatment	EE-84 (µM)				Celecoxib (µM)
%	0	10	30	50	40
Sub-G1	1.78 ± 0.91	1.48 ± 0.81	4.65 ± 2.42	8.34 ± 1.51	2.79 ± 1.90
G1	59.81 ± 2.29	59.59 ± 1.12	61.11 ± 1.58	58.40 ± 2.81	64.77 ± 3.09
S	18.02 ± 2.49	20.30 ± 1.68	20.99 ± 0.83	20.41 ± 1.84	15.00 ± 0.93
G2/M	20.39 ± 2.12	18.64 ± 0.75	13.25 ± 0.32	12.86 ± 1.46	17.44 ± 2.13
72 h Treatment	EE-84 (µM)				Celecoxib (µM)
%	0	10	30	50	40
Sub-G1	6.07 ± 2.88	4.08 ± 2.80	6.33 ± 0.74	13.03 ± 1.19	3.41 ± 2.04
G1	62.33 ± 2.13	60.83 ± 2.33	55.09 ± 2.26	52.03 ± 2.99	68.43 ± 4.67
S	15.50 ± 2.14	17.52 ± 4.24	21.55 ± 1.64	19.85 ± 1.33	11.20 ± 2.37
G2/M	16.10 ± 2.50	17.57 ± 0.90	17.03 ± 2.69	15.08 ± 2.89	16.96 ± 3.04

Results are the mean ± S.D. of three independent experiments.

2.2. Drug-Likeness of Compounds EE-84 and EE-115

Next, we examined the drug-likeness of the two compounds according to Lipinski's rule of five (Table 4) [13]. A molecule is orally active when there are no more than 5 H bond donors and no more than 10 H bond acceptors, when the molecular mass is less than 500 Daltons, and when the octanol–water partition coefficient LogP is not greater than 5. EE-115 did not violate any of the conditions mentioned above. For EE-84, The LogP corresponds to 5.91; however, this aplysinopsin derivative can still be considered a drug-like candidate since one exception is acceptable.

Table 4. In silico prediction for the drug-likeness of EE-84 and EE-115. Drug-likeness of the aplysinopsin derivatives were calculated and interpreted based on Lipinski's rule of five.

	EE-84	EE-115
Mass	500.00	254.00
Hydrogen bond donor	1	2
Hydrogen bond acceptor	5	4
LogP	5.91	1.85
Molar reactivity	142.51	74.54

2.3. Effect of EE-84 and EE-115 on Healthy Cells and Zebrafish Embryos

We then assessed the effect of EE-84 and EE-115 on healthy models. Even though EE-84 affected the proliferation of RPMI 1788 cells dose-dependently (Figure S4A), this modulation was evident at later times (as early as 72 h vs. 48 h in cancer cells), with a higher GI$_{50}$ (40.10 ± 3.79 in RPMI 1788 vs. 19.07 ± 0.80 µM after 72 h in K562 cells; Tables 1 and 5). Altogether, EE-84 generated significant differential toxicity of RPMI-1788/K562 cells at 40 and 50 µM (Figure 4A). On the other hand, EE-115 inhibited the growth of normal RPMI 1788 cells (Table 5) more than K562 cells (Figure S4A). Moreover, EE-84 did not significantly affect the viability of RPMI 1788 cells, whereas EE-115 reduced the viability of RPMI 1788 cells at the highest concentrations (Table S1 and Figure S4B). Altogether EE-84 appeared to have a more advantageous safety profile.

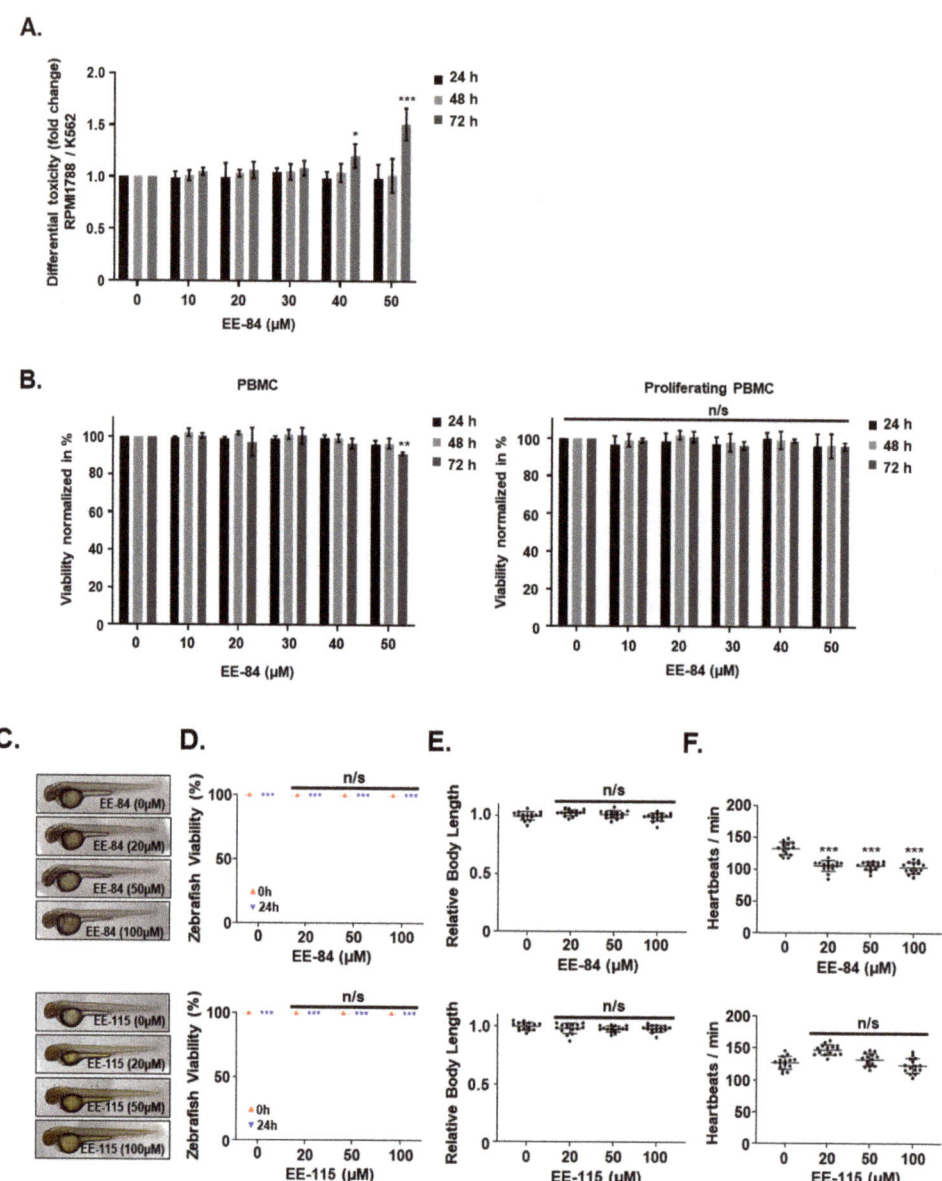

Figure 4. Effect of aplysinopsin derivatives on healthy cell models. (**A**) Differential toxicity (RPMI 788/K562) of EE-84 was determined by the trypan blue exclusion test. (**B**) Toxicity test of EE-84 in nonproliferating and proliferating PBMCs. After 24, 48, and 72 h of EE-84 treatment, viability was determined by the trypan blue exclusion test. Zebrafish toxicity assays were performed by treatment with aplysinopsins at indicated concentrations. (**C**) Representative pictures of zebrafish are shown. Zebrafish viability (**D**), relative body length (**E**), and heartbeats/min (**F**) were measured. Data represents a total of 15 fish per group. Trypan blue exclusion test data represents the mean ± SD of three independent experiments. Statistical analysis: two-way ANOVA with Dunnett's multiple comparison test (trypan blue exclusion test); * $p < 0.05$, ** $p < 0.01$, *** $p < 0.001$ compared to controls. Ordinary one-way ANOVA followed by Dunnett's post hoc test (Zebrafish assay) revealed significant differences indicated by *** $p < 0.001$ compared to control. n/s: not significant.

Table 5. GI$_{50}$ of aplysinopsins on RPMI 1788. GI$_{50}$ (µM) values were evaluated after indicated times of compound treatment.

Compound	GI$_{50}$ (µM)		
	24 h	48 h	72 h
EE-84	>50	>50	40.10 ± 3.79
EE-115	>50	30.36 ± 1.95	27.72 ± 2.30

GI$_{50}$ values were calculated after trypan blue staining and represent the mean ± S.D. of three independent experiments. GI$_{50}$ indicates the concentration required to cause 50% overall growth inhibition.

We generalized our findings and validated the absence of cytotoxic/cytostatic effects of EE-84 on nonproliferating and proliferating peripheral blood mononuclear cells (PBMCs) from healthy donors. In addition, EE-84 did not induce toxic effects in any of the two cell models (Figure 4B).

We then treated zebrafish embryos 24 h post-fertilization (hpf) to validate the in vivo safety profiles of the aplysinopsin compounds EE-84 and EE-115. The zebrafish were observed after 24 h of exposure to different concentrations of aplysinopsins. No significant morphological changes were notable at the different concentrations of the compounds used (Figure 4C). Concentrations up to 100 µM of EE-84 and EE-115 did not affect the survival rate (Figure 4D) or growth (Figure 4E) of the treated zebrafish. A moderate decrease in the heart rate (Figure 4F) was noted for EE-84.

Altogether, based on these results, we further investigated the molecular and cellular effects of EE-84, considering the observed differential toxicity.

2.4. EE-84 Induced Morphological Changes and Cell Stress Responses in CML Cells

EE-84 (50 µM) increased the cell size (Figure 5A) and the number of intracellular vacuoles up to 96 h. These morphological changes were quantified by flow cytometry (Figure 5B). Compared to DMSO-treated controls, EE-84-treated K562 cells showed a progressive increase in forward scatter values (FSC-H; a.u.) and side scatter (SSC-H; a.u.) as measurements of cell size and granularity, respectively. The increase in cell size and granularity and the cytostatic effects were considered part of a cellular stress response driving cells into senescence. We then examined the senescent-like phenotype using stress-associated (SA)-β-galactosidase staining. We measured increased cell size and SA-β-gal positive cells after treatment with EE-84 at 50 µM for 72 h. Doxorubicin (80 nM), known to induce senescence, was used as a bona fide control (Figure 5C).

In addition, morphological changes were examined by transmission electron microscopy (TEM). K562 cells treated with EE-84 underwent mitochondrial damage after 24, 48, and 72 h of compound exposure as well as mitophagy (Figure 5D). In addition, we assessed the mitochondrial metabolism in K562 after treatment with EE-84 at 30 µM for 72 h by using the Agilent Seahorse XFp Cell Mito Stress test. The oxygen consumption rate (OCR) significantly decreased after treatment with EE-84 compared to control (Figure 5E). Thus, our results confirmed that EE-84 induced cell stress and reduced mitochondrial activity in agreement with morphological alterations of the mitochondria observed by TEM.

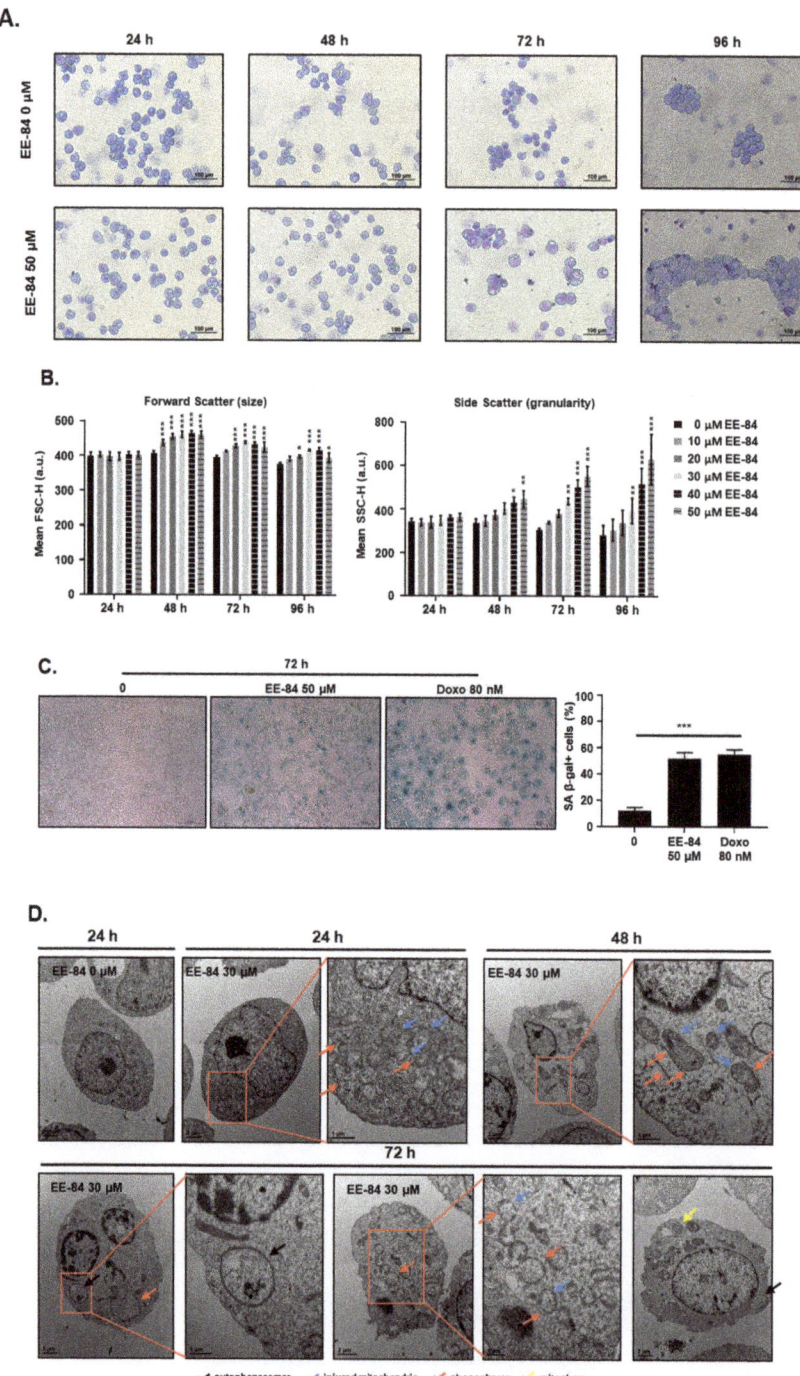

Figure 5. *Cont.*

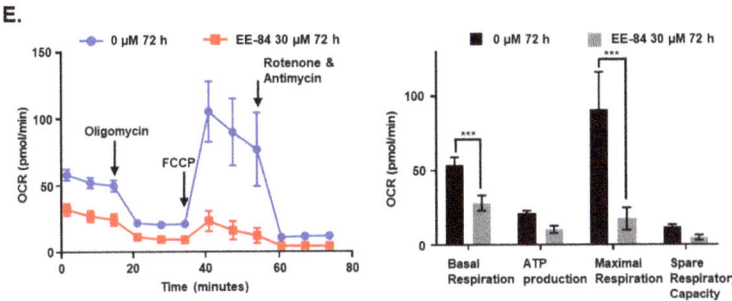

Figure 5. Morphological changes of K562 cells treated with EE-84. (**A**) K562 cells were treated with 50 µM EE-84 for 24, 48, 72, and 96 h. Light microscopy at magnification 200× was used for morphological observation. (**B**) K562 cells were treated with indicated concentrations of EE-84 for up to 96 h. At the indicated time points, cells were harvested and analyzed by flow cytometry using forward (relative cell sizes; FSC-H) and side scatter (granularity; SSC-H) measurements. For morphological analysis of EE-84, exposed K562 cell debris were excluded. (**C**) SA-β-gal staining of the K562 cells treated with 50 µM of EE-84 for 72 h. The quantitative analysis of the incidence of the cells with positive β-gal staining. Doxo: doxorubicin (80 nM). (**D**) Transmission electron microscopy at magnifications of 8000× or 10,000× (whole cells) and 20,000× or 25,000× (cell details). Cells were treated with 30 µM EE-84 and were exposed for up to 72 h. Phagophores, autophagosomes, injured mitochondria, and incidence of mitophagy were highlighted using red, black, blue, and yellow arrows, respectively. DMSO-treated K562 cells at 24 h were used as control. (**E**) Measurement of mitochondrial function in K562 cells. The experiments were conducted using the Seahorse XFp Cell Mito Stress test, and the OCR measurement is visualized. Results are the mean ± SD of three independent experiments. Statistical analysis was performed by two-way ANOVA, followed by Dunnett's multiple comparisons test (Cell size by FACS); by Tukey's multiple comparisons test (Senescence); by Sidak's multiple comparisons test (Seahorse XFp Cell Mito Stress test); * $p < 0.05$, ** $p < 0.01$, *** $p < 0.001$ compared to controls.

2.5. Autophagy and Endoplasmic Reticulum (ER) Stress Were Triggered by EE-84 as Cellular Stress Responses in K562 Cells

Autophagy is a catabolic pathway activated in response to different cellular stressors, such as damaged organelles, accumulation of misfolded or unfolded proteins, ER stress, and DNA damage [14]. Based on the TEM results, we then investigated the expression levels of the microtubule-associated protein-1 light chain 3 (LC3I) conversion to the phosphatidylethanolamine-conjugated form of LC3I (LC3II) by Western blot. Results showed that levels of LC3 II gradually increased over time after treatment with EE-84 at 30 µM in K562 at 24, 48, and 72 h, respectively (Figure 6A). In addition, we observed the formation of cytoplasmic vacuoles in EE-84 treated K562 cells after 48 h at 30 µM by Diff-Quik staining, suggestive of autophagy induction. To validate the involvement of EE-84 in autophagy induction, we post-treated bafilomycin A1 (Baf-A1), an inhibitor of the vacuolar-type H$^+$-ATPase which blocks the late phase of autophagy by preventing lysosomal acidification, at 40 nM for 8 h (cells were treated or not with EE-84 for 40 h before addition of Baf-A1 for 8 h), resulting in significant inhibition of vacuole formation after 48 h at 30 µM EE-84 (Figure 6B). To see the effect of autophagy inhibition on cell viability, we conducted a trypan blue assay test of EE-84 treated K562 cells with or without Baf-A1 post-treatment. 89.0% of cell viability was observed in EE-84 treated K562 cells with Baf-A1 post-treatment compared to 98.7% of cell viability in EE-84 treated K562 cells alone (Figure 6B).

In addition, studies have shown that autophagy and endoplasmic reticulum (ER) stress are closely related [8]. ER stress is considered a protective stress response in eukaryotic cells [15]. We then assessed whether EE-84 induces ER stress and subsequently regulates autophagy. We measured sensor proteins such as PERK, ATF6, and GRP78 that play a role in activating the unfolded protein response (UPR) in response to ER stress. PERK and phosphorylated eIF2α were significantly increased after treatment with EE-84 at 30 and 50 µM in K562 cells after 72 h. The abundance of ATF4, an effector of PERK and eIF2α, also increased, which indicated that the PERK-eIF2α-ATF4-CHOP pathway was activated under EE-84-induced ER stress (Figure 6C). Since GRP78 is involved in glycolysis [16], we then assessed the glycolytic flux levels in K562 after treatment with EE-84 at 50 µM for 72 h by using the Agilent seahorse XFp Glycolysis Stress test. The glycolysis and glycolytic capacity measured by the extracellular acidification rate (ECAR) significantly decreased after treatment with EE-84 compared to control (Figure 6D). We also confirmed the glycolytic flux levels in K562IR cells after treatment with EE-84 at 100 µM for 72 h. The results showed that the glycolytic capacity of ECAR also significantly decreased after treatment with EE-84 (Figure S5). Altogether, these data demonstrated that the prolonged treatment with EE-84 induced the PERK-eIF2α-ATF4-CHOP UPR pathway involved in EE-84-induced autophagy.

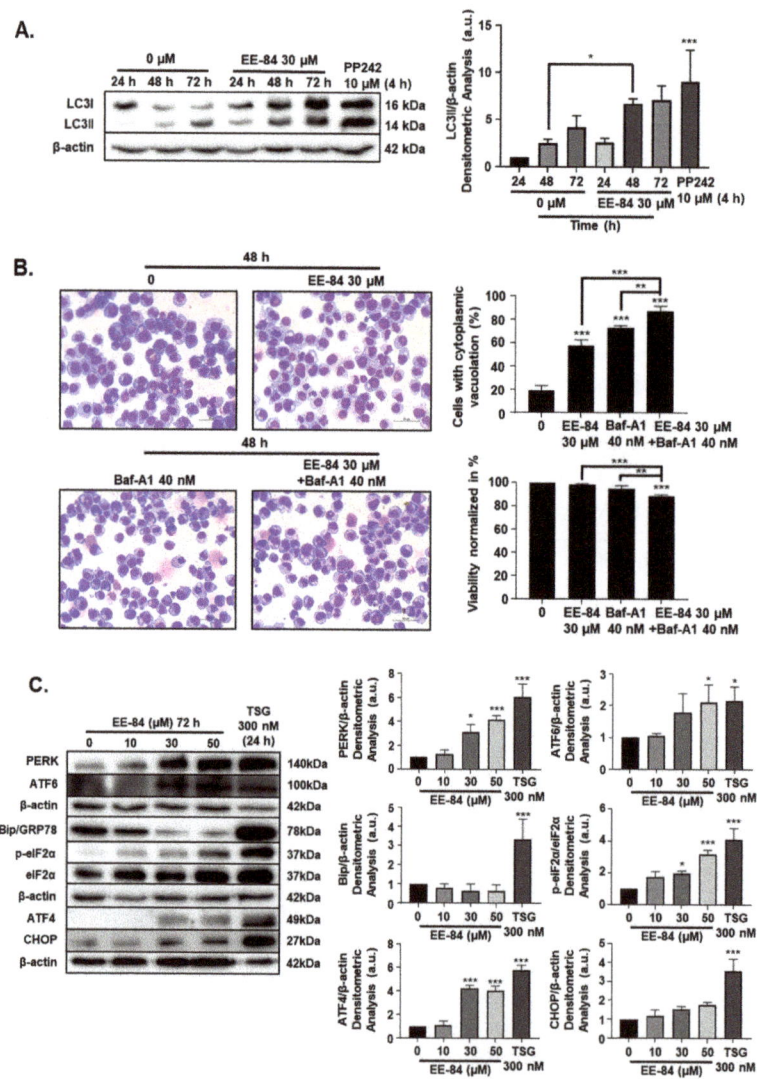

Figure 6. Cont.

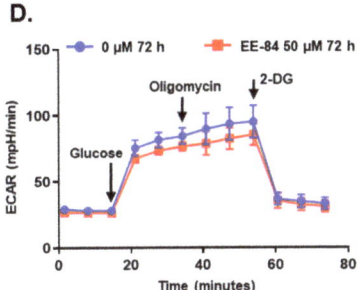 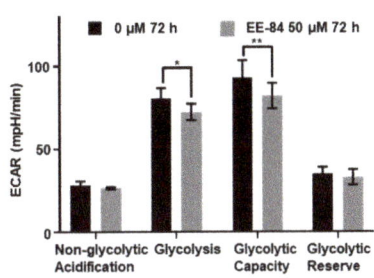

Figure 6. EE-84 induced autophagy and ER stress. (**A**) K562 cells were treated with 30 µM EE-84 for 24, 48, and 72 h. Western blot analysis of the LC3B protein. B-actin was used as a loading control. Quantification of LC3B protein bands through normalization by β-actin protein bands. (**B**) Diff-Quik staining of K562 cells after 48 h of EE-84 treatment (30 µM) with or without Baf-A1 post-treatment. Baf-A1: bafilomycin A1 (40 nM). (**C**) ER stress-related proteins were detected by Western blot analysis. B-actin was used as a loading control. After quantifying the bands, p-eiF2α levels were normalized to total eIF2α, and all other proteins were normalized to β-actin. TSG: thapsigargin (300 nM). (**D**) Measurement of glycolytic capacity in K562 cells. 2-DG: 2-deoxy-D-glucose. The experiments were conducted using the Seahorse XFp Glycolysis Stress test, and the flow chart and bar graph show the measurement of ECAR. Results are the mean ± SD of three independent experiments. Statistical analysis was performed by two-way ANOVA, followed by Tukey's multiple comparisons test (autophagy Western blot, Diff-Quik staining); by Dunnett's multiple comparisons test (ER stress Western blot); by Sidak's multiple comparisons test (Seahorse XFp Glycolysis Stress test); * $p < 0.05$, ** $p < 0.01$, *** $p < 0.001$ compared to controls.

2.6. EE-84 Sensitized K562 Cells against Mcl-1 Inhibitor A-1210477 and Showed Synergistic Cytotoxicity in K562 and K562IR Cells

Conditions of ER stress may promote Mcl-1 protein stabilization via mechanisms involving UPR and ATF4 upregulation [17,18]. Considering the cytostatic potential but limited cytotoxicity of EE-84 along with the induction of ER stress, we then investigated the expression levels of the antiapoptotic protein, Mcl-1, which may be responsible for the apoptotic blockage. Based on the increase of antiapoptotic Mcl-1 expression in EE-84-treated K562 cells after 24 h compared to control (Figure 7A), we speculated that the combined treatment of the specific Mcl-1 inhibitor A-1210477 with EE-84 might sensitize K562 cells to apoptotic cell death. Using subtoxic concentrations of EE-84 (20 and 30 µM) and A-1210477 (10 µM), we first assessed the combinatory effects of these compounds using Hoechst/PI staining after 24 h (Figure 7B). We observed 46.89 ± 21.84% and 56.00 ± 25.46% induction of apoptotic cell death in combinatory treatments. The combination index (CI) of each compound-pair was calculated, and the combinatory treatment showed a synergistic effect (Figure 7C and Table 6). We also compared viability between EE-84 alone and in combination with A-1210477 after 24 h (Table 7). Our results showed that the Mcl-1-specific inhibitor A-1210477 sensitized EE-84-treated K562 and K562IR cells. Next, we confirmed the apoptotic cell death mechanism triggered by the combination treatment. As shown in Figure 7D, about 14.5% of apoptotic cell death was induced by A-1210477 alone, whereas over 40% of apoptosis was observed by a combination of EE-84 and A-1210477 after 24 h. z-VAD pretreatment completely prevented apoptosis induction in K562 cells in single and combined treatments (Figure 7D). The caspase-dependent nature of cell death modality was also confirmed by Annexin V APC/PI staining after 24 h in K562 cells (Figure 7E). Results showed that EE-84 (30 µM) in combination with A-1210477 (10 µM) induced 23.03 ± 4.08% early apoptosis (AnnV+/PI−) and 23.07 ± 5.32% late apoptosis (AnnV+/PI+) in K562 cells after 24 h of treatment (Table 8). Again, zVAD completely protected against cell death in all instances. Imatinib (1 µM) was used as a control. In addition, the cytotoxic effect of subtoxic concentrations of EE-84 (30 and 50 µM) in combination with A-1210477 (20 µM) was also tested on K562IR cells after 24 h of treatment, using the trypan blue exclusion test (Figure 7F). Results showed that viability was reduced by 25.4% when cells were cotreated with 20 µM A-1210477 and 30 µM of EE-84. A co-treatment with 50 µM EE-84 and 20 µM A-1210477 induced 40% of cell death. We further confirmed the combinatory effects of these compounds using Annexin V APC/PI staining after 24 h in K562IR cells (Figure 7G). Altogether, our results indicated that the specific Mcl-1 inhibitor A-1210477 sensitized K562 and K562IR cells to EE-84, significantly increasing cell death induction. Since mitochondrial dysfunction can trigger apoptosis, we measured the percentage of mitochondrial membrane potential (MMP) loss due to the combined effects of EE-84 with A-1210477 in K562 after 24 h. Results showed that the percentage of MMP loss significantly increased in K562 after cotreatment with EE-84 and A-1210477 (Figure 7H). In addition, we confirmed the combination effects of EE-84 with A-1210477 in K562 by colony formation assays (CFA); EE-84 combined with A-1210477 reduced the number of colonies, the total surface area, and the average size of colonies in K562 (Figure 7I). The obtained values for the two compound combinations denoted synergism, and 30 µM of EE-84 with 10 µM of A-1201477 were selected for further investigations.

Table 6. Combination indexes obtained by Compusyn software after treatment of K562 with EE-84 and A-1201477.

EE-84 (µM)	A-1210477 (µM)	Fa	CI
20	10	0.483	0.66
30	10	0.563	0.57

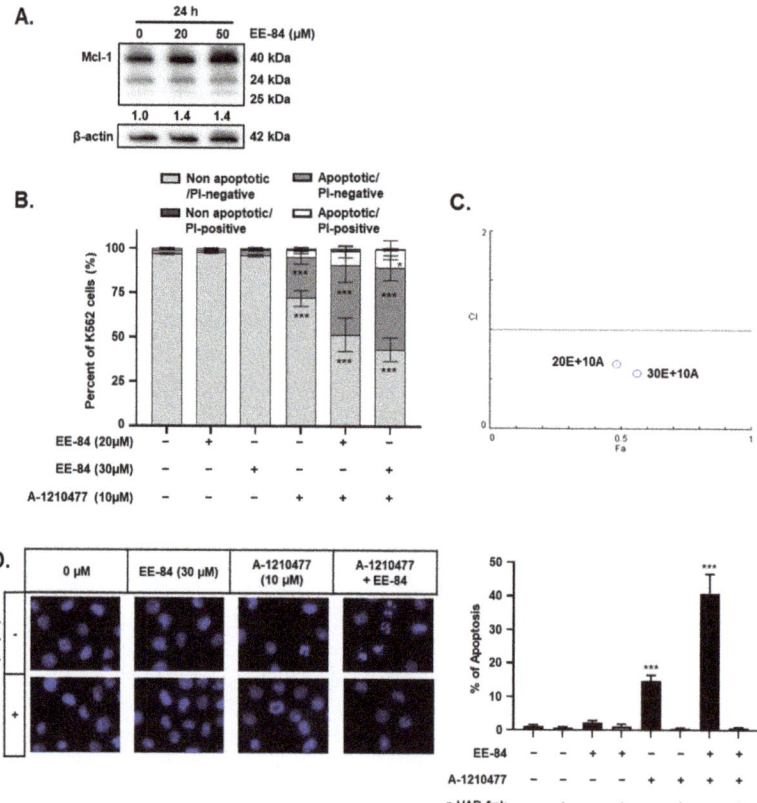

Figure 7. *Cont.*

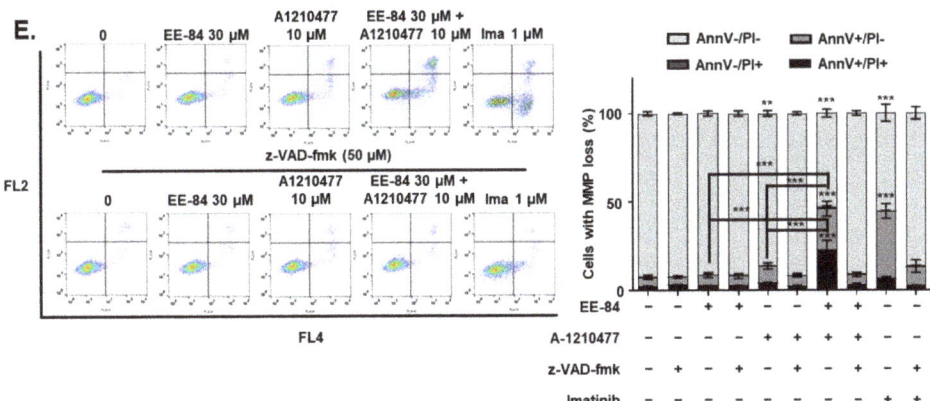

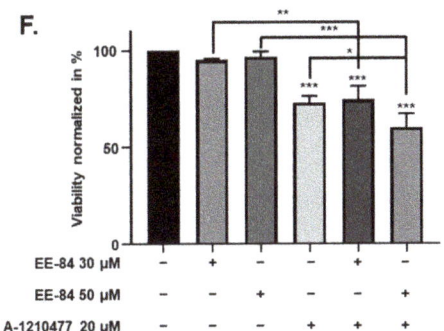

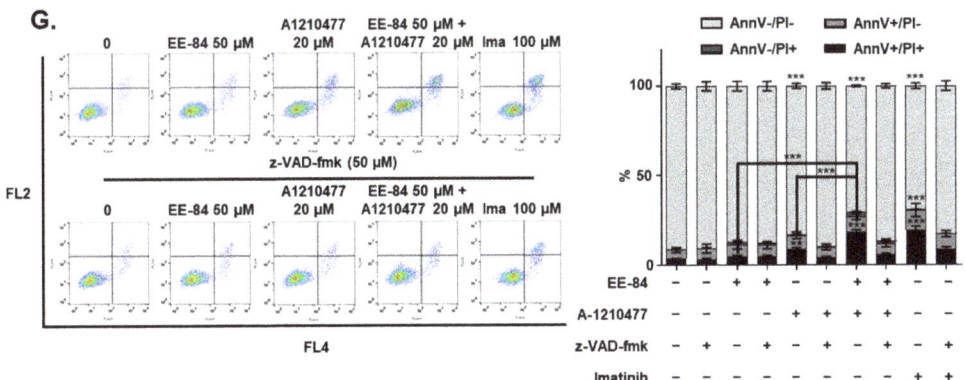

Figure 7. Cont.

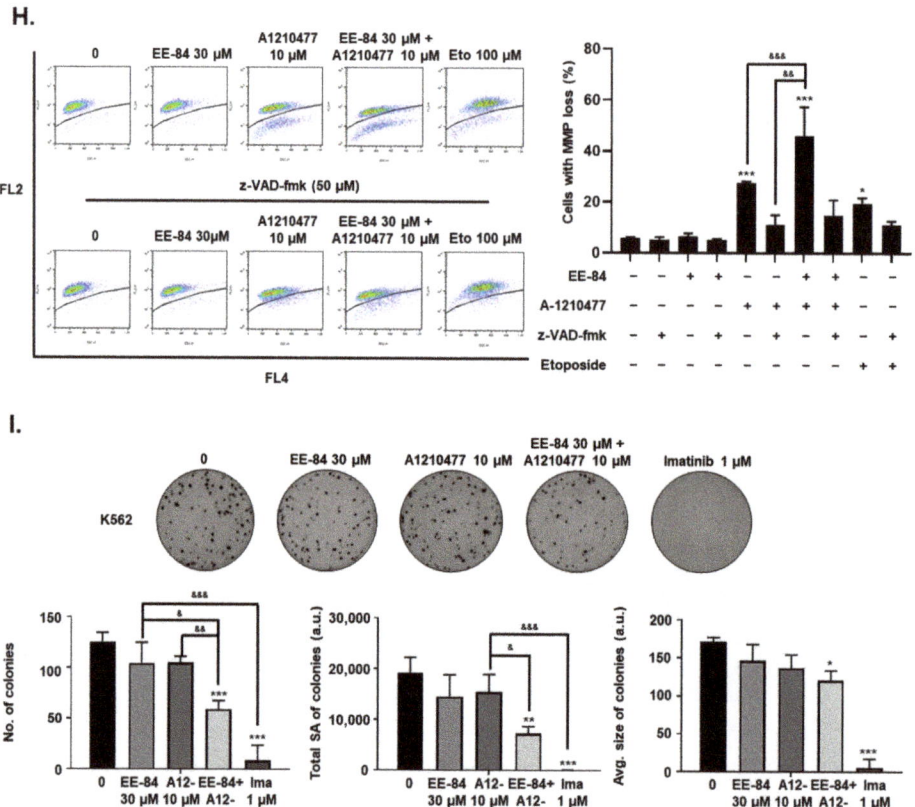

Figure 7. EE-84 sensitized CML cells to BH3 mimetics. (**A**) EE-84 increased expression levels of antiapoptotic protein Mcl-1 compared to DMSO-treated control. K562 cells were treated with varying concentrations of EE-84 for 24 h. The effects on Mcl-1 and β-actin were determined by Western blot analysis. Western blot data interpreted in terms of fold changes in protein expression compared to control at the corresponding time point. The values represented the average of three independent experiments. (**B**) Cotreatment analysis of 20 and 30 μM EE-84 with 10 μM A-1210477 using Hoechst 33258/PI staining showed an increase in apoptotic cell death compared to single treatments of compounds after 24 h in K562 cells. (**C**) The plot representing the fraction affected-combination index (Fa-CI) of the treatment of K562 cells with EE-84 and A-1210477 after 24 h was obtained with Compusyn software. (**D**) The optimal compound combination of 30 μM EE-84 and 10 μM A-1210477 was analyzed by Hoechst/PI staining. z-VAD-fmk was used as a pan-caspase inhibitor. (**E**) The compound combination of 30 μM EE-84 and 10 μM A-1210477 treated K562 cells after 24 h. After 24 h of treatment, the type of cell death triggered by EE-84 with or without A-1210477 was characterized by FACS after Annexin V APC/propidium iodide (PI) staining. Pictures are representative of three independent experiments (**left panel**), and the corresponding quantification (**right panel**) is shown. Ima: imatinib (1 μM). (**F**) K562IR cell viability by trypan blue exclusion assay. (**G**) Annexin V APC/PI staining of K562IR analyzed by FACS. Results are the mean ± SD of three independent experiments. (**H**) Mitochondrial membrane potential (MMP) of the combination of 30 μM EE-84 and 10 μM A-1210477 was analyzed by FACS, and the percentage of cells exhibiting MMP loss was calculated (**right panel**). z-VAD-fmk was used as a pan-caspase inhibitor. Eto: etoposide (100 μM). (**I**) Differential anti-leukemic effects observed by CFA after EE-84 treatments with A-1210477 on K562. Corresponding quantifications (the number of colonies, the total surface area of colonies, and the average size of colonies) are indicated on the right. Results are the mean ± SD of three independent experiments. Statistical analysis was performed by one-way or two-way ANOVA, followed by Dunnett's multiple comparisons test (Microscopy), by Tukey's multiple comparisons test (colony formation assay, MMP, Annexin V/PI); * $p < 0.05$, ** $p < 0.01$, *** $p < 0.001$ compared to controls, & $p < 0.05$, && $p < 0.01$, &&& $p < 0.001$ between indicated conditions.

Table 7. Viability of K562 and K562IR cells (%) after treatment with EE-84 alone or in combination with A-1210477. Viability (%) was calculated after indicated times of compound treatment.

Treatment	Viability (24 h) Cell Line	%
EE-84 (30 μM)	K562	98.0 ± 1.0
	K562IR	95.3 ± 0.6
EE-84 (50 μM)	K562	96.0 ± 0.7
	K562IR	97.0 ± 2.7
A-1210477 (10 μM)	K562	79.3 ± 1.5
A-1210477 (20 μM)	K562IR	73.0 ± 3.6
EE-84 (30 μM) + A-1210477 (10 μM)	K562	69.0 ± 3.0
EE-84 (30 μM) + A-1210477 (20 μM)	K562IR	74.7 ± 7.1
EE-84 (50 μM) + A-1210477 (20 μM)	K562IR	60.0 ± 7.2

Results are the mean ± S.D. of three independent experiments.

Table 8. Cell death induction (%) after treatment with EE-84 alone or in combination with A-1210477. (Data represent Figure 7E).

	0	EE-84 30 μM	A-1210477 10 μM	EE-84 30 μM + A-1210477 10 μM	Ima 1 μM
AnnV+/PI− (%)	5.36 ± 1.14	6.00 ± 1.43	9.31 ± 1.78	23.03 ± 4.08	37.77 ± 4.07
AnnV+/PI+ (%)	2.53 ± 0.28	2.98 ± 0.23	4.73 ± 0.17	23.07 ± 5.32	6.97 ± 0.88
Combined cell death (%)	7.90 ± 2.00	8.98 ± 2.14	14.04 ± 3.24	46.10 ± 0.02	44.74 ± 21.78
z-VAD-fmk (50 μM)					
	0	EE-84 30 μM	A-1210477 10 μM	EE-84 30 μM + A-1210477 10 μM	Ima 1 μM
AnnV+/PI− (%)	4.46 ± 0.68	5.33 ± 1.35	6.04 ± 0.99	5.24 ± 1.15	10.86 ± 3.57
AnnV+/PI+ (%)	3.61 ± 0.13	3.13 ± 0.21	2.81 ± 0.21	3.84 ± 0.28	2.93 ± 0.15
Combined cell death (%)	8.07 ± 0.60	8.46 ± 1.55	8.85 ± 2.28	9.08 ± 0.99	13.79 ± 5.60

Results are the mean ± S.D. of three independent experiments.

2.7. Synergistic Induction of Caspase-Dependent Apoptosis by Combination Treatment of EE-84 and A-1210477 in K562 Cells

The cytotoxic effect and caspase-dependent apoptotic activity of the combination treatment were also validated by quantification of intracellular ATP levels. ATP levels decreased significantly after combination treatments compared to the compounds alone (Figure 8A). The 1 h pretreatment of z-VAD-fmk showed an increase in cell viability with the single treatment of 10 μM A-1210477 and the combined treatment. The addition of the caspase inhibitor showed no significant difference in the ATP levels for the single treatment of 30 μM EE-84. To further validate our data, the activity of caspase-3/7 was measured. There was a significant increase in the caspase-3/7 activity by 5.52-fold after the combined treatment of EE-84 and the Mcl-1 inhibitor compared to the untreated control (Figure 8B). To examine the detailed mechanism by which the combined treatment acts, we studied the intrinsic and extrinsic apoptotic pathways in K562 cells by Western blot (Figure 8C–E). First, the expression level of caspase-8, a cysteine protease that initiates apoptotic signaling via the extrinsic pathway, was detected. Cleavage of pro-caspase-8 in the combined treatment was observed (Figure 8C). Our results showed a reduction of pro-caspase-9, the initiator caspase critical for the intrinsic pathway, concomitant with the appearance of a cleaved fragment at 18 kDa after the combined treatment. In line with the previous observation of increased caspase-3/7 activity for the combination treatment, we observed a strong cleavage of pro-caspase-3 and cleaved fragments of caspase-7 for the combined treatment (Figure 8D). Our evaluation of antiapoptotic Mcl-1 and Bcl-xL expression levels showed an increase of both in EE-84 (30 μM) and A-1210477 (10 μM) single treatments in K562 cells as well as in the combined treatment (Figure 8E).

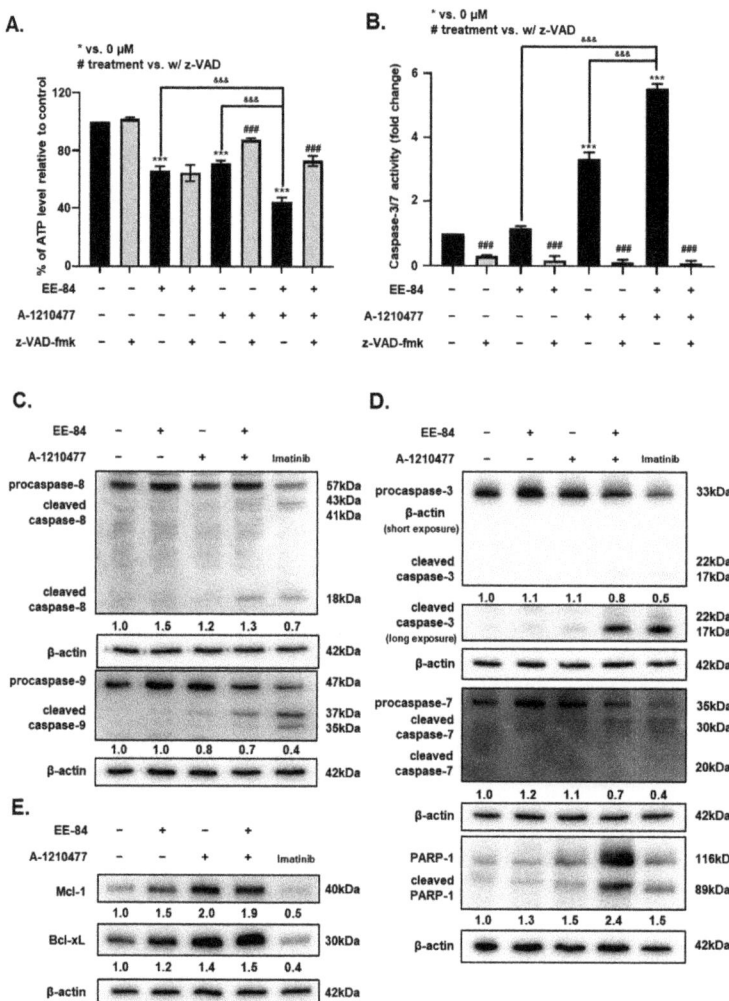

Figure 8. Caspase-dependent induction of apoptosis in K562 cells by EE-84 in synergism with the Mcl-1 inhibitor A-1210477. (**A**) K562 cell viability was determined by the measurement of cellular ATP content using the CellTiter-Glo assay. K562 cells were pretreated at the concentration of 50 µM z-VAD-fmk for 1 h before exposure to the compounds. (**B**) Effects of single or combination treatments of EE-84 and A-1210477 with or without z-VAD-fmk on caspase-3/7 activity in K562 cells. Three separate experiments were performed for both CellTiter-Glo and caspase-3/7 assays, and each condition was measured in triplicates. Values are the mean ± SD of three independent experiments. The asterisk indicates a value significantly different from the control. Statistical analysis was performed by one-way or two-way ANOVA, followed by Dunnett's multiple comparisons test (ATP assay, caspase-3/7 assay); *** $p < 0.001$ compared to controls; &&& $p < 0.001$ between indicated conditions; ### $p < 0.001$ compared to corresponding treatment without z-VAD-fmk. (**C–E**) Western blots showing expression levels of apoptosis-related proteins after single or combination treatments of EE-84 and A-1210477 in K562 cells. (**C**) Results of expression levels of initiator caspases, caspase-8 and -9; (**D**) expression levels of effector caspases, caspase-3 and -7, and PARP-1; (**E**) expression levels of antiapoptotic proteins Mcl-1 and Bcl-xL are displayed. Protein expression levels of procaspase-8, -9, -3, and -7 are quantified and expressed in fold changes relative to control. Protein expression levels of cleaved PARP-1, Mcl-1, and Bcl-xL are quantified and expressed in fold changes relative to control. The values represent the average of three independent experiments.

3. Discussion

Many products of marine organisms have been identified as modulators of cell death, exerting cytotoxic effects on cancer cells as activators of apoptosis, autophagy, or oncosis [19]. Currently, seven marine-based drugs have been approved, 23 compounds are undergoing phase I–III clinical trials, and thousands of compounds have been isolated from marine life and are undergoing preclinical studies [20]. Among these, four are used for cancer treatment: cytarabine (Cytosar-U®, Vitaris, Canonsburg, PA, USA), trabectedin (Yondelis®, PharmaMar, Colmenar Viejo, Madrid, Spain), eribulin mesylate (Halaven®, Eisai Inc., Tokyo, Japan) and the conjugated antibody brentuximab vedotin (Acentris®, Takeda Oncology, Cambridge, MA, USA) [21]. Cytosine arabinoside (cytarabine), originally isolated from the sponge *Cryptothethya crypa*, and now produced synthetically, is one of the most effective drugs to treat acute myeloid leukemia [21–23]. In addition, trabectedin, a marine metabolite of *Ecteinascidia turbinata*, is used for the treatment of soft tissue sarcoma [24]. However, despite the broad array of marine compounds clinically available or investigated, there is still an enormous library of natural products that remains untapped.

Aplysinopsins, a class of marine indole alkaloids, comprise two main distinct moieties—an indole and an imidazolidinone ring—and are isolated from a variety of marine organisms, including sponges [25], corals [26], anemone [27], and mollusks [28,29]. Aplysinopsins were first isolated by Kazlauskas et al., and initially identified as the major metabolite of eight Indo-Pacific sponge species of the genera *Thorecta* [12]. Since then, more aplysinopsin derivatives have been discovered and extracted from *Verongia spengeli, Dercitus* sp., *Smenospongia aurea, Verongular rigida, Dictyoceratida* sp., *Aplysinopsis reticulata, Aplysina* sp., *Hyrtios erecta*, and *Thorectandra* [28], among others. In line with the effort to identify new aplysinopsins with therapeutic potential, we report a set of synthetic aplysinopsin derivatives that possess anti-leukemic effects. In addition, aplysinopsin derivatives displayed a range of cytostatic effects, some inducing antiproliferating effects on myeloid leukemia cells more than others. We identified EE-84 as having the most potent antiproliferative effect in several chronic myeloid leukemia cell lines (K562, KBM5, MEG01, K562IR, and KBM5IR) as shown by trypan blue exclusion tests, CFAs, Hoechst/PI, and Annexin V/PI staining assays.

Identifying lead candidates from a library of compounds and characterizing their safety profiles by testing their toxicity in healthy models is essential in the drug discovery process. In addition, it helps predict clinical adverse effects in the future [28]. EE-84 showed differential toxicity in the noncancerous cell model, RPMI 1788, compared to K562, and was nontoxic to PBMCs. In the zebrafish model, EE-84 was also well-tolerated. The safe profile and drug-likeness of EE-84, supported by Lipinski's rule of five, warranted further investigation of this compound.

EE-84 induced morphological changes in K562 cells as shown by diff-Quik staining and TEM imaging. In parallel with the cytostatic effect, EE-84 triggered a significant increase in the cell size together with the appearance of mitochondrial damage after 48 h of treatment. Furthermore, evaluation of mitochondrial dysfunction by Agilent Seahorse XFp Cell Mito Stress test showed significant inhibition of mitochondrial function after 72 h of 30 µM treatment. Interestingly, EE-84-treated K562 cells displayed a senescent-like phenotype, suggesting an interplay between mitochondrial dysfunction and cellular senescence in the EE-84-induced antiproliferative effect.

Cellular senescence is one of the many defense mechanisms that cells undergo to combat extrinsic and/or intrinsic stresses by halting cell cycle progression. Drug-mediated cellular stress leading to senescence is often accompanied by senescence-associated secretory phenotype (SASP). Many studies revealed that in senescent cells, mitochondrial function is significantly affected [30]. For example, Galanos et al. showed perturbations in the mitochondrial morphology in p21-inducible precancerous and cancerous cellular models (Li-Fraumeni and Saos-2 cell lines), characterized by the enlargement of the mitochondria and the damaged morphology of cristae [31,32]. Mitochondria were elongated or branched, and the cristae were abnormally distributed or lost, suggesting a disturbance of mitochondrial dynamics in the senescent cell. Wiley et al. also reported a distinct type of senescence associated with mitochondrial damage called "Mitochondrial Dysfunction Associated-Senescence" (MiDAS). They observed that mitochondrial dysfunction induces senescence and differs from the senescence caused by genotoxic or oncogenic stress by analyzing the secretome [33].

Senolytic compounds specifically induce apoptosis in senescent cells [34]. Dasatinib has been approved to treat CML as one of the second-generation tyrosine kinase inhibitors used in imatinib resistance and/or intolerance [35]. The senolytic drug combination of dasatinib and quercetin decreased senescent cells in human adipose tissue [36]. In addition, BH3 mimetic ABT-263 (Navitoclax) also induced apoptosis in mouse senescent bone marrow hematopoietic stem cells (HSCs) as a potent senolytic drug [37]. Hence, these studies support the idea that EE-84 triggered a senescent-like phenotype in response to mitochondrial dysfunction, autophagy, and prolonged ER stress as cellular metabolic alteration. In the present study, we showed that EE-84 induces a senescent-like phenotype. Interestingly, the combination of BH3 mimetic A-1210477 with EE-84 further triggers canonical apoptotic cell death in K562 and K562IR. We speculate that under these conditions, Mcl-1 inhibitor A-1210477 may act as a senolytic compound able to eradicate imatinib-sensitive and resistant CML cells. The effect of EE-84 as a single agent points at the ability of this compound to act as a general stress inducer. New effective combinatorial anticancer treatments also include stress inducers forcing cancer cells to rely more on a prosurvival factor. Targeting this specific protein promotes the eradication of cancer cells. Interestingly, some of the cases reported do involve prosurvival Bcl-2 family proteins. Dexamethasone, for example, is leading to Bcl-2 dependence and sensitization to venetoclax in multiple myeloma by altering the balance between pro- and antiapoptotic Bcl-2 protein members (increased Bim and decreased Mcl-1 vs. Bcl-2 upregulation), making Bcl-2 expression essential for survival [38]. Kapoor and colleagues report that CLL chronically resistant to ibrutinib (a Bruton tyrosine kinase (BTK) inhibitor) are sensitized to venetoclax partly also by a STAT3-mediated Bcl-2 upregulation in resistant CLL, implying a shift in the type of Bcl-2 family protein dependence [39]. At this level of investigation, we might speculate that EE-84 contributes to a similar scenario. Mcl-1 protein upregulation (or stabilization?) might signalize an increased reliance of CML cells on Mcl-1 as part of a stress response induced by EE-84. Further investigations will be required to elucidate any modulatory effects of EE-84 on the expression level of proapoptotic Bcl-2 proteins. In this view, EE-84 might be a compound to consider in combinatorial regimens.

Next, we investigated whether autophagy and ER stress occur concurrently with inhibition of proliferation by EE-84 in K562 cells. Accumulation of LC3-II, a standard marker for autophagosomes, was detected increasingly over time after 24, 48, and 72 h of EE-84 treatment, as seen in our Western blotting results. There was a significant increase in the formation of cytoplasmic vacuoles after 48 h EE-84 treatment at 30 μM, and this phenomenon was abrogated by a post-treatment with Baf-A1. Furthermore, 98.7% of K562 cells were viable after 48 h EE-84 treatment alone; however, the viability of K562 cells significantly decreased with Baf-A1 post-treatment, implying that EE-84 drives the K562 cells to undergo autophagy as a cell survival mechanism. ER stress was also activated by EE-84, given that sensor proteins of UPR, such as PERK and ATF6, and downstream effectors such as CHOP and ATF4 were upregulated to varying degrees. GRP78 has been initially characterized as a glucose-regulated protein [16]. Our Western blot results showed decreased levels of GRP78. These results are in line with data obtained by using the Seahorse glycolysis stress test. We observed reduced glycolysis levels, supporting the hypothesis of an impairment of the glycolytic function by EE-84 treatment in K562 and K562IR cells. Altogether, EE-84 induced autophagy, ER stress, and mitochondrial alterations as cell stress reactions, further leading to apoptosis. Overall, EE-84 plays a potential role in inhibiting CML cell activities via induction of cellular stress modalities.

The evasion of apoptotic cell death by cancer cells can impair responses to anticancer therapy. Prosurvival B-cell lymphoma 2 (BCL-2) proteins play a role of perpetrators in this scenario because they prevent apoptosis by keeping the cell death effectors like BAX and BAK under control [40]. BH3 mimetics offer a solution to this as they are designed to inhibit antiapoptotic BCL2 family proteins, leading to BAX and BAK activation, and thus promoting apoptosis [41]. Mcl-1 became a popular therapeutic target because it is one of the most frequently amplified genes across all human cancers. Moreover, an increase in Mcl-1 expression is commonly associated with chemotherapy resistance [42]. This study evaluated the synergistic effect of EE-84, a cytostatic marine compound, with the Mcl-1 inhibitor A-1210477 against CML K562 and K562 imatinib-resistant cells. We showed that the cotreatment of the marine compound and the Mcl-1 inhibitor induced apoptotic cell death along with the activation of caspase activity. These results are in line with other studies in which BH3 mimetics like ABT199 showed synergism with cell stress inducers like cardiac glycosides [43,44] and coumarin derivatives [44].

In the present study, we investigated the preclinical use of aplysinopsins as anti-leukemic agents. Our results identify EE-84 as a potential drug candidate for CML as it possesses drug-like properties and is well-tolerated in healthy models in vitro and in vivo. Mechanistically, EE-84 induces antiproliferative effects associated with the complex interplay between mitochondrial dysfunction, a senescent-like phenotype, autophagy, and ER stress, potentially inducing a condition favorable for senolysis by synergizing with senolytic compounds. To potentiate the anti-leukemic effects of EE-84, we suggest the cotreatment of this aplysinopsin derivative with the BH3 mimetic A-1210477 in K562 and K562IR, as it significantly increases cell death of malignant cells. In conclusion, the combination of EE-84 with BH3 mimetics is efficient and highly synergistic. Future investigations will determine whether this combinatory approach can become a therapeutic opportunity against resistant forms of CML.

4. Materials and Methods

4.1. Chemistry

4.1.1. General Information

All reagents and solvents were of commercial grade. Melting points were determined on the digital melting point apparatus (Electro thermal 9100, Electro thermal Engineering Ltd., serial No. 8694, Rochford, UK) and are uncorrected. Elemental analyses were performed on a FlashSmart™ Elemental Analyzer (Thermo Scientific, Courtaboeuf, France) and were found within ±0.4% of the theoretical values. ^{1}H and ^{13}C NMR spectra were measured with a Bruker Avance spectrometer (Bruker, Germany) at 400 and 101 MHz, respectively, using TMS as the internal standard. Hydrogen coupling patterns are described as (s) singlet, (d) doublet, (t) triplet, (q) quartet, and (m) multiplet. The chemical shifts were defined as parts per million (ppm) relative to the solvent peak. The reaction progress was checked by pre-coated TLC Silica gel 0.2 nm F254 nm [Fluka], visualized under UV lamp 254 and 365 nm. 2-Cyanoacetohydrazide [45]; N-benzyl indoles [46] methyl creatinine [47]; 5-methoxy indole-3-aldehyde [48] were prepared as reported. 1-(2-Amino-5-methyl-4,5,6,7-tetrahydrobenzo[b]thiophen-3-yl)ethan-1-one [49] was provided by Ahmed B. Abdelwahab, Ph.D., UMR CNRS 7565 SRSMC, Université de Lorraine, 57070 Metz, France.

4.1.2. General Procedure for the Preparation of EE-31, EE-80, EE-84, EE-92

To a solution at 0 °C of oxalyl chloride (0.44 mL, 5.1 mmol) in dry ethyl ether (25 mL) was added dropwise a solution of indole (4.14 mmol) in dry ethyl ether (5 mL). The resulting solution was refluxed for 2 h. After removing the solvent under vacuo, the residue was dissolved in dry tetrahydrofuran (20 mL) and cooled to 0 °C. To the THF solution was added slowly the amine (9.73 mmol) in dry tetrahydrofuran (20 mL). After complete addition, 1 mL of triethylamine was added, and the reaction was left to stir overnight. The precipitate obtained was filtered off, washed several times with water, dried, and recrystallized from acetone.

2-(1-Benzyl-1H-Indol-3-yl)-N'-(2-Cyanoacetyl)-2-Oxoacetohydrazide EE-31

Yield 0.45g, 86%; mp 264–6 °C; ^{1}H NMR (400 MHz, DMSO) δ: 10.63 (s, 1H), 8.90 (s, 1H), 8.26 (s, 1H), 7.72–7.50 (m, 5H), 7.41–7.21 (m, 4H), 5.46 (s, 2H), 3.83 (s, 2H); 13C NMR (101 MHz, DMSO) δ: 162.16, 141.47, 136.79, 136.70, 129.14, 128.97, 128.56, 128.26, 128.01, 127.73, 127.65, 127.29, 126.98, 124.17, 123.56, 122.53, 121.92, 116.04, 112.14, 111.95, 50.28, 24.10; Anal. Calcd for $C_{20}H_{16}N_4O_3$ (360.37): C, 66.66; H, 4.48; N, 15.55; found: C, 66.87; H, 4.50; N, 15.42.

2-(1-Benzyl-5-Methoxy-1H-Indol-3-yl)-N′-(2-Cyanoacetyl)-2-Oxoacetohydrazide EE-80

Yield (0.31g, 63%); mp 199–201 °C; ^{1}H NMR (400 MHz, DMSO) δ: 10.62 (s, 1H), 8.78 (s, 1H), 7.76 (s, 1H), 7.57–7.43 (d, H), 7.41–7.20 (m, 5H), 7.06–6.77 (m, 2H), 5.44 (s, 2H), 3.87 (m, 3H), 3.33 (s, 2H); ^{13}C NMR (101 MHz, DMSO) δ 161.34, 162.32, 156.47, 136.51, 131.22, 128.74, 127.83, 127.60, 127.33, 115.52, 113.07, 112.52, 103.72, 55.37, 50.06, 23.80; Anal. Calcd for $C_{21}H_{18}N_4O_4$ (390.40): C, 64.61; H, 4.65; N, 14.35; found: C, 64.55; H, 4.70; N, 14.32.

(N-(3-Acetyl-4,5,6,7-Tetrahydro-5-Methylbenzo[b]Thiophen-2-yl)-2-(1-Benzyl-5-Methoxy-1H-Indol-3-yl)-2-Oxoacetamide EE-84

Yield (0.38g, 61%); mp 165–7 °C; ^{1}H NMR (400 MHz, CDCl$_3$) δ: 13.58 (s, 1H), 9.07 (s, 1H), 8.08 (d, J = 2.5 Hz, 1H), 7.35–6.90 (m, 8H), 5.38 (s, 2H), 3.92 (d, J = 6.4 Hz, 3H), 2.82–2.80 (dd, J = 16.1, 5.0 Hz, 1H), 2.58–2.55 (m, 2H), 2.41 (s, 3H), 1.91–1.87 (m, 2H), 1.15 (d, J = 6.4 Hz, 2H), 1.10 (d, J = 6.6 Hz, 3H); ^{13}C NMR (101 MHz, CDCl$_3$) δ: 196.38, 194.06, 164.12, 157.30, 140.94, 135.40, 131.26, 130.59, 130.42, 129.06, 128.98, 128.29, 128.24, 126.91, 123.08, 117.26, 115.78, 114.52, 111.48, 104.33, 55.81, 51.54, 36.56, 35.96, 31.01, 30.65, 29.25, 24.52, 21.76; Anal. Calcd for $C_{29}H_{28}N_2O_4S$ (500.61): C, 69.58; H, 5.64; N, 5.60; S, 6.40; found: C, 69.60; H, 5.56; N, 5.60; S, 6.48.

N′-(2-Cyanoacetyl)-2-(1-(2,4-Dichlorobenzyl)-5-Methoxy-1H-Indol-3-yl)-2-Oxoacetohydrazide EE-92

Yield (0.25g, 56%); mp 242–4 °C; 1H NMR (400 MHz, DMSO) δ: 10.74 (s, 1H), 10.39 (s, 1H), 8.70 (s, 1H), 7.75 (dd, J = 17.6, 2.3 Hz, 2H), 7.58–7.26 (m, 2H), 7.09–6.83 (m, 2H), 5.65 (s, 2H), 3.82 (s, 3H), 3.34 (s, 2H); 13C NMR (101 MHz, DMSO) δ: 180.68, 161.35, 156.58, 140.97, 133.49, 133.29, 132.90, 131.21, 130.50, 129.22, 127.88, 113.29, 112.27, 111.62, 103.79, 55.39, 47.52, 23.80; Anal. Calcd for C21H16Cl2N4O4 (459.28): C, 54.92; H, 3.51; Cl, 15.44; N, 12.20; found: C, 54.93; H, 3.46; Cl, 15.54; N, 12.33.

4.1.3. General Procedure for the Preparation of EE-115

1,3-Dimethyl creatinine (2.8 g, 22.7 mmol) and indole-3-aldehydes (22.7 mmol) were heated under reflux in piperidine (30 mL) for 4 h. After cooling, the reaction mixture was poured into water (200 mL) and then stirred for 30 min. The precipitate was filtered, washed several times with water, air dried and crystallized from methanol.

(Z)-5-((1H-Indol-3-yl)Methylene)-1,3-Dimethylimidazolidine-2,4-Dione (Aplysinopsin) EE-115 [50]

Yield 80%, mp 236–8 °C (reported mp 236 °C); ^{1}H NMR (400 MHz, CDCl$_3$) δ: 8.87 (d, J = 2.7 Hz, 1H), 8.54 (s, 1H), 7.85–7.66 (m, 1H), 7.45 (dd, J = 6.7, 1.4 Hz, 1H), 7.33–7.18 (m, 3H), 6.42 (s, 1H), 3.34 (s, 3H), 3.23 (s, 3H).

4.2. Cell Lines and Cell Cultures

The human chronic myeloid leukemia K562 (ATCC, CCL-243, Manassas, VA, USA), MEG01 (ATCC, CRL-2021, Manassas, VA, USA), and the normal B lymphocyte RPMI 1788 cell lines (KCLB, 10156, Seoul, Korea) were cultured in Roswell Park Memorial Institute (RPMI) 1640 medium (Lonza, Basel, Switzerland), supplemented with 10% heat-inactivated fetal bovine serum (FBS) (Biowest, Riverside, CA, USA) and 1% penicillin-streptomycin solution (100×) (GenDEPOT, Katy, TX, USA). KBM-5 cells were kindly donated by Dr. Bharat B. Aggarwal. Imatinib-resistant KBM5 cells (KBM5R) cells were obtained by sequentially increasing the concentration of imatinib from 0.25 to 1 µM imatinib in IMDM media supplemented with 10% (v/v) fetal calf serum and 1% (v/v) antibiotic–antimycotics [51]. Imatinib-resistant K562 (K562IR) cells were a gift of the Catholic University of Seoul and cultured in RPMI 1640 medium with 25 mM HEPES (Lonza) supplemented with 10% (v/v) FCS and 1% (v/v) antibiotic–antimycotics. Both resistant cell types were cultured with 1 µM of imatinib and washed three times before each experiment. Cells were maintained at 37 °C and 5% of CO_2 in a humified atmosphere. Mycoplasma detection by Mycoalert^{TM} (Lonza) was performed every 30 days, and cells were used within three months after thawing.

Peripheral blood mononuclear cells (PBMCs) were isolated by density gradient centrifugation using Ficoll-Hypaque (GE Healthcare, Roosendaal, The Netherlands) from freshly collected buffy coats as previously described [51], obtained from healthy adult human volunteers (Red Cross, Luxembourg City, Luxembourg) after ethical approval as well as written informed consent from each volunteer. After isolation, cells were incubated overnight at 2×10^6 cells/mL in RPMI 1640 (supplemented with 1% antibiotic–antimycotic and 10% FCS (BioWhittaker, Verviers, Belgium) at 37 °C and 5% CO_2 in a humidified atmosphere. The day after, cell concentration was adjusted at 1×10^6 cells/mL using the same fresh complete medium and then treated as indicated.

4.3. Compounds

Mcl-1 inhibitor, A-1210477 (S7790, Selleckchem, Seoul, Korea) was used in single and combination treatments. Etoposide (E1383, Sigma-Aldrich, Seoul, Korea), Imatinib (SML 1027, Sigma-Aldrich, St. Louis, MO, USA), and Celecoxib (PZ0008, Sigma-Aldrich, Seoul, Korea) were used as positive controls. Caspase inhibitor 1 (z-VAD-fmk, 187389-52-2, Calbiochem, Seoul, Korea) served to inhibit caspase-dependent apoptosis.

4.4. Cell Proliferation and Viability

Cell proliferation and viability were assessed by the trypan blue exclusion method (Lonza), and viable cells were counted using a hematocytometer (Marienfeld, Lauda-Königshofen, Germany). Differential toxicity was calculated by comparing the viability of RPMI 1788 cells to the viability of cancer cells (normal/cancer cells). The difference in viability was expressed in terms of fold change.

4.5. Colony Formation Assay

For 48 h pretreatment of EE-84 colony formation assays, approximately 3×10^5 cells were seeded in each well of a 24-well plate, treated with EE-84 at indicated concentrations, and incubated at 37 °C and 5% of CO_2 in a humidified atmosphere for 48 h. After 48 h, 1000 cells were counted and grown in a semisolid methylcellulose medium (Methocult H4230, StemCell Technologies Inc., Vancouver, BC, Canada) supplemented with 10% FBS. Colonies were detected after 10 days of culture by adding 1 mg/mL of 3-(4,5-dimethylthiazol-2-yl)-2,5-diphenyltetrazolium bromide (MTT) reagent (Sigma-Aldrich) and were analyzed by Image J 1.8.0 software (U.S. National Institute of Health, Bethesda, MD, USA).

4.6. Quantification of Apoptosis and Necrosis

The percentage of apoptotic cells was quantified as the fraction of cells showing fragmented nuclei, as assessed by fluorescence microscopy (Nikon, Tokyo, Japan) after staining with Hoechst 33342 (Sigma-Aldrich) and propidium iodide (Sigma-Aldrich). In addition, apoptosis was confirmed by Annexin V APC (Biolegend, 640919)/propidium iodide (BD Biosciences, 556547) staining and fluorescence-activated cell sorter (FACS) analysis according to the manufacturer protocol (BD Biosciences, 556547).

4.7. In Silico Drug Likeliness Properties

Lipinski's 'rule of five' for drug likeliness properties was evaluated using the SCFBio website (http://www.scfbio-iitd.res.in/).

4.8. Zebrafish Toxicity

For toxicity assays, embryos were treated with 0.003% phenylthiourea (PTU) 14 h before the assay to remove pigmentation. Then, 2 h before the assay, the embryo's shell was eliminated and then treated for up to 24 h with aplysinopsin compounds at indicated concentrations in 24-well plates. Viability and abnormal development were assessed after 24 h of treatment under light microscopy (Carl Zeiss Stereomicroscope DV4, Seoul, Korea). Pictures were taken by fixing embryos onto a glass slide with 3% methylcellulose (Sigma-Aldrich).

4.9. Cell Cycle Analysis

Cells were collected and fixed in 70% ethanol. DNA was stained with propidium iodide (PI) solution (1 µg/mL, Sigma-Aldrich, St. Louis, MO, USA) in 1XPBS (Biosesang, Seongnam, Korea) for 30 min at 37 °C, supplemented with RNase A (100 µg/mL, Roche, Basel, Switzerland). Samples were analyzed by flow cytometry using the FACSCalibur™ system, Becton Dickinson (BD) Biosciences (San Jose, CA, USA). Data were recorded statistically (10,000 events/sample) using the Cell Quest software (BD Biosciences) and analyzed using Flow-Jo 8.8.5 software (Tree Star, Inc., Ashland, OR, USA).

4.10. Cell Morphology/Wright-Giemsa Staining

Diff Quik staining was used to analyze the morphological features of compound-treated cells. Approximately 3×10^5 cells were seeded in each well of a 24-well plate and treated with EE-84 at the indicated concentrations for the indicated time. Cells were then spun onto a microscope glass slide for 5 min at $500 \times g$ using a cytopad with caps (Elitech Group Inc., Puteaux, France). Cells were fixed, air-dried, and then stained with the Diff-Quik staining kit (Sysmex, Kobe, Japan). The stained cells were examined, and images were captured with an inverted microscope (Nikon Eclipse Ti2).

4.11. SA-β-Gal Assay

The senescence-associated (SA)-β-Gal activity was measured as previously reported [52]. K562 cells treated with 80 nM doxorubicin 72 h were used as a positive control for senescence induction.

4.12. Analysis of Cell Size and Complexity (Granularity)

Flow cytometry acquisitions of FSC-H (forward) vs. SSC-H (size) were performed as a method to monitor the cell size and granularity (cell complexity) in untreated vs. EE-84-treated K562 (FACSCalibur™; BD Biosciences). Data (10,000 events) were recorded using the Cellquest Pro software (BD Biosciences) and further analyzed using FlowJo software (Treestar, Ashland, OR, USA).

4.13. Analysis of Mitochondrial Membrane Potential (MMP) Levels

To monitor mitochondrial membrane potential (MMP), cells were incubated at 37 °C for 30 min with 50 nM MitoTracker Red CMXRos (all from Molecular Probes, Invitrogen, Grand Island, NY, USA) and then analyzed by flow cytometry. Data were recorded statistically (10,000 events/sample) using the CellQuest Pro software. Data were analyzed using the Flow-Jo 8.8.7 software, and results were expressed as cells with MMP loss (%).

4.14. Transmission Electron Microscopy (TEM)

Cells were pelleted and fixed in 2.5% glutaraldehyde (Electron Microscopy Sciences, Hatfield, PA, USA) diluted in 0.1 M sodium cacodylate buffer, pH 7.2 (Electron Microscopy Sciences) overnight. Cells were then rinsed twice with sodium cacodylate buffer, postfixed for 2 h in 2% osmium tetroxide at room temperature, washed with distilled water, and stained with 0.5% uranyl acetate at 4 °C overnight. Samples were then dehydrated in successive ethanol washes, followed by infiltration of 1 (100% ethanol):1 (Spurr's resin). Samples were kept overnight embedded in 100% Spurr's resin, mounted in molds, and left to polymerize in an oven at 56 °C for 48 h. Ultrathin sections (70–90 nm) were cut with an ultramicrotome, EM UC7 (Leica Microsystems Ltd., Seoul, Korea). Sections were stained with uranyl acetate and lead citrate and subsequently viewed using a JEM1010 transmission electron microscope (JEOL Korea Ltd., Seoul, Korea).

4.15. Determination of the Oxygen Consumption Rate and Glycolysis Stress

The oxygen consumption rate (OCR) was measured using a Seahorse XFp Cell Mito Stress Assay (#103010-100, Agilent Technologies, Seoul, Korea) ran on a Seahorse XFp analyzer (Agilent Technologies, Seoul, Korea) according to the manufacturer's instructions. Briefly, cells were seeded at 30,000 cells per well and treated with EE-84 for 48 h in 175 µL medium. Before measurements, plates were equilibrated in a CO_2-free incubator at 37 °C for 1 h. The analysis was performed using 1.5 µM oligomycin, 0.5 µM carbonyl cyanide-4-(trifluoromethoxy)phenylhydrazone (FCCP), and 1 µM rotenone/antimycin A as indicated. Data were analyzed using the Seahorse XF Cell Mito Stress Test report generator software (Agilent). The extracellular acidification rate (ECAR) was measured in response to the sequential injection of 10 mM glucose, 2 µM oligomycin (H+-ATP-synthase inhibitor), and 50 mM 2-deoxy-d-glucose (2DG) (hexokinase inhibitor) to detect non-glycolytic acidification, glycolysis, maximal glycolytic capacity, and glycolytic reserve using a Seahorse XFp analyzer with a Glycolysis Stress Test kit (Agilent, Santa Clara, CA, USA).

4.16. Measurement of Intracellular ATP Content

To quantify metabolically active cells, intracellular ATP levels were measured by CellTiter-Glo Luminescent Cell Viability Assay (Promega, Cosmogenetech, Seoul, Korea) following the manufacturer's protocol.

4.17. Measurement of Caspase-3/7 Activity

According to the manufacturer's instructions, the activation of caspase-3/7 was measured using the Caspase-Glo 3/7 Assay (Promega, Madison, WI, USA). The caspase-3/7 reagent was added to the sample volume at a 1:1 ratio, and the cells were incubated for 1 h at room temperature. The luminescence of triplicate samples was measured using a microplate reader.

4.18. Whole-Cell Extracts and Western Blotting

For the preparation of whole-cell extracts, cells were harvested, washed in cold 1xPBS, and lysed in Mammalian Protein Extraction Reagent (M-PER^{TM}, Thermo Fisher, Waltham, MA, USA) supplemented with a 1× protease inhibitor cocktail (Complete, EDTA-free, Roche, Basel, Switzerland) according to the manufacturer's instructions. Protein concentration was measured using the Bradford assay. Proteins were aliquoted and stored at −80 °C. Afterward, proteins were subjected to sodium dodecyl sulfate (SDS)–polyacrylamide gel electrophoresis (PAGE) and transferred to PVDF membranes (GE Healthcare, Little Chalfont, UK). Membranes were incubated with selected primary antibodies: anti-caspase-7 (9494S), anti-caspase-9 (9502S), anti-caspase-8 (9746), anti-Mcl-1 (4572S), anti-LC3B (2775), ATF4 (11815), ATF6 (65880), Bip/GRP78 (C50B12), CHOP (L63F7), eIF2α (9722) and PERK (3192) from Cell Signaling (Danvers, MA, USA), anti-caspase-3 (sc-56053) and anti-PARP-1 (sc-53643) from Santa Cruz Biotechnology (Dallas, TX, USA), anti-Bcl-xL (610212) from BD Pharmingen (San Jose, CA, USA), eIF2a (Phospho-Ser51) (11279) from Signalway Antibody Co. (College Park, MD, USA) and anti-β-actin (5441) from Sigma Aldrich (St. Louis, MO, USA). Blots were probed in PBS-T containing the appropriate blocking agent (5% milk or 5% BSA) for 1 h. Membranes were prehybridized overnight with the indicated primary antibodies. After washing, blots were incubated with species-appropriate HRP-conjugated secondary antibody (Santa Cruz) in PBS-T containing 5% milk. Proteins of interest were detected with ECL Plus Western blotting Detection System reagent (GE Healthcare) using ImageQuant LAS 4000 mini system (GE Healthcare).

4.19. Statistical Analysis

Data are expressed as the mean ± SD and significance was estimated by using one-way or two-way ANOVA (analysis of variance) followed by either Dunnett's multiple comparison test or Sidak's multiple comparison test, unless otherwise stated, using Prism 8 software, GraphPad Software (La Jolla, CA, USA). *p*-values were considered statistically significant when $p < 0.05$. Legends are represented as follows: * $p < 0.05$, ** $p < 0.01$, *** $p < 0.001$.

5. Conclusions

Through the screening of several aplysinopsin analogs, we selected EE-84 as an interesting anti-leukemic agent. EE-84 exhibited a safety profile as it had minimal impact on healthy models in vitro and in vivo. We also found that the treatment of K562 with EE-84 induced an antiproliferative effect concomitant with autophagy and ER stress induction as well as senescence. In addition, mitochondrial dysfunction was observed in line with altered K562 cell morphology after EE-84 treatment. Treatment of EE-84 combined with the BH3 mimetic A-1210477 (specific for Mcl-1) potentialized apoptotic cell death. We suggest this cotreatment as a promising preclinical approach to therapeutic failure, specifically in resistant CML.

Supplementary Materials: The following are available online at https://www.mdpi.com/article/10.3390/md19060285/s1, Table S1: IC$_{50}$ of aplysinopsin analogs in the noncancerous cell line RPMI 1788. Figure S1: Effect on proliferation and viability of aplysinopsin-treated on K562 cells. Figure S2: ^{1}H NMR spectral data of (A) EE-31, (B) EE-80, (C) EE-84, (D) EE-92 and (E) EE-115. Figure S3: ^{13}C NMR spectral data of (A) EE-31, (B) EE-80, (C) EE-84, and (D) EE-92. Figure S4: Effect on the proliferation and viability of EE-84 and EE-115 on noncancerous cell line RPMI1 788. Figure S5: Measurement of glycolytic capacity in K562IR cells. Figure S6: EE-84 sensitizes K562IR cells to BH3 mimetics after 24 h.

Author Contributions: S.S. and S.K.: equally performed the experiments; S.S., S.K., B.O.-B., C.C. (Claudia Cerella), C.C. (Christo Christov), G.K., M.D. (Mario Dicato) and M.D. (Marc Diederich): analyzed/discussed the data; E.R.E.-S.: designed and prepared aplysinopsin and its analogs; G.K.: provided the compounds; S.K. and M.D. (Marc Diederich) conceived the experiments and wrote/edited the manuscript. All authors have read and agreed to the published version of the manuscript.

Funding: S.K., S.S. and M.D. (Marc Diederich) were supported by National Research Foundation (NRF) [Grant Number 019R1A2C1009231] and by a grant from the MEST of Korea for Tumor Microenvironment Global Core Research Center (GCRC) [Grant Number 2011-0030001]. Support from Brain Korea (BK21) FOUR program and Creative-Pioneering Researchers Program at Seoul National University [Funding number: 370C-20160062] are acknowledged. C.C. (Claudia Cerella) and B.O.-B. were supported by Télévie Luxembourg. LBMCC is supported by "Recherche Cancer et Sang" Foundation, "Recherches Scientifiques Luxembourg", "Een Häerz fir kriibskrank Kanner", Action Lions "Vaincre le Cancer", and Télévie Luxembourg. E.R.E.-S. was supported by French and Egyptian governments through a cofinanced fellowship granted by the French Embassy in Egypt (Institut Français d'Egypte) and the Science and Technology Development Fund (STDF).

Institutional Review Board Statement: The study was conducted in agreement with the guidelines of the Institutional Animal Care and Use Committee (IACUC) of Seoul National University.

Informed Consent Statement: PBMCs were obtained from Red Cross Luxembourg with informed consent obtained from all subjects (donators of PBMC blood products) involved in the study. Specifically, agreement LBMCC-2019-0001: Assessment of differential toxicity of new drugs or drug combinations in preclinical development in ex-vivo proliferating peripheral blood mononuclear cells vs. proliferating cancer cells, agreement LBMCC-2019-0002: Assessment of toxicity of new drugs or drug combinations in preclinical development in non-proliferating peripheral blood mononuclear cells (systemic acute toxicity).

Data Availability Statement: Data supporting reported results can be found here: https://data.mendeley.com/datasets/z2rkrgwbm9/2; https://data.mendeley.com/datasets/bs3r484nfn/1; https://data.mendeley.com/datasets/ym9mcsm2fg/1, accessed on 19 May 2021.

Conflicts of Interest: The authors declare no conflict of interest.

Abbreviations

AML	acute myeloid leukemia
Bcr-Abl	breakpoint cluster region-Abelson
BH	Bcl-2 homology domain
BSA	bovine serum albumin
CCyR	complete cytogenetic response
CFA	colony formation assay
CML	chronic myeloid leukemia
DMSO	dimethyl sulfoxide
FBS	fetal bovine serum
FDA	food and drug administration
FLT3	FMS-like tyrosine kinase 3
GI	growth inhibition
HPF	hours post fertilization
IC	inhibitory concentration
ITD	internal tandem duplication
LogP	octanol–water partition coefficient
MPER	mammalian protein extraction reagent
Mcl-1	myeloid cell leukemia 1
MMP	mitochondrial membrane potential
MTT	3-(4,5-dimethylthiazol-2-1)-2,5,-diphenyltetrazolium bromide
PARP-1	poly(ADP-ribose)polymerase
PBMC	peripheral blood mononuclear cell
PBS	phosphate buffered saline
PI	propidium iodide
PMSF	phenylmethylsulphonyl fluoride
PTU	phenylthiourea
RPMI	Roswell Park Memorial Institute
SA	surface area
SD	standard deviation
SDS-PAGE	sodium dodecyl sulfate polyacrylamide gel electrophoresis
TEM	transmission electron microscopy
TKD	tyrosine kinase domain
UPR	unfolded protein response

References

1. Kang, Z.-J.; Liu, Y.-F.; Xu, L.-Z.; Long, Z.-J.; Huang, D.; Yang, Y.; Liu, B.; Feng, J.-X.; Pan, Y.-J.; Yan, J.-S.; et al. The Philadelphia chromosome in leukemogenesis. *Chin. J. Cancer* **2016**, *35*, 1–15. [CrossRef] [PubMed]
2. Cheng, Y.-C.; Chang, J.-M.; Chen, C.-A.; Chen, H.-C. Autophagy modulates endoplasmic reticulum stress-induced cell death in podocytes: A protective role. *Exp. Biol. Med.* **2015**, *240*, 467–476. [CrossRef] [PubMed]
3. Bhamidipati, P.K.; Kantarjian, H.; Cortes, J.; Cornelison, A.M.; Jabbour, E. Management of imatinib-resistant patients with chronic myeloid leukemia. *Ther. Adv. Hematol.* **2012**, *4*, 103–117. [CrossRef] [PubMed]
4. Liu, Y.; Gong, W.; Yang, Z.Y.; Zhou, X.S.; Gong, C.; Zhang, T.R.; Wei, X.; Ma, D.; Ye, F.; Gao, Q.L. Quercetin induces protective autophagy and apoptosis through ER stress via the p-STAT3/Bcl-2 axis in ovarian cancer. *Apoptosis* **2017**, *22*, 544–557. [CrossRef]
5. Hetz, C.; Chevet, E.; Harding, H.P. Targeting the unfolded protein response in disease. *Nat. Rev. Drug Discov.* **2013**, *12*, 703–719. [CrossRef]
6. Kim, I.; Xu, W.; Reed, J.C. Cell death and endoplasmic reticulum stress: Disease relevance and therapeutic opportunities. *Nat. Rev. Drug Discov.* **2008**, *7*, 1013–1030. [CrossRef]
7. Murrow, L.; Debnath, J. Autophagy as a Stress-Response and Quality-Control Mechanism: Implications for Cell Injury and Human Disease. *Annu. Rev. Pathol. Mech. Dis.* **2013**, *8*, 105–137. [CrossRef]
8. Yin, H.; Zhao, L.; Jiang, X.; Li, S.; Huo, H.; Chen, H. DEV induce autophagy via the endoplasmic reticulum stress related unfolded protein response. *PLoS ONE* **2017**, *12*, e0189704. [CrossRef] [PubMed]
9. Molina, P.; Almendros, P.; Fresneda, P.M. Iminophosphorane-Mediated Imidazole Ring Formation—A New and General Entry to Aplysinopsin-Type Alkaloids of Marine Origin. *Tetrahedron* **1994**, *50*, 2241–2254. [CrossRef]

10. Segraves, N.L.; Crews, P. Investigation of brominated tryptophan alkaloids from two thorectidae sponges: Thorectandra and Smenospongia. *J. Nat. Prod.* **2005**, *68*, 1484–1488. [CrossRef]
11. Newman, D.J.; Cragg, G.M. Natural Products as Sources of New Drugs from 1981 to 2014. *J. Nat. Prod.* **2016**, *79*, 629–661. [CrossRef]
12. Kazlauskas, R.; Murphy, P.T.; Quinn, R.J.; Wells, R.J. Aplysinopsin, a new tryptophan derivative from a sponge. *Tetrahedron Lett.* **1977**, *18*, 61–64. [CrossRef]
13. Lipinski, C.A.; Lombardo, F.; Dominy, B.W.; Feeney, P.J. Experimental and computational approaches to estimate solubility and permeability in drug discovery and development settings. *Adv. Drug Deliv. Rev.* **2001**, *46*, 3–26. [CrossRef]
14. Radogna, F.; Dicato, M.; Diederich, M. Cancer-type-specific crosstalk between autophagy, necroptosis and apoptosis as a pharmacological target. *Biochem. Pharmacol.* **2015**, *94*, 1–11. [CrossRef]
15. Yoshida, H. ER stress and diseases. *FEBS J.* **2007**, *274*, 630–658. [CrossRef]
16. Li, Z.; Wang, Y.; Newton, I.P.; Zhang, L.; Ji, P.; Li, Z. GRP78 is implicated in the modulation of tumor aerobic glycolysis by promoting autophagic degradation of IKKbeta. *Cell Signal.* **2015**, *27*, 1237–1245. [CrossRef]
17. Jiang, C.C.; Lucas, K.; Avery-Kiejda, K.A.; Wade, M.; Debock, C.E.; Thorne, R.F.; Allen, J.; Hersey, P.; Zhang, X.D. Up-regulation of Mcl-1 Is Critical for Survival of Human Melanoma Cells upon Endoplasmic Reticulum Stress. *Cancer Res.* **2008**, *68*, 6708–6717. [CrossRef]
18. Hu, J.; Dang, N.; Menu, E.; De Bryune, E.; Xu, D.; Van Camp, B.; Van Valckenborgh, E.; Vanderkerken, K. Activation of ATF4 mediates unwanted Mcl-1 accumulation by proteasome inhibition. *Blood* **2012**, *119*, 826–837. [CrossRef]
19. Folmer, F.; Jaspars, M.; Dicato, M.; Diederich, M. Marine cytotoxins: Callers for the various dances of death. *Gastroenterol. Hepatol.* **2009**, *2*, S34–S50.
20. Malve, H. Exploring the ocean for new drug developments: Marine pharmacology. *J. Pharm. Bioallied Sci.* **2016**, *8*, 83–91. [CrossRef]
21. Jimenez, P.C.; Wilke, D.V.; Costa-Lotufo, L.V. Marine drugs for cancer: Surfacing biotechnological innovations from the oceans. *Clincs* **2018**, *73*, e482s. [CrossRef]
22. Roberts, W.K.; Dekker, C.A. A convenient synthesis of arabinosylcytosine (cytosine arabinoside). *J. Org. Chem.* **1967**, *32*, 816–817. [CrossRef] [PubMed]
23. Bergmann, W.; Feeney, R.J. Contributions to the Study of Marine Products. Xxxii. The Nucleosides of Sponges. I.1. *J. Org. Chem.* **2002**, *16*, 981–987. [CrossRef]
24. Mayer, A.M.; Glaser, K.B.; Cuevas, C.; Jacobs, R.S.; Kem, W.; Little, R.D.; McIntosh, J.M.; Newman, D.J.; Potts, B.C.; Shuster, D.E. The odyssey of marine pharmaceuticals: A current pipeline perspective. *Trends Pharmacol. Sci.* **2010**, *31*, 255–265. [CrossRef] [PubMed]
25. Hollenbeak, K.H.; Schmitz, F.J. Aplysinopsin: Antineoplastic tryptophan derivative from the marine sponge Verongia spengelii. *Lloydia* **1977**, *40*, 479–481.
26. Murata, M.; Miyagawa-Kohshima, K.; Nakanishi, K.; Naya, Y. Characterization of Compounds That Induce Symbiosis between Sea Anemone and Anemone Fish. *Science* **1986**, *234*, 585–587. [CrossRef]
27. Okuda, R.K.; Klein, D.; Kinnel, R.B.; Li, M.; Scheuer, P.J. Marine natural products: The past twenty years and beyond. *Pure Appl. Chem.* **1982**, *54*, 1907–1914. [CrossRef]
28. Bialonska, D.; Zjawiony, J.K. Aplysinopsins-Marine Indole Alkaloids: Chemistry, Bioactivity and Ecological Significance. *Mar. Drugs* **2009**, *7*, 166–183. [CrossRef]
29. Hu, J.F.; Schetz, J.A.; Kelly, M.; Peng, J.N.; Ang, K.K.; Flotow, H.; Leong, C.Y.; Ng, S.B.; Buss, A.D.; Wilkins, S.P.; et al. New antiinfective and human 5-HT2 receptor binding natural and semisynthetic compounds from the Jamaican sponge Smenospongia aurea. *J. Nat. Prod.* **2002**, *65*, 476–480. [CrossRef]
30. Yoon, Y.-S.; Yoon, D.-S.; Lim, I.K.; Yoon, S.-H.; Chung, H.-Y.; Rojo, M.; Malka, F.; Jou, M.-J.; Martinou, J.-C.; Yoon, G. Formation of elongated giant mitochondria in DFO-induced cellular senescence: Involvement of enhanced fusion process through modulation of Fis1. *J. Cell. Physiol.* **2006**, *209*, 468–480. [CrossRef]
31. Galanos, P.; Vougas, K.; Walter, D.; Polyzos, A.; Maya-Mendoza, A.; Haagensen, E.J.; Kokkalis, A.; Roumelioti, F.-M.; Gagos, S.; Tzetis, M.; et al. Chronic p53-independent p21 expression causes genomic instability by deregulating replication licensing. *Nat. Cell Biol.* **2016**, *18*, 777–789. [CrossRef] [PubMed]
32. Galanos, P.; Pappas, G.; Polyzos, A.; Kotsinas, A.; Svolaki, I.; Giakoumakis, N.N.; Glytsou, C.; Pateras, I.S.; Swain, U.; Souliotis, V.L.; et al. Mutational signatures reveal the role of RAD52 in p53-independent p21-driven genomic instability. *Genome Biol.* **2018**, *19*, 1–18. [CrossRef]
33. Wiley, C.D.; Velarde, M.C.; Lecot, P.; Liu, S.; Sarnoski, E.A.; Freund, A.; Shirakawa, K.; Lim, H.W.; Davis, S.S.; Ramanathan, A.; et al. Mitochondrial Dysfunction Induces Senescence with a Distinct Secretory Phenotype. *Cell Metab.* **2016**, *23*, 303–314. [CrossRef] [PubMed]
34. Petrova, N.V.; Velichko, A.K.; Razin, S.V.; Kantidze, O.L. Small molecule compounds that induce cellular senescence. *Aging Cell* **2016**, *15*, 999–1017. [CrossRef]
35. Keskin, D.; Sadri, S.; Eskazan, A.E. Dasatinib for the treatment of chronic myeloid leukemia: Patient selection and special considerations. *Drug Des. Dev. Ther.* **2016**, *10*, 3355–3361. [CrossRef]

36. Hickson, L.J.; Prata, L.G.L.; Bobart, S.A.; Evans, T.K.; Giorgadze, N.; Hashmi, S.K.; Herrmann, S.M.; Jensen, M.D.; Jia, Q.; Jordan, K.L.; et al. Senolytics decrease senescent cells in humans: Preliminary report from a clinical trial of Dasatinib plus Quercetin in individuals with diabetic kidney disease. *EBioMedicine* **2019**, *47*, 446–456. [CrossRef] [PubMed]
37. Chang, J.; Wang, Y.; Shao, L.; Laberge, R.-M.; DeMaria, M.; Campisi, J.; Janakiraman, K.; Sharpless, N.E.; Ding, S.; Feng, W.; et al. Clearance of senescent cells by ABT263 rejuvenates aged hematopoietic stem cells in mice. *Nat. Med.* **2016**, *22*, 78–83. [CrossRef]
38. Matulis, S.M.; Gupta, V.A.; Nooka, A.K.; Von Hollen, H.; Kaufman, J.L.; Lonial, S.; Boise, L.H. Dexamethasone treatment promotes Bcl-2 dependence in multiple myeloma resulting in sensitivity to venetoclax. *Leukemia* **2016**, *30*, 1086–1093. [CrossRef]
39. Kapoor, I.; Bodo, J.; Hill, B.T.; Hsi, E.D.; Almasan, A. Targeting BCL-2 in B-cell malignancies and overcoming therapeutic resistance. *Cell Death Dis.* **2020**, *11*, 1–11. [CrossRef]
40. Giam, M.; Huang, D.C.S.; Bouillet, P. BH3-only proteins and their roles in programmed cell death. *Oncogene* **2008**, *27*, S128–S136. [CrossRef]
41. Ni Chonghaile, T.; Letai, A. Mimicking the BH3 domain to kill cancer cells. *Oncogene* **2008**, *27*, S149–S157. [CrossRef]
42. Chonghaile, T.N. BH3 mimetics: Weapons of cancer cell destruction. *Sci. Transl. Med.* **2019**, *11*, eaaw5311. [CrossRef]
43. Cerella, C.; Gaigneaux, A.; Mazumder, A.; Lee, J.-Y.; Saland, E.; Radogna, F.; Farge, T.; Vergez, F.; Récher, C.; Sarry, J.-E.; et al. Bcl-2 protein family expression pattern determines synergistic pro-apoptotic effects of BH3 mimetics with hemisynthetic cardiac glycoside UNBS1450 in acute myeloid leukemia. *Leukemia* **2016**, *31*, 755–759. [CrossRef] [PubMed]
44. Lee, J.-Y.; Talhi, O.; Jang, D.; Cerella, C.; Gaigneaux, A.; Kim, K.-W.; Lee, J.W.; Dicato, M.; Bachari, K.; Han, B.W.; et al. Cytostatic hydroxycoumarin OT52 induces ER/Golgi stress and STAT3 inhibition triggering non-canonical cell death and synergy with BH3 mimetics in lung cancer. *Cancer Lett.* **2018**, *416*, 94–108. [CrossRef] [PubMed]
45. Klosa, J. Synthesis of various cyanoacetic acid hydrazide derivatives. VII. Synthesis of tuberculostatic agents. *Arch. Pharm. Ber. Dtsch. Pharm. Ges.* **1955**, *288*, 452–455. [CrossRef] [PubMed]
46. Ottoni, O.; Cruz, R.; Alves, R. Efficient and simple methods for the introduction of the sulfonyl, acyl and alkyl protecting groups on the nitrogen of indole and its derivatives. *Tetrahedron* **1998**, *54*, 13915–13928. [CrossRef]
47. Cummings, D.F.; Canseco, D.C.; Sheth, P.; Johnson, J.E.; Schetz, J.A. Synthesis and structure–affinity relationships of novel small molecule natural product derivatives capable of discriminating between serotonin 5-HT1A, 5-HT2A, 5-HT2C receptor subtypes. *Bioorg. Med. Chem.* **2010**, *18*, 4783–4792. [CrossRef]
48. James, P.N.; Snyder, H.R.; Boekelheide, V.; Knowles, R.N. Indole-3-Aldehyde. *Org. Synth.* **2003**, *39*, 30. [CrossRef]
49. Kirsch, G.; Abdelwahab, A.B.; Hanna, A.G. Synthesis of Novel 3-Acetyl-2-aminothiophenes and Investigation of their Behaviour in the Reaction with Vilsmeier–Haack Reagent. *Synthesis* **2016**, *48*, 2881–2888. [CrossRef]
50. Tymiak, A.A.; Rinehart, K.L.; Bakus, G.J. Constituents of Morphologically Similar Sponges-Aplysina and Smenospongia Species. *Tetrahedron* **1985**, *41*, 1039–1047. [CrossRef]
51. Mazumder, A.; Lee, J.-Y.; Talhi, O.; Cerella, C.; Chateauvieux, S.; Gaigneaux, A.; Hong, C.R.; Kang, H.J.; Lee, Y.; Kim, K.-W.; et al. Hydroxycoumarin OT-55 kills CML cells alone or in synergy with imatinib or Synribo: Involvement of ER stress and DAMP release. *Cancer Lett.* **2018**, *438*, 197–218. [CrossRef] [PubMed]
52. Schnekenburger, M.; Grandjenette, C.; Ghelfi, J.; Karius, T.; Foliguet, B.; Dicato, M.; Diederich, M. Sustained exposure to the DNA demethylating agent, 2′-deoxy-5-azacytidine, leads to apoptotic cell death in chronic myeloid leukemia by promoting differentiation, senescence, and autophagy. *Biochem. Pharmacol.* **2011**, *81*, 364–378. [CrossRef] [PubMed]

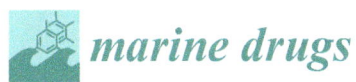

Article

Astaxanthin Reduces Stemness Markers in BT20 and T47D Breast Cancer Stem Cells by Inhibiting Expression of Pontin and Mutant p53

Yong Tae Ahn [1], Min Sung Kim [2], Youn Sook Kim [3] and Won Gun An [2],*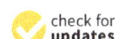

1. Research Institute for Longevity and Well-Being, Pusan National University, Busan 46241, Korea; sytahn@pusan.ac.kr
2. Division of Pharmacology, School of Korean Medicine, Pusan National University, Yangsan 50612, Korea; msk@pusan.ac.kr
3. Gene & Cell Therapy Research Center for Vessel-Associated Diseases, Pusan National University, Yangsan 50612, Korea; younskim@pusan.ac.kr
* Correspondence: wgan@pusan.ac.kr; Tel.: +82-51-510-8455

Received: 20 October 2020; Accepted: 17 November 2020; Published: 20 November 2020

Abstract: Astaxanthin (AST) is a product made from marine organisms that has been used as an anti-cancer supplement. It reduces pontin expression and induces apoptosis in SKBR3, a breast cancer cell line. Using Western blotting and qRT-PCR analyses, this study revealed that in the T47D and BT20 breast cancer cell lines, AST inhibits expression of pontin and mutp53, as well as the Oct4 and Nanog cancer stem cell (CSC) stemness genes. In addition, we explored the mechanism by which AST eradicates breast cancer cells using pontin siRNAs. Pontin knockdown by pontin siRNA reduced proliferation, Oct4 and Nanog expression, colony and spheroid formation, and migration and invasion abilities in breast cancer cells. In addition, reductions in Oct4, Nanog, and mutp53 expression following rottlerin treatment confirmed the role of pontin in these cells. Therefore, pontin may play a central role in the regulation of CSC properties and in cell proliferation following AST treatment. Taken together, these findings demonstrate that AST can repress CSC stemness genes in breast cancer cells, which implies that AST therapy could be used to improve the efficacy of other anti-cancer therapies against breast cancer cells.

Keywords: astaxanthin; T47D; BT20; pontin; mutp53; cancer stem cells; Oct4; Nanog; siRNA

1. Introduction

Breast cancer, most frequently found in women with menopause, develops from breast tissue and is characterized by uncontrolled cell growth, with the ability to metastasize to other tissues [1]. Risk factors for breast cancer include environmental mechanisms, genetic elements, and lifestyle components [2]. Current synthetic chemical anti-cancer agents are restricted to use for the removal of breast cancer due to their cytotoxic effects on normal host cells [3]. Thus, natural therapeutic products that inhibit cancer cell growth without excessive toxicity are under investigation to identify candidate therapeutics [4].

Many marine organisms and algae have the red pigment astaxanthin (AST), a xanthophyll carotenoid (3,3′-dihydroxy-beta, beta-carotene-4,4′-dione) [5]. AST has some effects against various types of cancer (e.g., oral, bladder, colon, blood, liver, lung, and breast). These effects are mediated by anti-proliferative, pro-apoptotic, antioxidant, anti-inflammatory, anti-invasion and migration, and anti-gap junctional intracellular communication mechanisms [6]. Potential molecular targets for AST in cancers include NF-kB, STAT3, P13K/AKT, MAPKs, PPAR, Nrf2, and pontin [6,7].

Pontin is a conserved ATPase of the AAA+ superfamily, with Walker A and B motifs, arginine fingers, and insertion domains that are conserved from yeast to humans [8]. The pontin gene is located on chromosome 3q21 and encodes a 456-amino-acid protein [9]. In association with its partner, reptin, pontin forms a multi-protein complex that is presumably involved in activities such as DNA damage sensing and repair, cell viability and death, gene transcription regulation, telomerase activity, and chromatin remodeling, protein assembly, and ribonucleoprotein complexes [10]. Pontin has limited homology to the bacterial helicase RuvB, which is involved in the resolution of Holliday junctions during recombination [11]. Pontin and reptin are both overexpressed in many cancer types, but only pontin is overexpressed in breast cancer cells [10]. There is some evidence that pontin reduces ATPase activity, thereby contributing to apoptotic activity in cancer cells [12]. Pontin was recently found to interact with mutant p53 (mutp53) to promote a gain of function mutation [13]. Pontin also serves as a cofactor for octamer-binding transcription factor 4 (Oct4) during the maintenance of mouse embryonic stem cells (ESCs) [14].

The tumor suppressor protein p53 plays an important role in the suppression of human cancers [15]. However, its function is sometimes impaired because of frequent mutations [16]. Furthermore, mutp53 is restricted to poorly differentiated tumors, whereas the overexpression of wild-type p53 is restricted to less-differentiated areas of tumors [17]. These findings have demonstrated that mutp53 is associated with cancer stem cell (CSC) formation and poor prognosis [18]. Recently, a correlation between mutp53 and CSC phenotype has been reported [19]. CSCs, also known as tumor-initiating cells, are a subpopulation of tumor cells that can generate heterogeneous progenies [20]. The proportion of CSCs in an overall cancer cell population is approximately 0.05–3%, but these cells are considered to be the fundamental barrier to operative cancer therapy due to their distinct cellular properties (e.g., self-renewal, differentiation, and tumor formation) [21]. CSCs are commonly identified in breast cancer using specific biomarkers including CD44, CD133, CD166, CD24, CD29, EpCAM, and aldehyde dehydrogenase 1 [22]. In addition, there is increasing evidence that mutp53 is involved in the expression of Oct4 and Nanog, which are crucial components for maintaining the pluripotency and self-renewal properties of normal stem cells and ESCs [14,23]. These genes promote each other's expression, control cancer progression, and are biomarkers of CSCs [24]. Oct4 belongs to the Pit-Oct-Unc (POU) family of transcriptional factors and plays a crucial role in stem cell differentiation and pluripotency by determining the fate of ESCs [25]. It also contributes to tumorigenesis and self-renewal through activation of its downstream target genes (e.g., Nanog, Sox2, and Klf4) [25]. Nanog is a homeobox domain transcription factor expressed in human cancers [26]. It plays a key role in malignant disease through effects on cell proliferation and traits such as clonogenic growth, tumorigenicity, invasiveness, and therapeutic resistance [26].

Previously, we reported that AST modulates pontin expression to cause apoptosis in breast cancer cells [7]. In this study, we explored how AST-targeted pontin functions in the obliteration of breast cancer cells and concluded that AST might impede breast cancer growth by reducing the populations of CSCs. These data demonstrate that the marine compound AST is a powerful anticancer agent.

2. Results

2.1. AST Reduces the Expression Levels of Pontin, mutp53, Oct4, and Nanog in T47D and BT20 Breast Cancer Cells, Inhibiting Their Proliferation

AST reduces pontin expression and mutp53 in the SKBR3 breast cancer cell line [7]. Moreover, the interaction between pontin and mutp53 promotes cancer migration and cancer stemness progression [13]. Thus, we investigated whether AST could affect cancer stemness properties in breast cancer cells. Because spheroid formation ability is a characteristic of CSCs [27], we investigated spheroid formation ability in SKBR3, T47D, and BT20 breast cancer cell lines. T47D and BT20 cells showed spheroid formation, whereas SKBR3 cells did not (Figure 1A). Because SKBR3 cells failed to form spheroids, we performed subsequent experiments with T47D and BT20 cells.

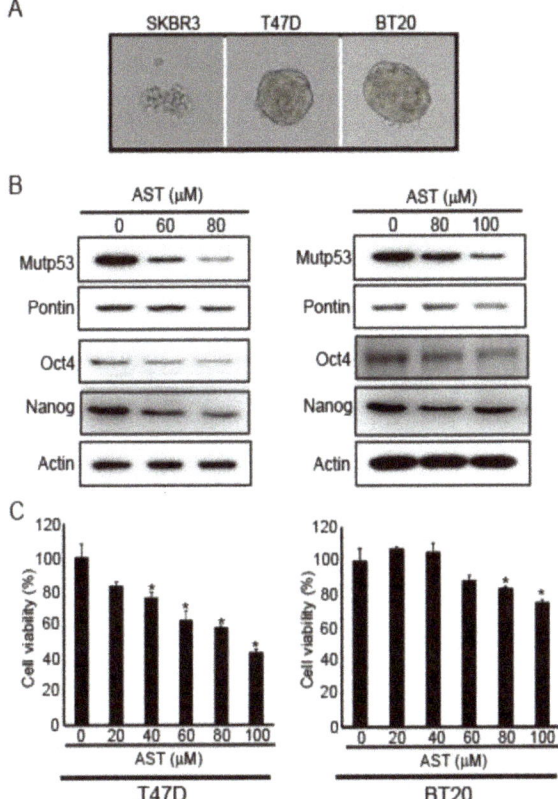

Figure 1. AST reduced the expression levels of pontin, mutp53, Oct4, and Nanog in T47D and BT20 breast cancer cell lines, thereby inhibiting cell proliferation. (**A**) Spheroid formation abilities of SKBR3, T47D, and BT20 breast cancer cell lines. (**B**) Expression levels of mutp53, pontin, Oct4, and Nanog were determined via Western blotting of T47D and BT20 cells after AST treatment. Actin was used as a loading control. (**C**) Cells were incubated for 48 h at 37 °C at the indicated concentrations of AST in a 96-well plate. Then, CCK-8 was added and the cells were incubated for 3 h at 37 °C. Absorbance was measured with a spectrophotometer at 450 nm. Data are expressed as the mean ± standard deviation (SD) of three independent experiments. * $p < 0.05$.

First, to determine whether AST could regulate the expression levels of pontin, mutp53, Oct4, and Nanog in T47D and BT20 cells, their levels were measured via Western blotting. As the concentration of AST increased, the expression levels of pontin, mutp53, Oct4, and Nanog decreased relative to control (Figure 1B). These findings indicate that AST can regulate CSC genes in both T47D and BT20 cells.

Next, cell viability was measured using a CCK-8 viability assay to determine whether AST would affect the growth of T47D and BT20 cells. Cell growth was clearly inhibited by AST treatment in a dose-dependent manner (Figure 1C). Therefore, AST can inhibit the proliferation of both T47D and BT20 breast cancer cell lines.

2.2. Pontin Knockdown Attenuates the Proliferation of T47D and BT20 Breast Cancer Cells

To determine whether pontin is necessary for the proliferation of breast cancer cells, we performed cell cycle arrest, Ki67 staining, and CCK8 viability assays following the induction of pontin silencing. As shown in Figure 2A, the cell cycle profiles of T47D cells treated with pontin siRNAs included significantly greater proportions of cells in the G0/G1 phase (siPontin1: 39.06% ± 0.57%, siPontin2: 41.07% ± 1.72%), compared to the control siRNA group (29.1% ± 0.7%). This trend was also evident in BT20 cells treated with pontin siRNAs (siPontin1; 37.06% ± 0.57%, siPontin2; 36.07% ± 1.72%), compared to the control siRNA group (28.0% ± 0.7%). Conversely, the proportions of cells in the G2/M phase after pontin siRNA transfection were significantly reduced in both cell lines. Therefore, pontin is a key molecule for the proliferation of breast cancer cells.

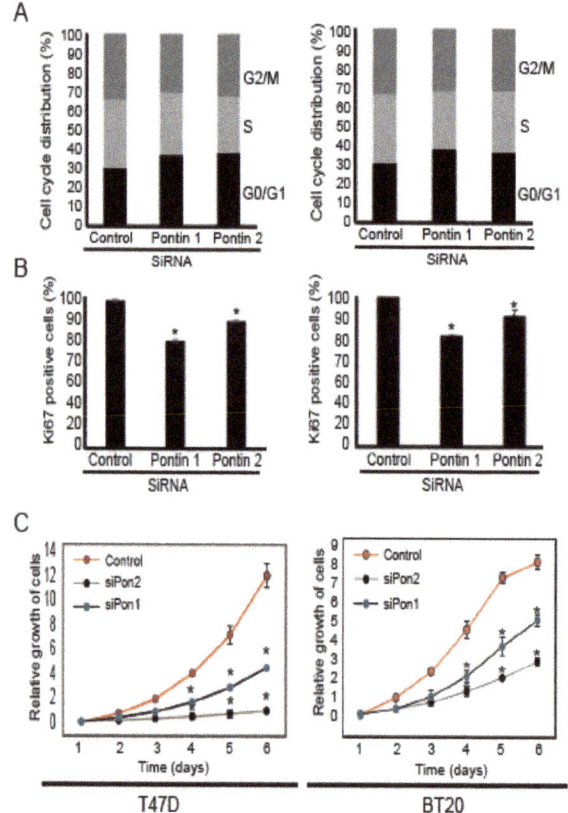

Figure 2. Pontin knockdown attenuated the proliferation of T47D and BT20 cells. (**A**) Cell cycle analyses of T47D and BT20 cells after targeted pontin knockdown. Cells were harvested 3 days after transfection of pontin siRNAs or control siRNA. Similar results were obtained from three independent experiments. (**B**) Ki67 incorporation was used to determine the proportions of cells in each cell cycle phase. Cells were harvested 3 days after transfection of control siRNA or pontin siRNAs. Proportions of Ki67-positive cells are shown. Results are expressed as the mean ± SD of three independent experiments. * $p < 0.05$. (**C**) Growth curves of T47D and BT20 cells after targeted pontin knockdown. Data are represented the mean ± SD of three independent experiments (* $p < 0.05$).

A Ki67 incorporation experiment showed reductions in the number of Ki67-positive cells following pontin siRNA treatment, compared to control siRNA (Figure 2B), indicating that pontin is an important molecule for cell proliferation. To examine whether downregulation of pontin would affect cancer cell growth, CCK8 viability assays were conducted (Figure 2C). The numbers of cells were significantly lower in pontin siRNA groups than in control siRNA groups after transfection.

Taken together, these data indicate that pontin depletion leads to defects in breast cancer cells, which implies that it plays a crucial role in the proliferation of breast cancer cells.

2.3. Pontin Knockdown Reduces the Levels of mutp53, Oct4, and Nanog in T47D and BT20 Breast Cancer Cells

Because AST reduced the expression levels of pontin, mutp53, Nanog, and Oct4, their levels were analyzed by Western blotting and quantitative reverse transcriptase polymerase chain reaction (qRT-PCR) analyses following pontin knockdown in T47D and BT20 cells. As shown in Figure 3A, after transfection of pontin siRNAs, the protein expression levels of mutp53, Nanog, and Oct4 were downregulated compared to control.

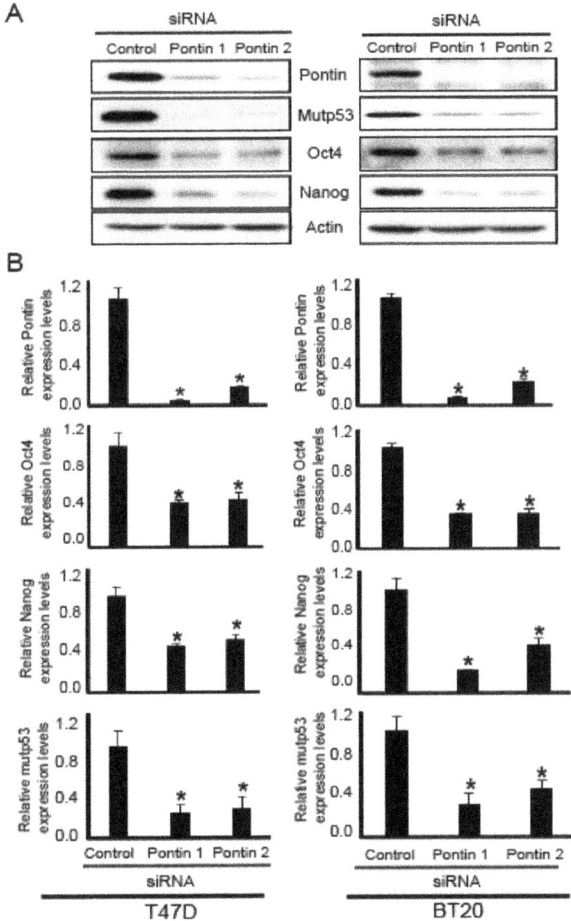

Figure 3. Effects of pontin-targeting siRNAs on expression levels of Oct4, Nanog, and mutp53 in T47D and BT20 breast cancer cell lines. Cells were transfected with pontin-targeting or control siRNA. (**A**) Cell lysates were prepared from T47D and BT20 cells, and the expression levels of Oct4, Nanog, and mutp53 were detected by Western blotting. (**B**) Total RNA was extracted, and the expression levels of Oct4, Nanog, and mutp53 were evaluated via qRT-PCR. All experiments were normalized by comparison with glyceraldehyde 3-phosphate dehydrogenase (GAPDH). Data represent the mean ± SD of three independent experiments (* $p < 0.05$).

To confirm the Western blotting results, the mRNA expression levels of pontin, mutp53, Nanog, and OCT4 in both T47D and BT20 cells were investigated via qRT-PCR. As shown in Figure 3B, pontin siRNA groups had reduced mRNA expression levels of pontin, mutp53, Nanog, and OCT4 in both

T47D and BT20 cells. These results suggest that pontin knockdown in T47D and BT20 cells can reduce the expression levels of mutp53, Nanog, and Oct4. Thus, pontin could be a crucial component of cancer stemness properties in T47D and BT20 breast cancer cell lines.

2.4. Pontin Knockdown Reduces Colony and Spheroid Formation Ability in T47D and BT20 Breast Cancer Cells

Pontin is a necessary cofactor for Oct4 during the maintenance of mouse ESCs [14]. Thus, pontin might regulate colony and spheroid formation in breast cancer cells because these abilities are essential CSC characteristics [27].

To test this hypothesis, colony formation assays were performed using T47D and BT20 cells transfected with pontin siRNAs. After 14 days in culture, the numbers of colonies formed by cells transfected with pontin siRNA were substantially reduced, compared to the numbers of T47D cells (Figure 4A) and BT20 cells (Figure 4B) transfected with control siRNA.

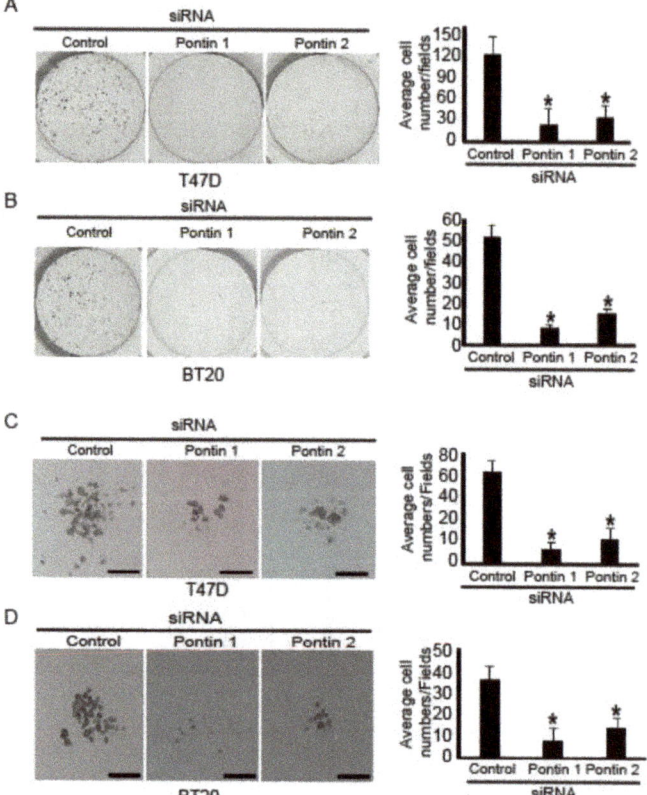

Figure 4. Pontin knockdown reduced colony and spheroid formation abilities in T47D and BT20 cells. Pontin knockdown with siRNA attenuated colony formation by (**A**) T47D and (**B**) BT20 cells. Left panel, representative images from a portion of field; right panel, quantification of average number of migrated cells/field. Pontin knockdown with siRNA attenuated spheroid formation by (**C**) T47D and (**D**) BT20 cells. Left panel, representative images from a portion of field; right panel, quantification of average number of migrated cells/field. Data represent the mean ± SD of three independent experiments (* $p < 0.05$).

Next, because CSCs have been shown to form floating spheres in culture [27], their abilities to form spheroids in vitro were measured after pontin knockdown. Control siRNA or pontin siRNAs were transfected into the cells, which then were grown in suspension with serum-free spheroid media for spheroid maintenance. After 7 days in culture, the numbers of spheroids formed in cells transfected with pontin siRNAs were considerably reduced, compared to the numbers of T47D cells (Figure 4C) and BT20 cells (Figure 4D) transfected with control siRNA.

Taken together, these results indicate that pontin knockdown in breast cancer cells might attenuate the properties of CSCs.

2.5. Pontin Knockdown Reduces Migration and Invasion Abilities in T47D and BT20 Breast Cancer Cells

Because specific depletion of pontin was able to change colony and spheroid formation abilities, other CSC abilities (e.g., migration and invasion) were presumably changed. To test this hypothesis, transwell migration and invasion assays were performed using cells transfected with pontin siRNAs or control siRNA. As shown in Figure 5, migration and invasion of breast cancer cells were inhibited by pontin knockdown, compared to controls. The migration inhibition rates of T47D and BT20 cells were 82% and 85%, respectively. The invasion inhibition rates of T47D and BT20 cells were 78% and 64%, respectively. These results suggest that pontin knockdown in breast cancer cells attenuates the properties of CSCs.

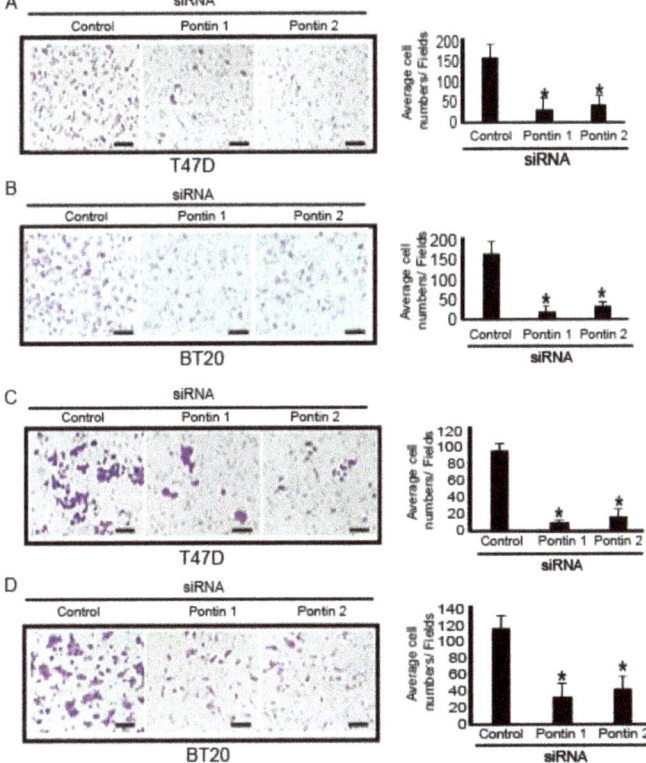

Figure 5. Pontin knockdown reduced migration and invasion in breast cancer cells. Pontin knockdown by siRNA attenuated migration of (**A**) T47D and (**B**) BT20 cells, as determined by transwell migration assays. Left panel, representative images from a portion of field; right panel, quantification of average number of migrated cells/field (×200 magnification). Pontin knockdown by siRNA attenuated invasion of (**C**) T47D and (**D**) BT20 cells, determined using Matrigel-coated transwell invasion assays. Left panel, representative images from a portion of field; right panel, quantification of average number of migrated cells/field (×200 magnification). Data represent the mean ± SD of three independent experiments (* $p < 0.05$).

2.6. Rottlerin Reduces Expression Levels of Oct4, Nanog, and mutp53 in T47D and BT20 Breast Cancer Cells

To further demonstrate the role of pontin in this study, rottlerin (a pontin-specific ATPase inhibitor) was used. The expression levels of mutp53, Nanog, and Oct4 under rottlerin treatment were measured via Western blotting and qRT-PCR analyses. As shown in Figure 6A, rottlerin diminished the expression levels of mutp53, Oct4, and Nanog in T47D and BT20 cells.

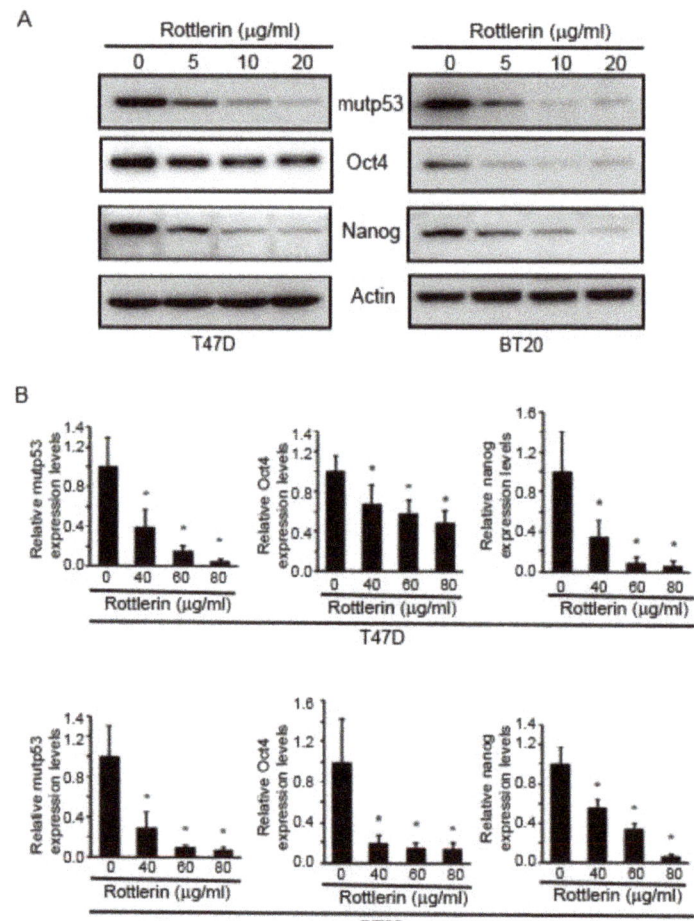

Figure 6. Rottlerin reduced expression levels of Oct4, Nanog, and mutp53 in T47D and BT20 breast cancer cell lines. Cell lysates were prepared from T47D and BT20 cells that had been subjected to rottlerin treatment. Expression levels of Oct4, Nanog, and mutp53 were detected via Western blotting analyses and qRT-PCR. (**A**) Cell lysates were prepared from T47D and BT20 cells, and the expression levels of Oct4, Nanog, and mutp53 were detected by Western blotting. (**B**) Total RNA was extracted, and the expression levels of Oct4, Nanog, and mutp53 were evaluated by qRT-PCR. All expression levels were normalized to GAPDH. Data represent the mean ± SD of three independent experiments (* $p < 0.05$).

To confirm these findings, the mRNA expression levels of mutp53, Nanog, and Oct4 in rottlerin-treated T47D and BT20 cells were investigated via qRT-PCR. With increasing rottlerin concentration, the mRNA expression levels of mutp53, Nanog, and Oct4 decreased in both T47D and BT20 cells (Figure 6B).

These results confirm that pontin regulates the expression levels of mutp53, Nanog, and Oct4 in breast cancer cells.

3. Discussion

AST obtained from marine organisms has powerful antioxidant, anti-inflammatory, and anti-cancer properties. In the present study, the anti-cancer effects of AST on breast cancer cells were investigated. Because AST regulates pontin expression and causes apoptosis in SKBR3 cells [7], its effects were further explored to identify the molecules that it regulates, as well as how pontin impedes breast cancer cell growth, using a pontin knockdown approach.

Pontin is an AAA+ ATPase that possesses both ATPase and DNA helicase activities [8,11]. Its overexpression has been observed in many cancers [28]. Its ATPase activity is important for cell proliferation in many tumors, including breast cancer and hepatocellular carcinoma [10]. In this study, pontin was found to participate in the proliferation of the T47D and BT20 breast cancer cell lines. Pontin is closely associated with various cell cycle-related genes, including E2F1 and RB [29]. The downregulation of pontin leads to cell cycle arrest, resulting in the accumulation of cells in the G1 phase and the reduction of cells in the S and G2/M phases [30]. In this study, pontin knockdown in T47 and BT20 cells led to a significant reduction in cell growth (Figure 2A). In addition, cell cycle analyses revealed that pontin siRNA induced G1 cell cycle arrest, indicating that pontin is a crucial component in breast cancer cell proliferation.

Pontin negatively regulates mutant p53 during cancer development [13]. It can also cause a gain of function in mutp53, supporting tumorigenesis [13]. Its interaction with mutp53 promotes cancer stemness properties such as proliferation, metastasis, and invasion [18]. A critical role for mutp53 in CSC production is supported by the association between tumors with mutp53 and the undifferentiated phenotypes in these tumors [17]. Moreover, mutp53 has been shown to encourage a stem-like phenotype in breast cancers [31], while undifferentiated breast tumors express specific stemness genes [32,33]. Therefore, pontin was presumed to regulate specific stemness genes and markers by mediating mutp53 activity. Pontin and mutp53 are considered important regulatory components within the CSC circuitry. Additional studies are needed to determine whether pontin can regulate the expression of Oct4 and Nanog through a mutp53-related mechanism and to determine how it selectively regulates the expression of mutp53 and stemness genes in cancer cells.

CSCs have unique stemness properties concerning self-renewal, differentiation, and proliferative capacities. Notably, they exhibit robust expression of stemness genes including Oct4 and Nanog [34]. In CSCs, the expression of Nanog and Oct4 is associated with a more aggressive tumor phenotype [35]. Therefore, CSCs are presumed to promote the growth and development of most human malignancies. Nanog is expressed in cancer cells, where it enhances tumorigenesis by activating CSCs [36]. Moreover, Nanog and mutp53 are co-expressed in cancer cells [37]. Oct4 plays a key role in stem cell differentiation and pluripotency by determining the fate of ESCs [25]. Notably, pontin depletion causes downregulation of Oct4 in ESCs [14]. Pontin serves as a co-activator for Oct4-dependent long intergenic non-coding RNA transcription [14], indicating that it regulates Oct4 and Nanog expression. Here, we confirmed that AST repressed Oct4 and Nanog expression in T47D and BT20 cells.

Drug resistance is a well-known characteristic of CSCs [38]. CSCs possess high aldehyde dehydrogenase 1 activity and express CD44 but not CD24 [39–41]. Aldehyde dehydrogenase 1 overexpression is associated with poor prognosis and cancer recurrence after chemotherapy [42]. Furthermore, mutp53-dependent drug resistance is mediated by enhanced CSC properties [42]. CSCs can undergo cell cycle arrest, thereby resisting chemotherapy and radiotherapy [43]. Notably, tumor invasion and recurrence after radiotherapy and chemotherapy have been attributed to CSCs [44]. Therefore, therapeutic targeting of CSCs may improve the prognosis of patients with cancer [45]. Our findings imply that AST might be useful for the treatment of breast cancer because of its ability to repress CSC genes.

In conclusion, AST is a robust antioxidant that blocks the proliferation of T47D and BT20 breast cancer cells. It also inhibits the expression of pontin, mutp53, Oct4, and Nanog, which constitute CSC stemness genes in T47D and BT20 cells. In addition, the use of pontin siRNA in this study revealed the mechanisms by which AST eradicates breast cancer cells. Pontin knockdown reduced cell proliferation, Oct4 and Nanog expression, colony and spheroid formation, and migration and invasion in both T47D and BT20 cells. In addition, the reduction of Oct4, Nanog, and mutp53 expression levels following rottlerin treatment confirmed the role of pontin in these cells. Therefore, pontin might play a central role in the regulation of CSC properties and the proliferation of cancer cells, following addition of AST. Taken together, our findings suggest that AST could eradicate CSCs and serve as a powerful treatment for breast cancer. Further studies are needed to elucidate how AST represses the expression of CSC genes at the transcriptional or translational levels, what quantities of AST provide optimal cancer treatment effects, and the relationship between pontin and hsp90 during AST treatment for breast cancer.

4. Materials and Methods

4.1. Chemicals and Antibodies

Dulbecco's modified Eagle medium (DMEM), fetal bovine serum (FBS), and Dulbecco's phosphate-buffered saline (DPBS) were purchased from Gibco (Grand Island, NY, USA). Monoclonal antibodies specific for pontin, Oct4, Nanog, p53, and actin were obtained from Cell Signaling Technology (Danvers, MA, USA).

4.2. Cell Culture and Transfection

Human breast cancer cell lines SKBR3, T47D, and BT20 (American Type Culture Collection, Manassas, VA, USA) were cultured in DMEM containing 10% (v/v) FBS and 1% (v/v) penicillin-streptomycin (Gibco) at 37 °C in a 5% CO_2 incubator. Cells were subcultured by enzymatic digestion with trypsin– ethylenediaminetetraacetic acid (EDTA) (0.25% trypsin and 1 mM EDTA) solution when they reached approximately 80% confluency. For siRNA targeting knockdown, siRNA oligos against pontin were purchased from Integrated Bioneer Corporation (Daejeon, Korea). Pontin-targeting siRNA sequences were as follows: siRNA-1, 5'-CAUGGGAGGAUAUGGCAAA-3'; siRNA-2, 5'-GAGGAUAUGGCAAAACCAU-3'. The control siRNA sequence was as follows: 5'-CCUACGCCACCAAUUUCGU-3'. The Neon Transfection System (Invitrogen) was used for electroporation to transfect T47D and BT20 cells with pontin siRNAs or control siRNA. Briefly, 2×10^6 cells in buffer R were electroporated in 100 µL tips with 500 ng of siRNA, then plated with culture media in a 100 mm culture plate. The electroporation parameters were cell-line-specific (T47D: 1400 V, 20 mA, two pulses; BT20:1300 V, 20 mA, one pulse). For rottlerin treatment, cells were treated with various concentrations of rottlerin (Calbiochem, Billerica, MA, USA) for 12 h.

4.3. Cell Proliferation Assay

Cell proliferation was determined using a CCK-8 assay (Dojindo, Tokyo, Japan). For growth rate analyses, control and pontin knockdown cells were seeded with culture medium in 96-well plates (SPL Life Sciences, Seoul, Korea) at a density of 5×10^3 cells per well. After incubation for 24 h at 37 °C, CCK-8 in culture medium was added to each well and cells were incubated for 2 h at 37 °C. The optical density was read at 450 nm using an ELISA reader (Tecan Group Ltd., Männedorf, Switzerland). Results were expressed as the mean ± SD of three independent experiments.

4.4. Cell Cycle Analyses

For cell cycle analyses, the Muse® Cell Cycle Assay Kit (Millipore, Burlington, MA, USA) was used to determine the proportions of cells in each cell cycle phase. In brief, cells were transfected with pontin siRNAs or control siRNA, then harvested and fixed in 70% ethanol at −20 °C for 12 h. After fixation, the cells were washed twice with DPBS and stained with cell cycle solution for 20 min at room temperature in the dark. Then, the cells were counted using a Muse Cell Analyzer (Millipore).

In addition, the Muse® Ki67 Proliferation Kit (Millipore) was used to measure the populations of proliferating cells. Briefly, harvested cells were washed three times in ice-cold DPBS and suspended in fixation solution for 15 min. Then, they were transferred to permeabilization solution and incubated for 15 min. Next, they were washed three times in ice-cold DPBS and suspended in assay buffer with the hKi67-PE antibody for 15 min. Finally, they were counted using a Muse Cell Analyzer.

4.5. Western Blotting Analyses

Cells were collected by centrifugation at 4 °C, washed three times in ice-cold DPBS, and suspended in Radioimmunoprecipitation assay (RIPA) lysis buffer (50 mM Tris (pH 7.5), 2 mM EDTA, 100 mM NaCl, 1% NP-40) containing protease inhibitor cocktail (Sigma-Aldrich, St. Louis, MO, USA). Then, cell lysates were centrifuged at 13,000 rpm for 15 min at 4 °C, and the protein concentrations were determined using a bicinchoninic acid protein assay kit (Thermo Fisher Scientific, Rockford, IL, USA). Equal amounts of total protein (30 µg) were resolved by 8–12% SDS–PAGE and proteins were transferred to polyvinylidene difluoride (PVDF) membranes (Millipore). The membranes were blocked with 5% (*v/v*) skim milk in Tris-buffered saline with Tween (TBS-T; 50 mM Tris, 150 mM NaCl, and 0.1% Tween-20), incubated with specific primary antibodies in blocking buffer overnight at 4 °C, washed three times in TBS-T, and incubated for 1 h at room temperature with horseradish peroxidase-conjugated secondary antibody. Immunoreactive bands were developed using an enhanced chemiluminescence detection system (ECL Plus, Thermo Fisher Scientific).

4.6. Tumor Spheroid Formation Assay

T47D and BT20 cells were transfected with siRNA oligos targeting pontin or control for 24 h. Harvested cells from SKBR3, T47D, and BT20 cells or transfected T47D and BT20 cells were suspended in 24-well ultra-low attachment surface plates at 400 cells per well in spheroid media (serum-free DMEM/F12 media supplemented with 20 ng/mL hEGF, 10 ng/mL β-FGF, 2% B-27 supplement, and penicillin-streptomycin solution). Following 2 weeks of cultivation, spheroid formation was assessed using an Olympus IX51 microscope (Olympus, Waltham, MA, USA). Results were recorded for at least three independent experiments.

4.7. Cell Invasion Assay

Transwell chambers were used to examine cell invasion capability. T47D and BT20 cells were transfected with pontin-targeting or control siRNA oligos for 48 h. For transwell assays, the transwell chambers were coated with 100 µL BD Biosciences Matrigel™ overnight in a cell incubator. Then, transfected cells were trypsinized and resuspended at 1×10^5 cells in 200 µL serum-free medium. The resuspended cells were placed into the upper chambers of a 24-well transwell plate (8 mm pore size; Corning Inc., Corning, NY, USA). The lower chambers were filled with 700 µL complete medium with 10% FBS. Following incubation for 24 h at 37 °C, non-invading cells were removed from the upper chamber with a cotton swab. Invading cells on the lower surface of the inserts were fixed with 4% paraformaldehyde and stained with 1% crystal violet. Three random fields for each insert were counted at 200× magnification. Data were recorded as the mean ± SD of at least three independent experiments.

4.8. Cell Migration Assay

The migration assay was performed using transwell chambers. T47D and BT20 cells were transfected with pontin-targeting or control siRNA oligos for 48 h. Then, transfected cells were trypsinized and resuspended at 2×10^4 cells in 200 µL serum-free medium. The resuspended cells were placed into the upper chambers of a 24-well transwell plate (8 mm pore size; Corning Inc.). The lower chambers were filled with 700 µL complete medium with 10% FBS. Following incubation for 24 h at 37 °C, non-invading cells were removed from the upper chamber with a cotton swab. Invading cells on the lower surface of the inserts were fixed with 4% paraformaldehyde and stained with 1% crystal violet. Three random fields for each insert were counted at 200× magnification. Data were recorded as the mean ± SD of at least three independent experiments.

4.9. RNA Isolation and qRT-PCR

Total RNA was extracted using an RNeasy mini kit (Qiagen, Hilden, Germany) from T47D and BT20 cells transfected with pontin-targeting or control siRNA oligos, in accordance with the manufacturer's instructions. Total RNA was reverse-transcribed into cDNA using Superscript II Reverse Transcriptase (Invitrogen, Carlsbad, CA, USA), in accordance with the manufacturer's instructions. The cDNA was amplified by qPCR in an ABI 7500 real-time PCR system (Applied Biosystems, Foster City, CA, USA) using the SYBR Select Master Mix kit (Applied Biosystems) and with gene-specific primers. The thermocycling conditions were initial denaturation at 95 °C for 15 min, followed by 30 cycles of 95 °C for 20 s, 58 °C for 40 s, and 72 °C for 1 min. The results were normalized by comparison with the housekeeping gene GAPDH. The primer sequences used in this study were as follows: pontin forward, 5′-TGA AGA GCA CTA CGA AGA CG-3′; pontin reverse, 5′-AAC AAG ACA GCT CTT CCA GC-3; mutp53 forward, 5′-AGA AAA CCT ACC AGG GCA GC-3′; mutp53 reverse, 5′-CTC CGT CAT GTG CTG TGA CT-3′; Oct4 forward, 5′-CGA CTA TGC ACA ACG AGA GG-3′; Oct4 reverse, 5′-AGA GTG GTG ACG GAG ACA G-3′; Nanog forward, 5′-TCT TCC TAC CAC CAG GGA TG-3′; Nanog reverse, 5′-ATG CAG GAC TGC AGA GAT TC-3′; GAPDH forward 5′-ATA TGA TTC CAC CCA TGG CAA-3′; and GAPDH reverse, 5′-GAT GAT GAC CCT TTT GGC TCC-3. The expressions of genes including Pontin, mutp53, Oct4, and nanog were quantified using the $\Delta\Delta Ct$ method.

4.10. Statistical Analyses

Statistical analyses were performed using SPSS Statistics Ver. 23 (IBM Corp., Armonk, NY, USA). Results are presented as the mean ± SD. Comparisons were performed using independent *t*-tests. p values < 0.05 were considered statistically significant.

Author Contributions: Conceptualization, Y.T.A., M.S.K. and W.G.A.; Methodology, M.S.K., Y.S.K. and Y.T.A.; Data analysis, Y.T.A., Y.S.K. and W.G.A.; Data curation and graphing, M.S.K. and Y.S.K.; Writing—original draft preparation, M.S.K., Y.T.A.; Writing—review and editing, Y.T.A. and W.G.A.; Supervision, W.G.A. All authors have read and agreed to the published version of the manuscript.

Funding: This research was supported by the Basic Science Research Program through the National Research Foundation of Korea (NRF) funded by the Ministry of Education (NRF-2018R1D1A3B07049092).

Conflicts of Interest: The authors declare no conflict of interest.

References

1. Lavery, J.F.; Clarke, V.A. Causal attributions, coping strategies, and adjustment to breast cancer. *Cancer Nurs.* **1996**, *19*, 20–28. [CrossRef] [PubMed]
2. Sun, Y.S.; Zhao, Z.; Yang, Z.N.; Xu, F.; Lu, H.J.; Zhu, Z.Y.; Shi, W.; Jiang, J.; Yao, P.P.; Zhu, H.P. Risk Factors and Preventions of Breast Cancer. *Int. J. Biol. Sci.* **2017**, *13*, 1387–1397. [CrossRef]
3. Singh, P.; Ngcoya, N.; Kumar, V. A Review of the Recent Developments in Synthetic Anti-Breast Cancer Agents. *Anticancer Agents Med. Chem.* **2016**, *16*, 668–685. [CrossRef]
4. Sparreboom, A.; Scripture, C.D.; Trieu, V.; Williams, P.J.; De, T.; Yang, A.; Beals, B.; Figg, W.D.; Hawkins, M.; Desai, N. Comparative preclinical and clinical pharmacokinetics of a cremophor-free, nanoparticle albumin-bound paclitaxel (ABI-007) and paclitaxel formulated in Cremophor (Taxol). *Clin. Cancer Res.* **2005**, *11*, 4136–4143. [CrossRef]
5. Fassett, R.G.; Coombes, J.S. Astaxanthin: A potential therapeutic agent in cardiovascular disease. *Mar. Drugs* **2011**, *9*, 447–465. [CrossRef]
6. Zhang, L.; Wang, H. Multiple Mechanisms of Anti-Cancer Effects Exerted by Astaxanthin. *Mar. Drugs* **2015**, *13*, 4310–4330. [CrossRef]
7. Kim, M.S.; Ahn, Y.T.; Lee, C.W.; Kim, H.; An, W.G. Astaxanthin Modulates Apoptotic Molecules to Induce Death of SKBR3 Breast Cancer Cells. *Mar. Drugs* **2020**, *18*, 266. [CrossRef]

8. Tucker, P.A.; Sallai, L. The AAA+ superfamily—A myriad of motions. *Curr. Opin. Struct. Biol.* **2007**, *17*, 641–652. [CrossRef] [PubMed]
9. Bauer, A.; Huber, O.; Kemler, R. Pontin, an interaction partner of β-catenin, binds to the TATA box binding protein. *Proc. Natl. Acad. Sci. USA* **1998**, *95*, 14787–14792. [CrossRef] [PubMed]
10. Mao, Y.Q.; Houry, W.A. The Role of Pontin and Reptin in Cellular Physiology and Cancer Etiology. *Front. Mol. Biosci.* **2017**, *58*, 1–24. [CrossRef]
11. Makino, Y.; Mimori, T.; Koike, C.; Kanemaki, M.; Kurokawa, Y.; Inoue, S.; Kishimoto, T.; Tamura, T. TIP49, homologous to the bacterial DNA helicase RuvB, acts as an autoantigen in human. *Biochem. Biophys. Res. Commun.* **1998**, *245*, 819–823. [CrossRef]
12. Wang, X.; Huang, X.; Wu, C.; Xue, L. Pontin/Tip49 negatively regulates JNK-mediated cell death in *Drosophila*. *Cell Death Discov.* **2018**, *4*, 74. [CrossRef] [PubMed]
13. Zhao, Y.; Zhang, C.; Yue, X.; Li, X.; Liu, J.; Yu, H.; Belyi, V.A.; Yang, Q.; Feng, Z.; Hu, W. Pontin, a new mutant p53-binding protein, promotes gain-of-function of mutant p53. *Cell Death Differ.* **2015**, *22*, 1824–1836. [CrossRef] [PubMed]
14. Boo, K.; Bhin, J.; Jeon, Y.; Kim, J.; Shin, H.-J.R.; Park, J.-E.; Kim, K.; Kim, C.R.; Jang, H.; Kim, I.-H.; et al. Pontin functions as an essential coactivator for Oct4-dependent lincRNA expression in mouse embryonic stem cells. *Nat. Commun.* **2016**, *6*, 6810. [CrossRef]
15. Liu, J.; Zhang, C.; Hu, W.; Feng, Z. Tumor suppressor p53 and its mutants in cancer metabolism. *Cancer Lett.* **2015**, *356*, 197–203. [CrossRef] [PubMed]
16. Liu, J.; Zhang, C.; Feng, Z. Tumor suppressor p53 and its gain-of-function mutants in cancer. *Acta Biochim. Biophys. Sin.* **2014**, *46*, 170–179. [CrossRef]
17. Prabhu, V.V.; Allen, J.E.; Hong, B.; Zhang, S.; Cheng, H.; El-Deiry, W.S. Therapeutic targeting of the p53 pathway in cancer stem cells. *Expert. Opin. Ther. Targets* **2012**, *16*, 1161–1174. [CrossRef]
18. Aloni-Grinstein, R.; Shetzer, Y.; Kaufman, T.; Rotter, V. p53: The barrier to cancer stem cell formation. *FEBS Lett.* **2014**, *588*, 2580–2589. [CrossRef]
19. Solomon, H.; Dinowitz, N.; Pateras, I.S.; Cooks, T.; Shetzer, Y.; Molchadsky, A.; Charni, M.; Rabani, S.; Koifman, G.; Tarcic, O.; et al. Mutant p53 gain of function underlies high expression levels of colorectal cancer stem cells markers. *Oncogene* **2018**, *37*, 1669–1684. [CrossRef]
20. Plaks, V.; Kong, N.; Werb, Z. The cancer stem cell niche: How essential is the niche in regulating stemness of tumor cells? *Cell Stem Cell* **2015**, *16*, 225–238. [CrossRef]
21. Ingangi, V.; Minopoli, M.; Ragone, C.; Motti, M.L.; Carriero, M.V. Role of microenvironment on the fate of disseminating cancer stem cells. *Front. Oncol.* **2019**, *9*, 82. [CrossRef] [PubMed]
22. Chiotaki, R.; Polioudaki, H.; Theodoropoulos, P.A. Stem cell technology in breast cancer: Current status and potential applications. *Stem Cells Cloning* **2016**, *9*, 17–29. [PubMed]
23. Boiani, M.; Schöler, H.R. Regulatory networks in embryo-derived pluripotent stem cells. *Nat. Rev. Mol. Cell Biol.* **2005**, *6*, 872–881. [CrossRef]
24. Ezeh, U.I.; Turek, P.J.; Reijo, R.A.; Clark, A.T. Human embryonic stem cell genes OCT4, NANOG, STELLAR, and GDF3 are expressed in both seminoma and breast carcinoma. *Cancer* **2005**, *104*, 2255–2265. [CrossRef] [PubMed]
25. Scholer, H.R.; Ruppert, S.; Suzuki, N.; Chowdhury, K.; Gruss, P. New type of POU domain in germ line-specific protein Oct-4. *Nature* **1990**, *344*, 435. [CrossRef] [PubMed]
26. Jeter, C.R.; Yang, T.; Wang, J.; Chao, H.-P.; Tang, D.G. Concise Review: NANOG in Cancer Stem Cells and Tumor Development: An Update and Outstanding Questions. *STEM Cells* **2015**, *33*, 2381–2390. [CrossRef] [PubMed]
27. Abbaszadegan, M.R.; Bagheri, V.; Razavi, M.S.; Momtazi, A.A.; Sahebkar, A.; Gholamin, M. Isolation, identification, and characterization of cancer stem cells: A review. *J. Cell Physiol.* **2017**, *232*, 2008–2018. [CrossRef] [PubMed]
28. Lauscher, J.C.; Elezkurtaj, S.; Dullat, S.; Lipka, S.; Gröne, J.; Buhr, H.J.; Huber, O.; Kruschewski, M. Increased Pontin expression is a potential predictor for outcome in sporadic colorectal carcinoma. *Oncol. Rep.* **2012**, *28*, 1619–1624. [CrossRef] [PubMed]
29. Tarangelo, A.; Lo, N.; Teng, R.; Kim, E.; Le, L.; Watson, D.; Furth, E.; Raman, P.; Ehmer, U.; Viatour, P. Recruitment of Pontin/Reptin by E2f1 amplifies E2f transcriptional response during cancer progression. *Nat. Commun.* **2015**, *6*, 10028. [CrossRef] [PubMed]

30. Yuan, X.-S.; Wang, Z.-T.; Hu, Y.-J.; Bao, F.-C.; Yuan, P.; Zhang, C.; Cao, J.-L.; Wang, L.; Hu, J. Downregulation of RUVBL1 inhibits proliferation of lung adenocarcinoma cells by G1/S phase cell cycle arrest via multiple mechanisms. *Tumour Biol.* **2016**, *37*, 16015–16027. [CrossRef]
31. Spike, B.T.; Wahl, G.M. p53, Stem cells, and reprogramming: Tumor suppression beyond guarding the genome. *Genes Cancer* **2011**, *2*, 404–419. [CrossRef] [PubMed]
32. Pei, J.; Wang, Y.; Li, Y. Identification of key genes controlling breast cancer stem cell characteristics via stemness indices analysis. *J. Transl. Med.* **2020**, *18*, 74. [CrossRef] [PubMed]
33. Sin, W.C.; Lim, C.L. Breast cancer stem cells—From origins to targeted therapy. *Stem Cell Investig.* **2017**, *4*, 96. [CrossRef] [PubMed]
34. Aponte, P.M.; Caicedo, A. Stemness in cancer: Stem cells, cancer stem cells, and their microenvironment. *Stem Cells Int.* **2017**, *2017*, 5619472. [CrossRef]
35. Rasti, A.; Mehrazma, M.; Madjd, Z.; Abolhasani, M.; Zanjani, L.S.; Asgari, M. Co-expression of cancer stem cell markers OCT4 and NANOG predicts poor prognosis in renal cell carcinomas. *Sci. Rep.* **2018**, *8*, 11739. [CrossRef]
36. Chambers, I.; Colby, D.; Robertson, M.; Nichols, J.; Lee, S.; Tweedie, S.; Smith, A. Functional expression cloning of Nanog, a pluripotency sustaining factor in embryonic stem cells. *Cell* **2003**, *113*, 643–655. [CrossRef]
37. Lee, H.-J.; Kang, Y.-H.; Lee, J.-S.; Byun, J.-H.; Kim, U.-K.; Jang, S.-J.; Rho, G.-J.; Park, B.-W. Positive expression of NANOG, mutant p53, and CD44 is directly associated with clinicopathological features and poor prognosis of oral squamous cell carcinoma. *BMC Oral Health* **2015**, *15*, 153. [CrossRef]
38. Prieto-Vila, M.; Takahashi, R.U.; Usuba, W.; Kohama, I.; Ochiya, T. Drug resistance driven by cancer stem cells and their niche. *Int. J. Mol. Sci.* **2017**, *18*, 2574. [CrossRef]
39. Yan, Y.; Zuo, X.; Wei, D. Concise review: Emerging role of CD44 in cancer stem cells: A promising biomarker and therapeutic target. *Stem Cells Transl. Med.* **2015**, *4*, 1033–1043. [CrossRef]
40. Deng, X.; Apple, S.; Zhao, H.; Song, J.; Lee, M.; Luo, W.; Wu, X.; Chung, D.; Pietras, R.J.; Chang, H.R. CD24 expression and differential resistance to chemotherapy in triple-negative breast cancer. *Oncotarget* **2017**, *8*, 38294–38308. [CrossRef]
41. Nozaki, Y.; Tamori, S.; Inada, M.; Katayama, R.; Nakane, H.; Minamishima, O.; Onodera, Y.; Abe, M.; Shiina, S.; Tamura, K.; et al. Correlation between c-Met and ALDH1 contributes to the survival and tumor-sphere formation of ALDH1 positive breast cancer stem cells and predicts poor clinical outcome in breast cancer. *Genes Cancer* **2017**, *8*, 628–639. [CrossRef] [PubMed]
42. Kida, K.; Ishikawa, T.; Yamada, A.; Shimada, K.; Narui, K.; Sugae, S.; Shimizu, D.; Tanabe, M.; Sasaki, T.; Ichikawa, Y.; et al. Effect of ALDH1 on prognosis and chemoresistance by breast cancer subtype. *Breast Cancer Res. Treat.* **2016**, *156*, 261–269. [CrossRef] [PubMed]
43. Cojoc, M.; Mäbert, K.; Muders, M.H.; Dubrovska, A. A role for cancer stem cells in therapy resistance: Cellular and molecular mechanisms. *Semin. Cancer Biol.* **2015**, *31*, 16–27. [CrossRef] [PubMed]
44. Peitzsch, C.; Tyutyunnykova, A.; Pantel, K.; Dubrovska, A. Cancer stem cells: The root of tumor recurrence and metastases. *Semin. Cancer Biol.* **2017**, *44*, 10–24. [CrossRef] [PubMed]
45. Singh, A.; Settleman, J. EMT, cancer stem cells and drug resistance: An emerging axis of evil in the war on cancer. *Oncogene* **2010**, *29*, 4741–4751. [CrossRef]

Publisher's Note: MDPI stays neutral with regard to jurisdictional claims in published maps and institutional affiliations.

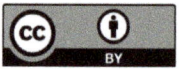

© 2020 by the authors. Licensee MDPI, Basel, Switzerland. This article is an open access article distributed under the terms and conditions of the Creative Commons Attribution (CC BY) license (http://creativecommons.org/licenses/by/4.0/).

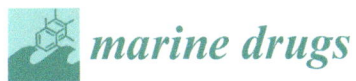

Article

Anti-Tumor Effects of Astaxanthin by Inhibition of the Expression of STAT3 in Prostate Cancer

Shao-Qian Sun, You-Xi Zhao, Si-Yu Li, Jing-Wen Qiang and Yi-Zhi Ji *

Biochemical Engineering College, Beijing Union University, Beijing 100023, China; shaoqian168@sina.com (S.-Q.S.); zhaoyouxi@buu.edu.cn (Y.-X.Z.); emmalee0316@163.com (S.-Y.L.); JKstrong99@163.com (J.-W.Q.)
* Correspondence: 20167003@buu.edu.cn; Tel.: +86-10-52072148

Received: 7 July 2020; Accepted: 29 July 2020; Published: 7 August 2020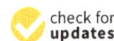

Abstract: Astaxanthin is a natural product gaining increasing attention due to its safety and anti-cancer properties. In this study, we investigated the mechanisms of the anti-cancer effects of astaxanthin on prostate cancer (PCa) cell lines using aggressive PCa DU145 cells. Also an instantaneous silenced cell line (si-STAT3) derived from DU145 and a control cell line (si-NK) were used for the MTT and colony formation assays to determine the role of astaxanthin in proliferation and colony formation abilities. Flow cytometry assays were used to detect the apoptosis of tumor cells. Migration and invasion assays detected the weakening of the respective abilities. Western blot and RT-PCR tests detected the levels of STAT3 protein and mRNA. Astaxanthin resulted in suppression of the proliferation of DU145 cells and the level of STAT3. The treatment of DU145 cells with astaxanthin decreased the cloning ability, increased the apoptosis percentage and weakened the abilities of migration and invasion of the cells. Furthermore, astaxanthin reduced the expression of STAT3 at protein and mRNA levels. The effects were enhanced when astaxanthin and si-STAT3 were combined. The results of animal experiments were consistent with the results in cells. Thus, astaxanthin inhibits the proliferation of DU145 cells by reducing the expression of STAT3.

Keywords: prostate cancer; astaxanthin; STAT3; proliferation; colony formation; apoptosis; migration; invasion

1. Introduction

Prostate cancer is one of the most frequently diagnosed malignancies in men, with increasing incidence in China [1,2]. Surgery, radiotherapy, chemotherapy and endocrine therapy are curative treatment options for prostate cancer [3]. However, after receiving endocrine therapy or surgery, 80–90% of patients develop hormone resistance within 3–4 years. In patients tolerant to endocrine therapy, increasing the doses of radiotherapy and chemotherapy can, rarely, improve the treatment effect, and severe toxicity and side effects cannot be avoided [4]. In addition, whether radiotherapy or chemotherapy resistance appeared after a period of treatment was elucidated using aggressive prostate cancer cells [5]. Thus, finding a drug that effectively inhibits prostate cancer is clinically significant.

Signal transducer and activator of transcription 3 (STAT3) is one of the critical members of the signal transducer and activator of transcription family and is composed of about 770 amino acids [6,7]. STAT3 activation plays a major role in mediating cell proliferation, differentiation, invasion, metastasis, inflammation, apoptosis and other biological cell processes [8–12]. Some studies have shown that compared to normal cells, the 705 site of the C-amino terminal tyrosine in STAT3 is continuously and abnormally activated in about 70% of tumor cells [8,12,13]. This protein is aberrantly activated in prostate cancer and contributes to the promotion of metastatic progression [14,15]. Therefore, STAT3 plays a major role in the occurrence and development of prostate cancer by effectively blocking the activation of related pathways, which is a novel method of cancer treatment.

About 67% of anti-cancer drugs are derived from natural products or natural product derivatives [16]. Astaxanthin is a natural product that is safe and possesses anti-cancer properties. It is primarily found in marine organisms such as algae, phytoplankton and shrimp. It is the final form of carotenoid synthesis with a strong ability to quench singlet oxygen and clear free radicals [17–19]. Recently, many in vivo and in vitro studies have confirmed that astaxanthin inhibits the growth of various tumor cells, such as neuroblastoma, lung cancer, gastric cancer, oral cancer, colon cancer, breast cancer, bladder cancer, liver cancer and leukemia [20–26]. Anti-cancer effects include anti-proliferation [27], enhancing apoptosis [27], anti-oxidation [28,29], anti-inflammation [28,30], preventing migration and invasion, and so on [31]. Although the mechanisms of astaxanthin mediating anti-cancer action have not yet been fully clarified, a number of molecular targets of astaxanthin have been proposed, which may explain the anti-tumor effects of this drug, such as NF-κB, STAT3, PI3K/AKT, MAPKs, PPARγ, and so on [31–34]. However, whether astaxanthin suppresses prostate cancer through STAT3 is yet to be elucidated.

Herein, whether astaxanthin can effectively inhibit the proliferation, cloning ability, invasion and migration ability and increase the apoptosis of DU145 cells by inhibiting the expression of STAT3 and its related proteins at protein and mRNA levels is evaluated.

2. Results

2.1. Astaxanthin Inhibits the Proliferation of DU145 Cells and Reduces the Expression of STAT3

To explore the effects of astaxanthin on the proliferation of DU145, we conducted the MTT assay. DU145 cells were cultured in the presence of different concentrations of astaxanthin. The results showed that astaxanthin significantly suppressed the proliferation of DU145 cells, and the inhibition of proliferation was dose-dependent. Astaxanthin suppressed cell proliferation at 50, 100 and 200% as compared to the control at the rates of 27, 38 and 50%, respectively (Figure 1A). These results indicate that astaxanthin inhibits DU145 cells, and the IC50 (half-inhibitory concentration) was <200 μM.

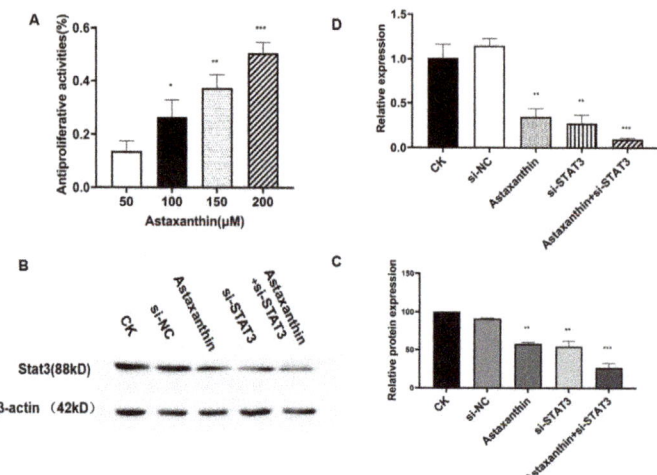

Figure 1. Cell proliferation assay and Western blotting using prostate cancer DU145 cells. (**A**) Cells were pretreated with 0, 50, 100 and 200 μM astaxanthin for 48 h. Proliferation was measured by MTT assay. Data are presented as the average of three experiments (±SD), * $p < 0.05$, ** $p < 0.01$, and *** $p < 0.001$. (**B**) DU145 cells were pretreated with 200 μM astaxanthin for 24 h. Western blotting results show that 200 μM astaxanthin reduces the level of STAT3. (**C**) Relative protein expression analysis. * $p < 0.05$, ** $p < 0.01$, and *** $p < 0.001$. (**D**) Relative mRNA expression analysis. ** $p < 0.01$, and *** $p < 0.001$.

To explore whether astaxanthin was a potential inhibitor, we examined the expression of STAT3 in protein (Figure 1B,C) and mRNA levels (Figure 1D). The results indicated that astaxanthin is a potential inhibitor of STAT3 and downregulates its expression at both protein and mRNA levels.

2.2. Astaxanthin Reduces the Colony Formation Ability of DU145 Cells

CK was the blank control. The expression of STAT3 in DU145 was lowered by siRNA-STAT3, and siRNA-NC was the blank control to si-STAT3. After 48 h post-transfection, 200 µM was administered for 24 h.

The colony formation assay revealed that astaxanthin, siRNA-STAT3 and astaxanthin+siRNA-STAT3 reduced the number of colonies of DU145 cells (Figure 2A,B). The colony inhibition rates of astaxanthin, siRNA-STAT3 and astaxanthin+siRNA-STAT3 treatments were 48, 46 and 83%, respectively. Therefore, the results suggest that astaxanthin effectively inhibits the cloning ability of DU145 cells, while the effect of astaxanthin+si-STAT3 was as high as 83% (Figure 2C).

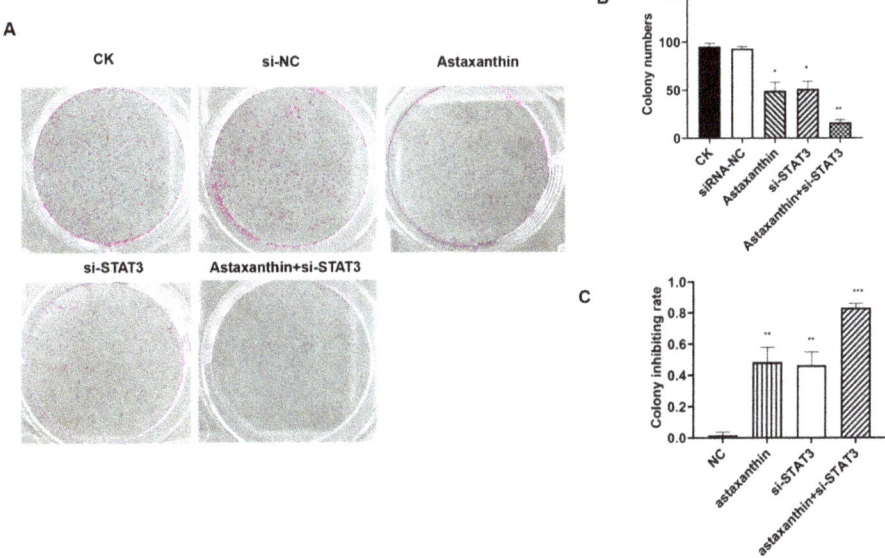

Figure 2. Colony inhibition rate analysis. The experiments were conducted on five groups. CK was the blank control group. The astaxanthin group was pretreated with astaxanthin for 24 h. The si-STAT3 group was transfected with siRNA-STAT3 for 48 h, and the siRNA-NC group was the blank control to si-STAT3. Astaxanthin+si-STAT3 group was transfected with a si-STAT3 plasmid for 48 h and treated with astaxanthin for 24 h. (**A**) Clone formation experiments were carried out. (**B,C**) Colony numbers were measured, and colony inhibition rates were calculated. The results show that astaxanthin inhibits the cloning ability of DU145 cells, while the effect of astaxanthin combined with si-STAT3 is superior. Data are presented as the average of three experiments (±SD), * $p < 0.05$, ** $p < 0.01$, *** $p < 0.001$.

2.3. Astaxanthin Induces Apoptosis on DU145 Cells

To determine whether astaxanthin induces apoptosis, we used Annexin V-Fluorescein and a PI double staining assay. The experiments were divided into five groups: CK (blank control), astaxanthin, siRNA-NC (blank control to si-STAT3), si-STAT3 and astaxanthin+siRNA-STA3 (Figure 3A).

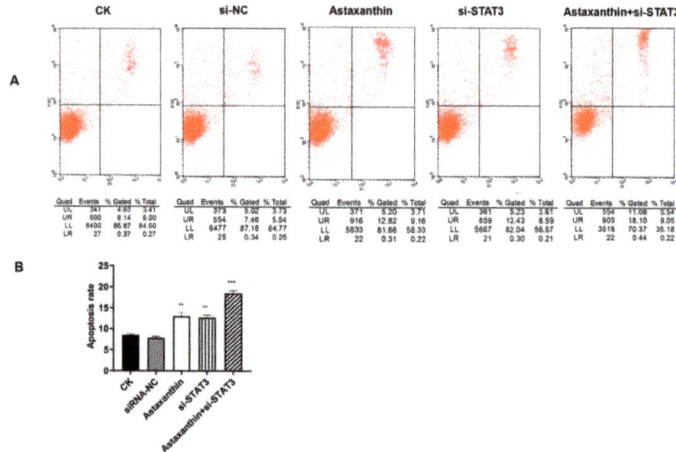

Figure 3. Effects of astaxanthin on apoptosis in DU145 cells. The experiments were divided into five groups. CK was the blank control group. The astaxanthin group was pretreated with astaxanthin for 24 h. The si-STAT3 group was transfected with siRNA-STAT3 for 48 h, and the siRNA-NC group was the blank control to si-STAT3. The astaxanthin+si-STAT3 group was transfected with a si-STAT3 plasmid for 48 h and then treated with astaxanthin for 24 h. (**A**) The progression of the apoptotic cells and the respective phase were analyzed with Annexin V-FITC assay. (**B**) The apoptosis rate was analyzed. The results show that both astaxanthin and si-STAT3 promote the apoptosis of DU145 cells, while the effect of astaxanthin combined with si-STAT3 is enhanced. Data are presented as the average of three experiments (±SD), ** $p < 0.01$ and *** $p < 0.001$.

As shown in Figure 3B, compared to the CK group, treatment of DU145 cells with 200 μM astaxanthin for 24 h increased the percentage of apoptotic cells from 8.5% to 13.1%. The group containing si-STAT3 increased the percentage of apoptosis to 12.7%. However, the percentage of apoptosis was highest at 18.5% when combining astaxanthin with si-STAT3.

2.4. Astaxanthin Decreases the Migration and Invasion of DU145 Cells

Excessive migration and invasion are critical characteristics of tumor cells. We analyzed changes in the migration and invasion of DU145 cells with astaxanthin, si-STAT3 and astaxanthin combined with si-STAT3. As shown in Figure 4, astaxanthin and si-STAT3 decreased the migration and invasion of DU145 cells. When cells were treated with astaxanthin, about 41% of cells could not pass from one chamber to another ($p < 0.01$), and 36% cells could not pass through the transwell membrane as compared to the control group. When cells were treated with si-STAT3, the migration inhibition rate was 40%, and the invasion inhibition rate was 34%. In addition, the combination of astaxanthin and si-STAT3 increased the migration and invasion rates to 71% and 56% respectively.

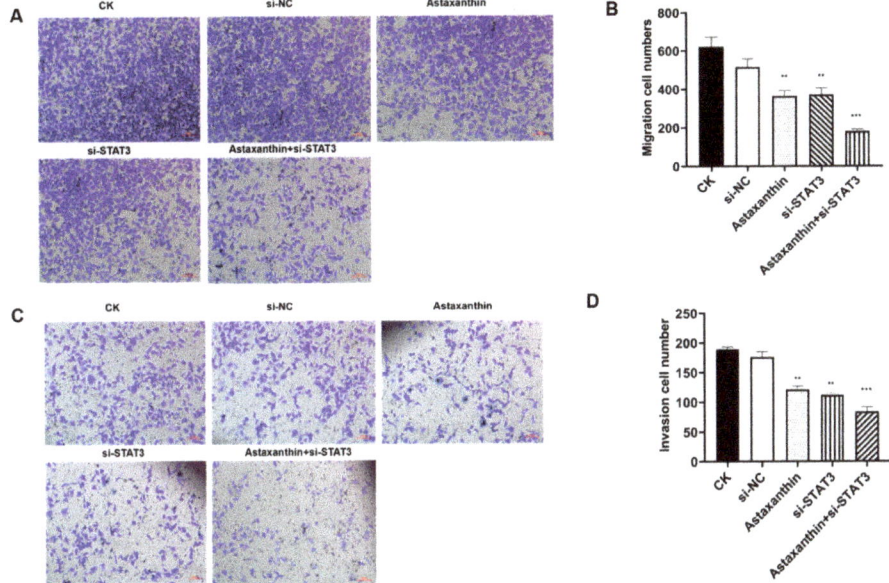

Figure 4. Astaxanthin influences the migration and invasion of DU145 cells. The groups are as described in Figure 2. (**A**) Image of the migratory transwell assay. (**B**) Both astaxanthin and si-STAT3 suppress the migration of DU145 cells, while the effect of astaxanthin combined with si-STAT3 is superior. Data are presented as the average of three experiments (±SD), ** $p < 0.01$ and *** $p < 0.001$. (**C**) Image of the invasive transwell assay. (**D**) Both astaxanthin and si-STAT3 suppress the invasion of DU145 cells, while the effect of astaxanthin combined with si-STAT3 is enhanced. Data are presented as the average of three experiments (±SD), ** $p < 0.01$ and *** $p < 0.001$.

2.5. Astaxanthin Reduces the Expression of STAT3 and the Combination of Astaxanthin and Silent STAT3 Increases the Reducing Effects

To explore whether the inhibitory effects produced by astaxanthin were due to the STAT3-related pathway, we examined the expression of JAK2, Caspase3, Caspase9, NF-κB, BAX and BCL-2. As shown in Figure 5A, astaxanthin downregulates the protein expression of JAK2, BCL-2 and NF-κB and upregulates the protein expression of BAX, Caspase3 and Caspase9. These results indicate that the effects of inhibiting proliferation, increasing apoptosis and weakening migration and invasion of astaxanthin could reduce the expression of STAT3 and the related pathway proteins. Thus, the combination of astaxanthin and si-STAT3 improved the anti-tumor effects.

RT-PCR (Figure 5B) analyses also confirmed that anti-tumor effects by astaxanthin were due to the suppression function of STAT3 and the related pathway gene. Astaxanthin downregulates the gene expression of JAK2, BCL-2 and NF-κB and upregulates the gene expression of BAX, Caspase3 and Caspase9.

This profile revealed that the lower expression of STAT3 caused by astaxanthin effectuated anti-tumor functions.

2.6. Impact of Astaxanthin on the Growth of Xenograft Tumors

Next, we explored whether the inhibitory effects of astaxanthin were operative in xenograft tumors. Five xenograft models were established in nude mice. Both astaxanthin and si-STAT3 suppressed the growth of tumors. These suppression effects were enhanced when astaxanthin and si-STAT3 were combined (Figure 6A,B), supporting the cell-based observation that astaxanthin exerts a significant inhibitory effect on tumor growth. These results described the effect of astaxanthin by suppressing the expression of STAT3, thereby resulting in the inhibition of xenograft tumors and confirming the hypothesis derived from cell-based experiments.

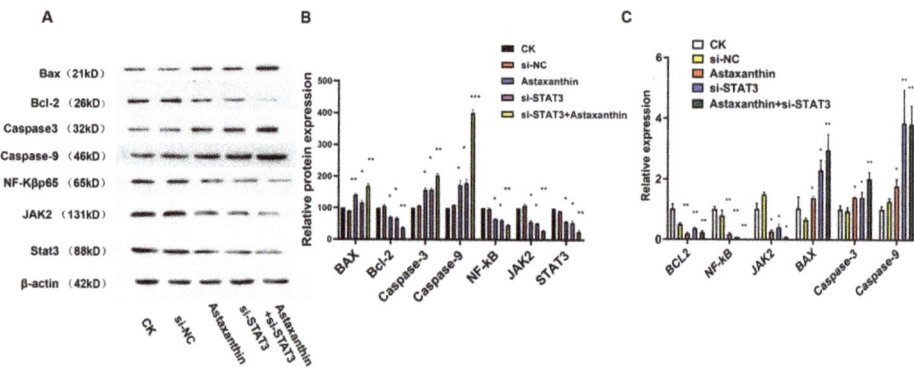

Figure 5. Astaxanthin influences the expression of STAT3. mRNA expression was consistent with that of the protein. (**A**) Western blotting results showed that astaxanthin suppresses the expression of STAT3 and the related proteins JAK2, NF-Kβp65 and Bcl-2, and it increases the levels of Caspase9, Bax and Caspase3. (**B**) Relative protein expression analysis. * $p < 0.05$, ** $p < 0.01$, and *** $p < 0.001$. (**C**) RT-PCR also confirmed that astaxanthin suppresses the expression of STAT3 and the related genes JAK2, NF-κBp65 and Bcl-2, and it increases the expression of Bax, Caspase3 and Caspase9. * $p < 0.05$ and ** $p < 0.01$.

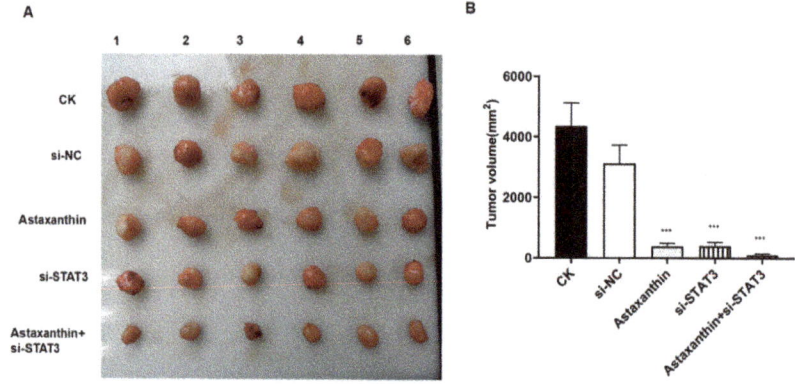

Figure 6. Astaxanthin inhibits the growth of DU145 tumor xenografts in nude mice. (**A**) Representative observations of the growth of the five groups. (**B**) Both astaxanthin and si-STAT3 effectively compress the tumor growth, while the effect of astaxanthin combined with si-STAT3 is superior. Data are presented as the average of three experiments (±SD), *** $p < 0.001$.

3. Discussion

Herein, we used aggressive prostate cancer DU145 cells and found that astaxanthin inhibits their proliferation and suppresses the expression of STAT3. In addition, the cloning ability of the cells can be reduced. Interestingly, astaxanthin promotes apoptosis of DU145 cells, while the ability of migration and invasion is reduced. The combination of astaxanthin and si-STAT3 exhibits a pronounced reduction effect.

Prostate cancer is a malignant tumor of the urogenital system in elderly men, and the incidence and death rate of the disease are rising. In the USA and European countries, prostate cancer is the highest incidence of malignant tumors and the second leading cause of mortality. In China, the incidence of prostate cancer also shows a clear upward trend [1,2]. Primary treatments for prostate cancer include radical surgery, hormone therapy, radiotherapy and chemotherapy. However, resistance to these treatments remains a poorly elucidated phenomenon rendering the tumor excessively aggressive [3–5]. Therefore, finding a drug that can effectively suppress aggressive tumor cells is clinically crucial.

Accumulating evidence demonstrates that STATs play a major role in the process of tumor formation, especially STAT3 [35,36]. Activated STAT3 is involved in tumorigenesis by regulating multiple pathways, such as apoptosis suppressor genes (Mcl-l, Bcl-x L and Survivin), cell cycle regulators (Cyclin Dl/D2 and C-myc), angiogenesis factors (vascular endothelial growth factor (VEGF)) and tumor metastasis-related genes (matrix metalloproteinases (MMPs)) [37,38]. STAT3 is an oncogene with functional activation closely related to the occurrence of prostate cancer. In addition, it shows abnormal expression or increased activity in human leukemia, multiple myeloma, squamous cell carcinoma of the head and neck, breast cancer and prostate cancer. This signaling pathway has been confirmed as an effective molecular target for various human tumor interventions [39,40]. Several molecules of the STAT3 pathway, especially the genes regulated by STAT3, are related to the occurrence and development of tumors. Hence, treating cancer by targeting STAT3 via inhibition of the activation or expression of the molecule, to block the signal transmission pathways of the tumor cells, seems an optimal approach.

About 67% of anti-cancer drugs are derived from natural products or natural product derivatives [16], while >200 natural product-derived drugs are in the preclinical or clinical development stage [41]. In recent years, several studies have reported that natural products and their derivatives, such as alantolactone and 6,7-dimethoxycoumarin, affect the progress of tumors or inflammation by regulating the protein activity or transcription level of the STAT3 signaling pathway. These findings provide new directions for the discovery of new drugs [42–45]. Although it has been shown that many STAT3 inhibitors have anti-tumor effects in vitro, screening out inhibitors with high efficiency, low toxicity and fewer side effects is rather challenging, and further animal experiments have studied less in relation to the pharmacology and toxicology of related inhibitors. Currently, only a few inhibitors are under clinical evaluation [46–48]. Therefore, inhibitors with high efficiency, low toxicity and fewer side effects need to be developed urgently.

Astaxanthin is a natural product that is safe for use and has anti-cancer properties. However, whether it can suppress prostate cancer through STAT3 is not yet elucidated. In the current study, we found that astaxanthin inhibits the proliferation of DU145 prostate cancer cells by reducing the level of STAT3.

Nevertheless, the present study has several limitations. First, in addition to inhibiting levels of STAT3, there may be other mechanisms of the inhibiting effects of astaxanthin on tumor cells. In this study, we explored only STAT3 and the related pathways, thereby necessitating the analysis of other participating genes. Second, we explored the inhibiting effects of astaxanthin on aggressive prostate cancer cells. However, whether it can reduce the resistance to radiotherapy or chemotherapy necessitates further studies.

Furthermore, astaxanthin was found to inhibit proliferation and cloning formation, promote apoptosis and weaken the invasion and migration ability of DU145 cells. Western blotting and RT-PCR confirmed that astaxanthin not only reduces the expression of STAT3, but also that of the related molecules at protein and mRNA levels. Together, the effects described above were significant when astaxanthin was combined with si-STAT3. The results of animal experiments were consistent with those of cell experiments (Figure 7).

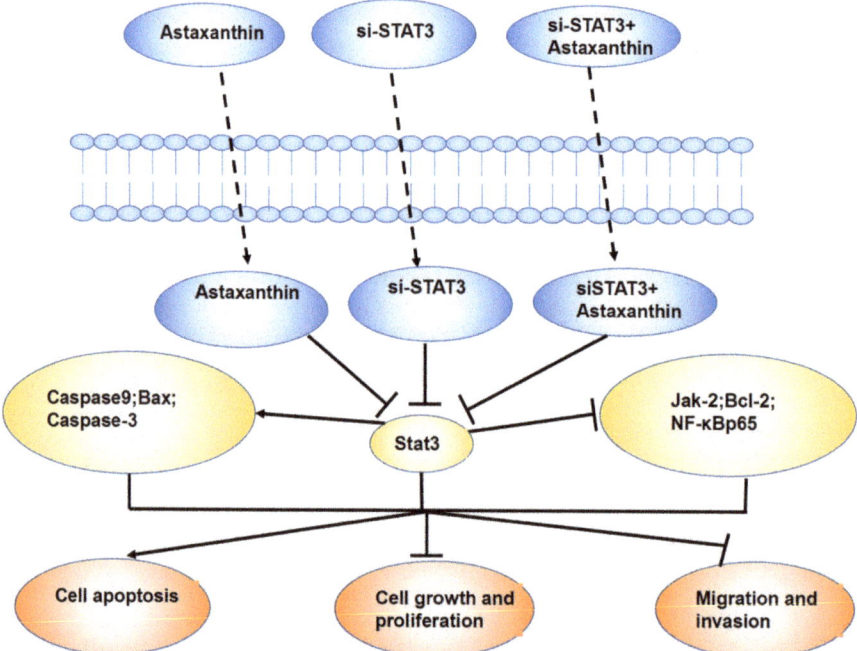

Figure 7. Schematic representation of the mechanism of action of astaxanthin on prostate cancer DU145. Astaxanthin inhibits DU145 tumor cells by reducing the levels of STAT3 and its related proteins. When astaxanthin and si-STAT3 are combined, the effects are better.

4. Materials and Methods

4.1. Cell culture and Reagents

The DU145 prostate cancer cell line was provided by the Urinary Surgery Department of the First Affiliated Hospital of Peking University and cultured in RPMI 1640 medium (M&C Gene Technology, Beijing, China) supplemented with 10% fetal bovine serum (FBS, Gibco, Auckland, New Zealand). The cells were maintained in a humidified incubator with 5% CO_2 at 37 °C. Astaxanthin was purchased from Sigma–Aldrich (St. Louis, MO, USA).

4.2. MTT Assay

A density of 10^3–10^4 DU145 cells/well were seeded into 96-well plates. A volume of 100 μL fresh culture medium containing different concentrations of drugs was added and incubated for 48 h, following which 20 μL of MTT solution (5 mg/mL in phosphate-buffered saline (PBS), pH = 7.4) was added to each well, and incubation continued for an additional 4 h. Finally, 150 μL DMSO was added to each well, and the absorbance was measured at 490 nm on the ELISA reader (Cayman Chemical, Ann Arbor, MI, USA).

4.3. Colony Assay

Drug treatment: The corresponding groups were transfected with siRNA-STAT3 and siRNA-NC, respectively, and 48 h post-transfection, 200 μM astaxanthin drug was administered for 24 h.

Clone formation: The culture was continued for 10–14 days. The cells were then harvested in PBS, fixed with 4% paraformaldehyde for 20 min and stained with 0.1% crystal violet for 20 min.

4.4. Flow Cytometry Assay

Annexin V-FITC/PI assay was used. The cells from each group were harvested and stained with 5 μL Annexin V-FITC/PI staining solution in the dark for 5 min. The rate of apoptosis was detected by flow cytometry (Columbus 2.4, PerkinElmer, Waltham, MA, USA).

4.5. Cell Migration and Cell Invasion Assay

Detection of cell migration: The cells of each group were collected, resuspended in 2% serum medium and inoculated in the upper transwell chamber, while 10% serum was added to the lower chamber. The cells were fixed with 4% paraformaldehyde after 16 h of incubation. Subsequently, the cells in the upper layer of the chamber membrane were wiped with a cotton swab, stained with crystal violet for 20 min, washed twice with PBS, dried, and images were then captured.

Detection of cell invasion: The cells of each group were collected, resuspended in 2% serum medium and inoculated in the upper transwell chamber (the upper chamber pretreated with Matrigel), while the lower chamber was supplemented with 10% serum medium. After 16 h of culture, 4% paraformaldehyde was used to fix the cells, the upper cell membrane was wiped with a cotton swab, stained with crystal violet for 20 min, washed twice with PBS, and images were acquired after drying.

4.6. Western Blot

Protein expression in DU145 cells treated with either CK (control) or si-NK, astaxanthin or si-STAT3, or astaxanthin and si-STAT3 was evaluated using Western blotting. DU145 cells were seeded in 6-well plates and cultured to 80% confluency. The cells were then treated with CK (control) or si-NK, astaxanthin or si-STAT3, or astaxanthin and si-STAT3 for 24 h, followed by protein extraction. An equivalent of 30 μg protein was subjected to SDS-PAGE and Western blotting. The primary antibodies were diluted as follows: Bcl-2(26 kDa) 1:1000 (ab692, Abcam, Cambrige, MA, USA), Bax (21 kDa) 1:1000 (ab7977, Abcam, Cambrige, MA, USA), Caspase3 (32 kDa) 1:1000 (ab32351, Abcam, Cambrige, MA, USA), Caspase9 (46 kDa) 1:1000 (ab32539, Abcam, Cambrige, MA, USA), NF-κB p65 (65 kDa) 1:1000 (ab76302, Abcam, Cambrige, MA, USA), JAK2 (131 kDa) 1:1000 (ab92552, Abcam, Cambrige, MA, USA) and Stat3 (88 kDa) 1:1000 (ab119352, Abcam, Cambrige, MA, USA). Each Western blotting assay was repeated at least two times.

4.7. RT-PCR

Total RNA was extracted using Baosai lysis reagent (Baosai, Hangzhou, China; RE02050), and 1 μg was reverse-transcribed using the RevertAid First Strand cDNA synthesis kit (Baosai; RT02020), according to the manufacturer's instructions. For qRT-PCR, 25–50 ng of cDNA was used as the template for PCR amplification using the fluorescence quantification kit (Baosai; PM10003). Primers for PCR amplification were as follows: Bcl2-F: CCCCGTTGCTTTTCCTCTG; Bcl2-R: CATCACTATCTCCCGGTTATCG; Bax-F: TTTCCGAGTGGCAGCTG; Bax-R: CAAAGTAGAAAAGGGCGACAAC; Casp3-F: CCCATTTCCTACAGAACGACC; Casp3-R: CATCAATGAATCTAAAGTGCGGG; Casp9-F: CCTAGAAAACCTTACCCCAGTG; Casp9-R: TCAAGAGCACCGACATCAC; NF-κB-F: ACCCTGACCTTGCCTATTTG; NF-κB-R: GCTTGGCGGATTAGCTCTTT; JAK2-F: AGTAAAGATGCCTTCTGGTGAA; JAK2-R: TCCATTTCCAAGTTCTCCACT; STAT3-F: GGGACACTGGGTGAGAGTTA; STAT3-R: CACACACACACAAGCCATC; actin-F: GGTGGTCTCCTCTGACTTCAACA; actin-R: GTTGCTGTAGCCAAATTCGTTGT.

4.8. Construction of DU145 Tumor Model

In the first group, DU145 cells were cultured up to the logarithmic phase, and 2×10^7 cells were inoculated in the left armpit of each of 20 nude mice. In the second group, 10 inoculated nude mice were transfected with blank vector for 24 h, while the third group of cells was transfected with the interference vector si-STAT3. At 24 h post-interference, 20 nude mice were inoculated. After 2 weeks of inoculation and culture, 12 tumor-bearing nude mice were randomly selected from the first group and divided into two groups. Six were given saline and the other six were given astaxanthin solution. In the second group, six tumor-bearing nude mice were selected for continuous culture. In the third group, 12 tumor-bearing nude mice were randomly selected and divided into two groups: six were given intragastric astaxanthin solution and the other six were continued in culture.

Group A: Blank control group, intragastric administration of normal saline; Group B: Blank transfection group; Group C: Astaxanthin at a dose of 200 mg/kg administered intragastrically once a day. Nude mice weighed approximately 20 g, the drug concentration was 40 mg/mL, and 100 μL suspension was administered by gastric perfusion; Group D: Interference group; Group E: Interfered with the astaxanthin gavage group. Nursing mice were sacrificed after continuous gavage for 3 weeks, tumor tissues were removed and weighed and images captured.

4.9. Ethics Statement

All experiment procedures were conducted in strict accordance with the appropriate institutional guidelines for animal research. The protocol was approved by the Committee on the Ethics of Animal Experiments of Beijing Union University. The approval number is: CIHFBUU-ZYZDS-B01-15-01.

4.10. Statistical Analysis

The Student's *t*-test was used to determine the statistical difference between the means of two groups and data. A p-value < 0.05 indicated statistical significance.

5. Conclusions

Astaxanthin can effectively inhibit the proliferation and cloning formation of DU145, promote the apoptosis of the DU145 cells and weaken the invasion and migration ability of DU145. In addition, astaxanthin can not only reduce the expression of STAT3 but also the expression of the related proteins of STAT3 in protein and mRNA levels. When astaxanthin and si-STAT3 were combined, all the effects were improved. The results of animal experiments are consistent with the results of cell experiments.

Thus, we concluded that astaxanthin inhibits DU145 tumor cells by reducing the level of STAT3. It may be a prospective drug that can effectively suppress aggressive tumor cells.

Author Contributions: Conceived and designed the experiments: Y.-Z.J. Performed the experiments: S.-Q.S. Analyzed the data: Y.-Z.J.; Y.-X.Z.; S.-Y.L. and J.-W.Q. Wrote the paper: S.-Q.S. All authors have read and agreed to the published version of the manuscript.

Funding: This work was supported by grants from Scientific Research Common Program of Beijing Municipal Commission of Education (No. KM201911417013) and Premium Funding Project for Academic Human Resources Development in Beijing Union University (No. BPHR2019DZ04).

Conflicts of Interest: The authors declare no conflict of interest.

References

1. Siegel, R.L.; Miller, K.D.; Jemal, A. Cancer statistics, 2016. *CA A Cancer J. Clin.* **2016**, *66*, 7–30. [CrossRef] [PubMed]
2. Chen, W.; Zheng, R.; Baade, P.D.; Zhang, S.; Zeng, H.; Bray, F.; Jemal, A.; Yu, X.Q.; He, J. Cancer statistics in China, 2015. *CA A Cancer J. Clin.* **2016**, *66*, 115–132. [CrossRef] [PubMed]
3. Attard, G.; Parker, C.; Eeles, R.A.; Schroder, F.; Tomlins, S.A.; Tannock, I.; Drake, C.G.; de Bono, J.S. Prostate cancer. *Lancet* **2016**, *387*, 70–82. [CrossRef]
4. Fu, W.; Madan, E.; Yee, M.; Zhang, H. Progress of molecular targeted therapies for prostate cancers. *Biochim. Biophys. Acta* **2012**, *1825*, 140–152. [CrossRef] [PubMed]
5. Wong, Y.N.; Ferraldeschi, R.; Attard, G.; de Bono, J. Evolution of androgen receptor targeted therapy for advanced prostate cancer. *Nat. Rev. Clin. Oncol.* **2014**, *11*, 365–376. [CrossRef] [PubMed]

6. Luwor, R.B.; Stylli, S.S.; Kaye, A.H. The role of Stat3 in glioblastoma multiforme. *J. Clin. Neurosci.* **2013**, *20*, 907–911. [CrossRef]
7. Zammarchi, F.; de Stanchina, E.; Bournazou, E.; Supakorndej, T.; Martires, K.; Riedel, E.; Corben, A.D.; Bromberg, J.F.; Cartegni, L. Antitumorigenic potential of STAT3 alternative splicing modulation. *Proc. Natl. Acad. Sci. USA* **2011**, *108*, 17779–17784. [CrossRef]
8. Yue, P.; Turkson, J. Targeting STAT3 in cancer: How successful are we? *Expert Opin. Investig. Drugs* **2009**, *18*, 45–56. [CrossRef]
9. Lu, K.; Fang, X.S.; Feng, L.L.; Jiang, Y.J.; Zhou, X.X.; Liu, X.; Li, P.P.; Chen, N.; Ding, M.; Wang, N.; et al. The STAT3 inhibitor WP1066 reverses the resistance of chronic lymphocytic leukemia cells to histone deacetylase inhibitors induced by interleukin-6. *Cancer Lett.* **2015**, *359*, 250–258. [CrossRef]
10. Liu, Y.F.; Lu, Y.M.; Qu, G.Q.; Liu, Y.; Chen, W.X.; Liao, X.H.; Kong, W.M. Ponicidin induces apoptosis via JAK2 and STAT3 signaling pathways in gastric carcinoma. *Int. J. Mol. Sci.* **2015**, *16*, 1576–1589. [CrossRef]
11. McCann, G.A.; Naidu, S.; Rath, K.S.; Bid, H.K.; Tierney, B.J.; Suarez, A.; Varadharaj, S.; Zhang, J.; Hideg, K.; Houghton, P.; et al. Targeting constitutively-activated STAT3 in hypoxic ovarian cancer, using a novel STAT3 inhibitor. *Oncoscience* **2014**, *1*, 216–228. [CrossRef] [PubMed]
12. Tai, W.T.; Chu, P.Y.; Shiau, C.W.; Chen, Y.L.; Li, Y.S.; Hung, M.H.; Chen, L.J.; Chen, P.L.; Su, J.C.; Lin, P.Y.; et al. STAT3 mediates regorafenib-induced apoptosis in hepatocellular carcinoma. *Clin. Cancer Res.* **2014**, *20*, 5768–5776. [CrossRef] [PubMed]
13. Gao, L.; Li, F.; Dong, B.; Zhang, J.; Rao, Y.; Cong, Y.; Mao, B.; Chen, X. Inhibition of STAT3 and ErbB2 suppresses tumor growth, enhances radiosensitivity, and induces mitochondria-dependent apoptosis in glioma cells. *Int. J. Radiat. Oncol. Biol. Phys.* **2010**, *77*, 1223–1231. [CrossRef]
14. Mora, L.B.; Buettner, R.; Seigne, J.; Diaz, J.; Ahmad, N.; Garcia, R.; Bowman, T.; Falcone, R.; Fairclough, R.; Cantor, A.; et al. Constitutive activation of Stat3 in human prostate tumors and cell lines: Direct inhibition of Stat3 signaling induces apoptosis of prostate cancer cells. *Cancer Res.* **2002**, *62*, 6659–6666. [PubMed]
15. Abdulghani, J.; Gu, L.; Dagvadorj, A.; Lutz, J.; Leiby, B.; Bonuccelli, G.; Lisanti, M.P.; Zellweger, T.; Alanen, K.; Mirtti, T.; et al. Stat3 promotes metastatic progression of prostate cancer. *Am. J. Pathol.* **2008**, *172*, 1717–1728. [CrossRef] [PubMed]
16. Ghantous, A.; Gali-Muhtasib, H.; Vuorela, H.; Saliba, N.A.; Darwiche, N. What made sesquiterpene lactones reach cancer clinical trials? *Drug Discov. Today* **2010**, *15*, 668–678. [CrossRef]
17. Ge, X.X.; Xing, M.Y.; Yu, L.F.; Shen, P. Carotenoid intake and esophageal cancer risk: A meta-analysis. *Asian Pac. J. Cancer Prev.* **2013**, *14*, 1911–1918. [CrossRef]
18. Larsson, S.C.; Bergkvist, L.; Naslund, I.; Rutegard, J.; Wolk, A. Vitamin A, retinol, and carotenoids and the risk of gastric cancer: A prospective cohort study. *Am. J. Clin. Nutr.* **2007**, *85*, 497–503. [CrossRef]
19. Cui, L.; Liu, X.; Tian, Y.; Xie, C.; Li, Q.; Cui, H.; Sun, C. Flavonoids, flavonoid subclasses, and esophageal cancer risk: A meta-analysis of epidemiologic studies. *Nutrients* **2016**, *8*, 350. [CrossRef]
20. Naguib, Y.M. Antioxidant activities of astaxanthin and related carotenoids. *J. Agric. Food Chem.* **2000**, *48*, 1150–1154. [CrossRef]
21. Wakabayashi, K.; Hamada, C.; Kanda, R.; Nakano, T.; Io, H.; Horikoshi, S.; Tomino, Y. Oral astaxanthin supplementation prevents peritoneal fibrosis in rats. *Perit. Dial. Int.* **2015**, *35*, 506–516. [CrossRef] [PubMed]
22. Salehi, M.; Moradi-Lakeh, M.; Salehi, M.H.; Nojomi, M.; Kolahdooz, F. Meat, fish, and esophageal cancer risk: A systematic review and dose-response meta-analysis. *Nutr. Rev.* **2013**, *71*, 257–267. [CrossRef] [PubMed]
23. Qu, X.; Ben, Q.; Jiang, Y. Consumption of red and processed meat and risk for esophageal squamous cell carcinoma based on a meta-analysis. *Ann. Epidemiol.* **2013**, *23*, 762–770. [CrossRef] [PubMed]
24. Jiang, G.; Li, B.; Liao, X.; Zhong, C. Poultry and fish intake and risk of esophageal cancer: A meta-analysis of observational studies. *Asia Pac. J. Clin. Oncol.* **2016**, *12*, e82–e91. [CrossRef] [PubMed]
25. Roerecke, M.; Shield, K.D.; Higuchi, S.; Yoshimura, A.; Larsen, E.; Rehm, M.X.; Rehm, J. Estimates of alcohol-related oesophageal cancer burden in Japan: Systematic review and meta-analyses. *Bull. World Health Organ.* **2015**, *93*, 329–338. [CrossRef] [PubMed]
26. Singh, S.; Sharma, A.N.; Murad, M.H.; Buttar, N.S.; El-Serag, H.B.; Katzka, D.A.; Iyer, P.G. Central adiposity is associated with increased risk of esophageal inflammation, metaplasia, and adenocarcinoma: A systematic review and meta-analysis. *Clin. Gastroenterol. Hepatol.* **2013**, *11*, 1399–1412. [CrossRef]
27. Song, X.D.; Zhang, J.J.; Wang, M.R.; Liu, W.B.; Gu, X.B.; Lv, C.J. Astaxanthin induces mitochondria-mediated apoptosis in rat hepatocellular carcinoma CBRH-7919 cells. *Biol. Pharm. Bull.* **2011**, *34*, 839–844. [CrossRef]

28. Franceschelli, S.; Pesce, M.; Ferrone, A.; De Lutiis, M.A.; Patruno, A.; Grilli, A.; Felaco, M.; Speranza, L. Astaxanthin treatment confers protection against oxidative stress in U937 cells stimulated with lipopolysaccharide reducing O2- production. *PLoS ONE* **2014**, *9*, e88359. [CrossRef]
29. Kim, K.N.; Heo, S.J.; Kang, S.M.; Ahn, G.; Jeon, Y.J. Fucoxanthin induces apoptosis in human leukemia HL-60 cells through a ROS-mediated Bcl-xL pathway. *Toxicol. In Vitro* **2010**, *24*, 1648–1654. [CrossRef]
30. Speranza, L.; Pesce, M.; Patruno, A.; Franceschelli, S.; de Lutiis, M.A.; Grilli, A.; Felaco, M. Astaxanthin treatment reduced oxidative induced pro-inflammatory cytokines secretion in U937: SHP-1 as a novel biological target. *Mar. Drugs* **2012**, *10*, 890–899. [CrossRef]
31. Nagendraprabhu, P.; Sudhandiran, G. Astaxanthin inhibits tumor invasion by decreasing extracellular matrix production and induces apoptosis in experimental rat colon carcinogenesis by modulating the expressions of ERK-2, NFkB and COX-2. *Investig. New Drugs* **2011**, *29*, 207–224. [CrossRef] [PubMed]
32. Kowshik, J.; Baba, A.B.; Giri, H.; Deepak Reddy, G.; Dixit, M.; Nagini, S. Astaxanthin inhibits JAK/STAT-3 signaling to abrogate cell proliferation, invasion and angiogenesis in a hamster model of oral cancer. *PLoS ONE* **2014**, *9*, e109114. [CrossRef] [PubMed]
33. Palozza, P.; Torelli, C.; Boninsegna, A.; Simone, R.; Catalano, A.; Mele, M.C.; Picci, N. Growth-inhibitory effects of the astaxanthin-rich alga Haematococcus pluvialis in human colon cancer cells. *Cancer Lett.* **2009**, *283*, 108–117. [CrossRef] [PubMed]
34. Zhang, X.; Zhao, W.E.; Hu, L.; Zhao, L.; Huang, J. Carotenoids inhibit proliferation and regulate expression of peroxisome proliferators-activated receptor gamma (PPARgamma) in K562 cancer cells. *Arch. Biochem. Biophys.* **2011**, *512*, 96–106. [CrossRef] [PubMed]
35. Ni, Z.; Lou, W.; Leman, E.S.; Gao, A.C. Inhibition of constitutively activated Stat3 signaling pathway suppresses growth of prostate cancer cells. *Cancer Res.* **2000**, *60*, 1225–1228.
36. Song, J.I.; Grandis, J.R. STAT signaling in head and neck cancer. *Oncogene* **2000**, *19*, 2489–2495. [CrossRef]
37. Kanda, N.; Seno, H.; Konda, Y.; Marusawa, H.; Kanai, M.; Nakajima, T.; Kawashima, T.; Nanakin, A.; Sawabu, T.; Uenoyama, Y.; et al. STAT3 is constitutively activated and supports cell survival in association with survivin expression in gastric cancer cells. *Oncogene* **2004**, *23*, 4921–4929. [CrossRef]
38. Itoh, M.; Murata, T.; Suzuki, T.; Shindoh, M.; Nakajima, K.; Imai, K.; Yoshida, K. Requirement of STAT3 activation for maximal collagenase-1 (MMP-1) induction by epidermal growth factor and malignant characteristics in T24 bladder cancer cells. *Oncogene* **2006**, *25*, 1195–1204. [CrossRef]
39. Buettner, R.; Mora, L.B.; Jove, R. Activated STAT signaling in human tumors provides novel molecular targets for therapeutic intervention. *Clin. Cancer Res.* **2002**, *8*, 945–954.
40. Nam, S.; Buettner, R.; Turkson, J.; Kim, D.; Cheng, J.Q.; Muehlbeyer, S.; Hippe, F.; Vatter, S.; Merz, K.H.; Eisenbrand, G.; et al. Indirubin derivatives inhibit Stat3 signaling and induce apoptosis in human cancer cells. *Proc. Natl. Acad. Sci. USA* **2005**, *102*, 5998–6003. [CrossRef]
41. Lin, Y.; Wang, F.; Zhang, G.L. Natural products and their derivatives regulating the janus kinase/signal transducer and activator of transcription pathway. *J. Asian Nat. Prod. Res.* **2014**, *16*, 800–812. [CrossRef] [PubMed]
42. Chun, J.; Li, R.J.; Cheng, M.S.; Kim, Y.S. Alantolactone selectively suppresses STAT3 activation and exhibits potent anticancer activity in MDA-MB-231 cells. *Cancer Lett.* **2015**, *357*, 393–403. [CrossRef] [PubMed]
43. Park, S.; Kim, J.K.; Oh, C.J.; Choi, S.H.; Jeon, J.H.; Lee, I.K. Scoparone interferes with STAT3-induced proliferation of vascular smooth muscle cells. *Exp. Mol. Med.* **2015**, *47*, e145. [CrossRef] [PubMed]
44. Chen, X.; Du, Y.; Nan, J.; Zhang, X.; Qin, X.; Wang, Y.; Hou, J.; Wang, Q.; Yang, J. Brevilin A, a novel natural product, inhibits janus kinase activity and blocks STAT3 signaling in cancer cells. *PLoS ONE* **2013**, *8*, e63697. [CrossRef]
45. Zhang, T.; Li, S.; Li, J.; Yin, F.; Hua, Y.; Wang, Z.; Lin, B.; Wang, H.; Zou, D.; Zhou, Z.; et al. Natural product pectolinarigenin inhibits osteosarcoma growth and metastasis via SHP-1-mediated STAT3 signaling inhibition. *Cell Death Dis.* **2016**, *7*, e2421. [CrossRef]
46. Lin, L.; Benson, D.M., Jr.; DeAngelis, S.; Bakan, C.E.; Li, P.K.; Li, C.; Lin, J. A small molecule, LLL12 inhibits constitutive STAT3 and IL-6-induced STAT3 signaling and exhibits potent growth suppressive activity in human multiple myeloma cells. *Int. J. Cancer* **2012**, *130*, 1459–1469. [CrossRef]

47. Ball, D.P.; Lewis, A.M.; Williams, D.; Resetca, D.; Wilson, D.J.; Gunning, P.T. Signal transducer and activator of transcription 3 (STAT3) inhibitor, S3I-201, acts as a potent and non-selective alkylating agent. *Oncotarget* **2016**, *7*, 20669–20679. [CrossRef]
48. Okusaka, T.; Ueno, H.; Ikeda, M.; Mitsunaga, S.; Ozaka, M.; Ishii, H.; Yokosuka, O.; Ooka, Y.; Yoshimoto, R.; Yanagihara, Y.; et al. Phase 1 and pharmacological trial of OPB-31121, a signal transducer and activator of transcription-3 inhibitor, in patients with advanced hepatocellular carcinoma. *Hepatol. Res.* **2015**, *45*, 1283–1291. [CrossRef]

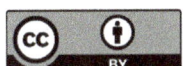

© 2020 by the authors. Licensee MDPI, Basel, Switzerland. This article is an open access article distributed under the terms and conditions of the Creative Commons Attribution (CC BY) license (http://creativecommons.org/licenses/by/4.0/).

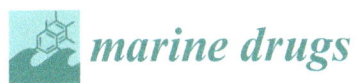

Article

Exploring the Mechanism of Flaccidoxide-13-Acetate in Suppressing Cell Metastasis of Hepatocellular Carcinoma

Yu-Jen Wu [1,2,3,†], Wen-Chi Wei [4,†], Guo-Fong Dai [3], Jui-Hsin Su [5], Yu-Hwei Tseng [4] and Tsung-Chang Tsai [6,*]

1. Department of Beauty Science, Meiho University, Pingtung 91202, Taiwan; x00002180@meiho.edu.tw
2. Department of Food and Nutrition, Meiho University, Pingtung 91202, Taiwan
3. Yu Jun Biotechnology Co., Ltd., Kaohsiung 807, Taiwan; fwind101@gmail.com
4. National Research Institute of Chinese Medicine, Taipei 112, Taiwan; jackwei@nricm.edu.tw (W.-C.W.); mayeeshat@nricm.edu.tw (Y.-H.T.)
5. National Museum of Marine Biology and Aquarium, Pingtung 94450, Taiwan; x2219@nmmba.gov.tw
6. Antai Medical Care Corporation Antai Tian-Sheng Memorial Hospital, Pingtung 92842, Taiwan
* Correspondence: a088186@mail.tsmh.org.tw; Tel.: +886-8-8329966 (ext. 5523); Fax: +886-8-8329977
† These authors contributed equally to this work.

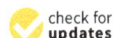

Received: 17 May 2020; Accepted: 12 June 2020; Published: 15 June 2020

Abstract: Hepatocellular carcinoma (HCC) is the most common liver or hepatic cancer, accounting for 80% of all cases. The majority of this cancer mortality is due to metastases, rather than orthotopic tumors. Therefore, the inhibition of tumor metastasis is widely recognized as the key strategy for successful intervention. A cembrane-type diterpene, flaccidoxide-13-acetate, isolated from marine soft coral *Sinularia gibberosa*, has been reported to have inhibitory effects against RT4 and T24 human bladder cancer invasion and cell migration. In this study, we investigated its suppression effects on tumor growth and metastasis of human HCC, conducting Boyden chamber and Transwell assays using HA22T and HepG2 human HCC cell lines to evaluate invasion and cell migration. We utilized gelatin zymography to determine the enzyme activities of matrix metalloproteinases MMP-2 and MMP-9. We also analyzed the expression levels of MMP-2 and MMP-9. Additionally, assays of tissue inhibitors of metalloproteinase-1/2 (TIMP-1/2), the focal adhesion kinase (FAK)/phosphatidylinositide-3 kinases (PI3K)/Akt/mammalian target of the rapamycin (mTOR) signaling pathway, and the epithelial-mesenchymal transition (EMT) process were performed. We observed that flaccidoxide-13-acetate could potentially inhibit HCC cell migration and invasion. We postulated that, by inhibiting the FAK/PI3K/Akt/mTOR signaling pathway, MMP-2 and MMP-9 expressions were suppressed, resulting in HCC cell metastasis. Flaccidoxide-13-acetate was found to inhibit EMT in HA22T and HepG2 HCC cells. Our study results suggested the potential of flaccidoxide-13-acetate as a chemotherapeutic candidate; however, its clinical application for the management of HCC in humans requires further research.

Keywords: flaccidoxide-13-acetate; hepatocellular carcinoma; invasion; migration; epithelial-mesenchymal transition

1. Introduction

Among the primary liver cancers, hepatocellular carcinoma (HCC) is especially common, and the majority of liver cancer deaths can be attributed to HCC [1]. Worldwide, it ranks sixth in terms of cancer incidence and is one of the deadliest types of cancer [2]. Countries in Asia and sub-Saharan Africa, in particular, suffer severely from this epidemic, patients in China, North and South Korea, Vietnam, and sub-Saharan African countries accounting for almost 82% of liver cancer cases [3]. Hepatitis B and C viruses are the main etiological factors in the Asia-Pacific region, chronic hepatitis B (CHB) infections being the major cause of liver cancer [3,4]. In addition, antiviral medication for CHB and hepatitis C (CHC) is a proven treatment by which to reduce the incidence of HCC [5]. Currently, HCC treatment options include surgical resection, radiotherapy, trans-arterial chemoembolization, radioembolization, targeted therapy, and liver transplantation, depending on the tumor progression [6,7]. Recent advances in surgical treatments and loco regional therapies have significantly improved the short-term survival of HCC patients [8]. However, the recurrence or metastasis of HCC remain serious concerns, representing an unmet need that warrants the development of new drugs for patients with malignant HCC. Marine organisms offer one of the richest sources of leading candidates for drug development due to the highly diversified marine environment [9]. Since the 1960s, the isolation and identification of many novel compounds have been performed. Marine-based drugs to combat cancer and other diseases have been developed and introduced in clinical settings [10,11]. Existing in warm seawater bodies, soft corals possess unique and abundant secondary metabolites that have been investigated with regards to various biological activities, such as anti-inflammatory and anticancer effects [12,13].

A cembrane-type diterpenoid, flaccidoxide-13-acetate, isolated from marine soft coral *Sinularia gibberosa*, has been suggested to induce apoptosis in human bladder cancer cells [14]. To our knowledge, its effect on HCC remains to be confirmed. This study aimed to fill the gap by investigating the inhibitory effects of this compound on the tumor growth and metastasis of human HCC.

2. Results

2.1. Cytotoxic Activity of Flaccidoxide-13-acetate against HA22T and HepG2 Cells

We used a methylthiazole tetrazolium (MTT) assay to measure the cytotoxic effects of flaccidoxide-13-acetate at different concentrations (0, 2, 4, 6, and 8 µM) on human HCC cell lines HA22T and HepG2, the results of which are shown in Figure 1. Flaccidoxide-13-acetate was found to inhibit the cell viability of HA22T and HepG2 cells in a dose-dependent manner (* $p < 0.01$ and # $p < 0.05$) (Figure 1). Only at 8 µM did HA22T and HepG2 cells exhibit a cell viability below 80% (Figure 1). Therefore, we selected lower concentrations (2–8 µM) for uses in all subsequent experiments.

2.2. Flaccidoxide-13-acetate Reduces Cellular Migration and Invasion in HA22T and HepG2 Cells

The cell–matrix interaction and cell motility play crucial roles in determining the metastatic properties of cancer cells. To investigate the inhibitory properties of flaccidoxide-13-acetate on the tumor growth and metastasis of human HCC, we conducted Boyden and Transwell chamber assays in HA22T and HepG2 human HCC cell lines to evaluate cell migration and invasion. Flaccidoxide-13-acetate was found to inhibit the cell migration of HA22T and HepG2 cells in a dose-dependent manner. After treatments of HA22T and HepG2 cells with 8-µM flaccidoxide-13-acetate for 24 h, the cell migratory capacities dropped to 85% and 80%, respectively (Figure 2). Similar reductions were observed in the invasive capacities of both cell lines (Figure 3).

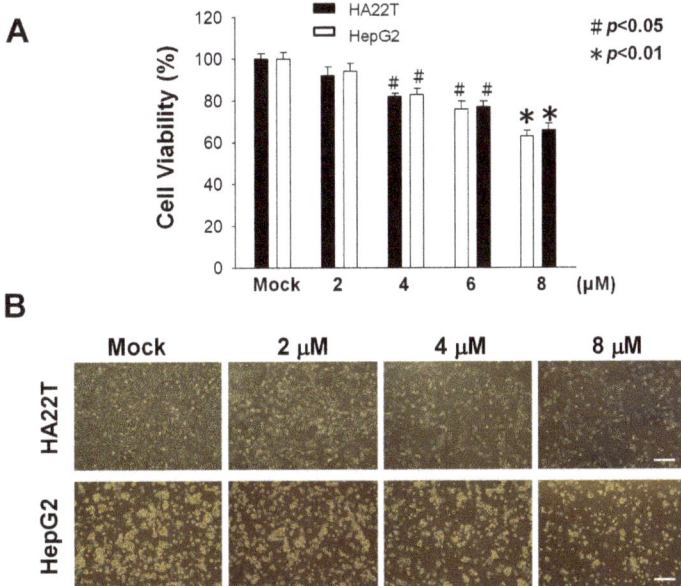

Figure 1. Cell viabilities of HA22T and HepG2 cells treated with flaccidoxide-13-acetate and a control (Mock: DMSO as the vehicle) after 24 h. (**A**) Cytotoxic effects on HA22T and HepG2 cells treated with flaccidoxide-13-acetate exhibiting a dose-dependent manner (# $p < 0.05$ and * $p < 0.01$). (**B**) Morphologies of HA22T and HepG2 cells after 24 h of incubation with 0–8-μM flaccidoxide-13-acetate. Scale bar = 20 μm. The results were obtained from three individual experiments.

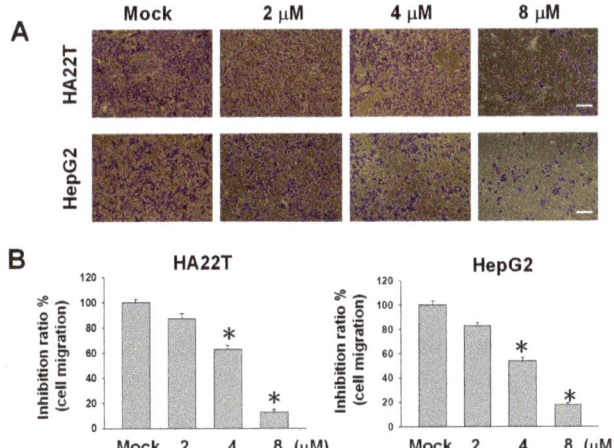

Figure 2. Effects of the flaccidoxide-13-acetate treatment on HA22T and HepG2 cell migrations after treatment for 24 h. (**A**) Images of the migrations of flaccidoxide-13-acetate-treated HA22T and HepG2 cells as compared with controls (Mock: DMSO as the vehicle). Each image was representative of three individual experiments. (**B**) Inhibition ratios of flaccidoxide-13-acetate-treated HA22T and HepG2 cells as compared with controls (* $p < 0.01$). Data were calculated from three individual experiments. Scale bar = 20 μm.

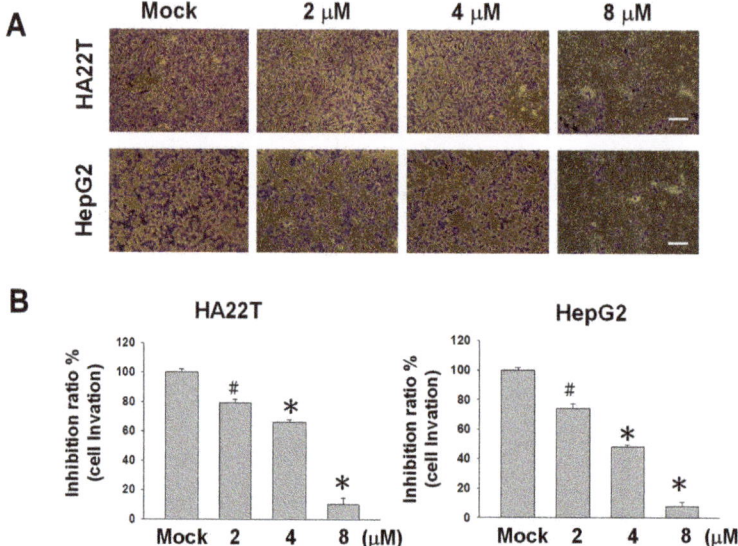

Figure 3. Effects of 24-h flaccidoxide-13-acetate treatments on HA22T and HepG2 cell invasions. (**A**) Images of the invasions of flaccidoxide-13-acetate-treated HA22T and HepG2 cells as compared with the control (Mock: DMSO as the vehicle control). Each image was representative of three individual experiments. (**B**) Inhibition ratios of flaccidoxide-13-acetate-treated HA22T and HepG2 cells as compared with the controls (# $p < 0.05$ and * $p < 0.01$). Data were calculated from three individual experiments. Scale bar = 20 µm.

2.3. Flaccidoxide-13-acetate Reduced the uPA and MMP-2/-9 Activities and Regulated the Expressions of MMP-2/-9, uPA, TIMP-1, and TIMP-2 in HA22T and HepG2 Cells

To investigate the enzymatic activities of MMP-2, MMP-9, and uPA produced from HA22T and HepG2 cells, gelatin zymography was used. We cultured HA22T and HepG2 cells in a serum-free media with flaccidoxide-13-acetate (0, 2, 4, 6, and 8 µM) for 24 h and collected the conditioned media to determine the activities of MMP-2, MMP-9, and the urokinase plasminogen activator (uPA). Flaccidoxide-13-acetate was found to inhibit the activities of MMP-2, MMP-9, and uPA, exhibiting a dose-dependent effect, as shown in Figure 4A. To clarify the roles of the endogenous tissue inhibitors of metalloproteinases (TIMPs) and serine protease uPA in regulating the activities of MMP-2, MMP-9, and MMP-13 after treatments with flaccidoxide-13-acetate, we performed Western blotting to measure the extent to which flaccidoxide-13-acetate regulated the expressions of the MMP-2, MMP-9, MMP-13, uPA, TIMP-1, and TIMP-2 proteins. We observed declines in the protein levels of MMP-2, MMP-9, MMP-13, and uPA, while, on the contrary, the expressions of TIMP-1 and TIMP-2 increased in HA22T and HepG2 cells after treatments with flaccidoxide-13-acetate for 24 h (Figure 4B).

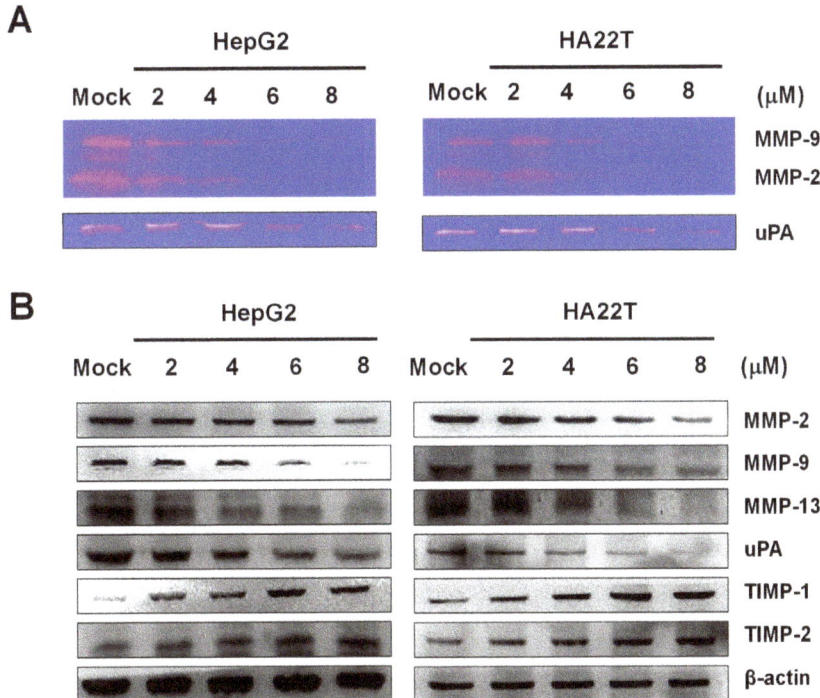

Figure 4. Activities of MMP-2/-9 and uPA and the protein levels of MMP-2, MMP-9, MMP-13, uPA, TIMP-1, and TIMP-2 after treatments of the HA22T and HepG2 cells with flaccidoxide-13-acetate at different concentrations for 24 h. (**A**) Images of the gelatin zymography of MMP-2/-9 and uPA activities. (**B**) Expression levels of MMP-2, MMP-9, MMP-13, uPA, TIMP-1, and TIMP-2. Mock: DMSO as the vehicle control.

2.4. Flaccidoxide-13-acetate Inhibited the FAK/PI3K/Akt/mTOR Signaling Pathway

Focal adhesion kinase (FAK) is cytoplasmic protein kinase in the cytoplasm. The overactivation of FAK has been recognized to promote the progression and metastasis of tumors via the regulation of cell motility, survival, and proliferation. To investigate the inhibitory effects of flaccidoxide-13-acetate on the FAK activity and downstream signaling pathways in HA22T and HepG2 cells, we adopted the Western blotting technique to measure the extent to which flaccidoxide-13-acetate regulated the expressions of FAK, PI3K, AKT, mTOR, p-PI3K, mTOR, and p-mTOR proteins. Declines in the protein levels of FAK, p-PI3K, mTOR, and p-mTOR were observed (Figure 5).

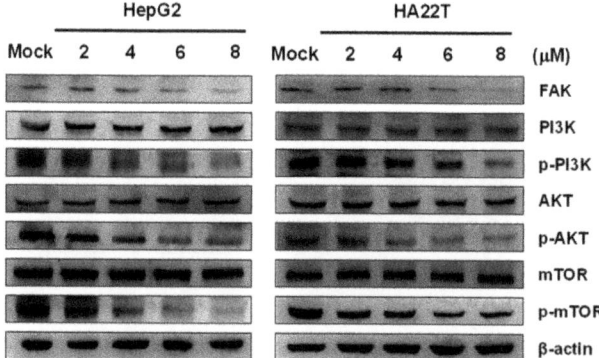

Figure 5. Effects of flaccidoxide-13-acetate on the FAK/PI3K/Akt/mTOR signaling pathway in HA22T and Hep G2 cells. Protein expression levels of FAK, PI3K, Akt, and mTOR and the phosphorylation of PI3K, Akt, and mTOR after treatments with flaccidoxide-13-acetate for 24 h. β-actin: loading control. Mock: DMSO as the vehicle control.

2.5. Flaccidoxide-13-acetate Inhibited the Epithelial-to-Mesenchymal Transition (EMT)

EMT is a process in which epithelial cells lose adherence and become mesenchymal cells, playing a significant role in tumor metastasis. During EMT, Snail, a key transcription factor for EMT, inhibits E-cadherin transcription, and vimentin regulates β-catenin translocation.

In order to investigate whether flaccidoxide-13-acetate inhibited EMT in HA22T and HepG2 cells, Western blotting was used to measure the expressions of cytosolic β-catenin, N-cadherin, E-cadherin, vimentin, and nucleic Snail. The results showed increases in the protein levels of N- and E-cadherin, while, on the contrary, those of β-catenin, vimentin, and Snail decreased in HA22T and HepG2 cells after treatments with flaccidoxide-13-acetate (Figure 6).

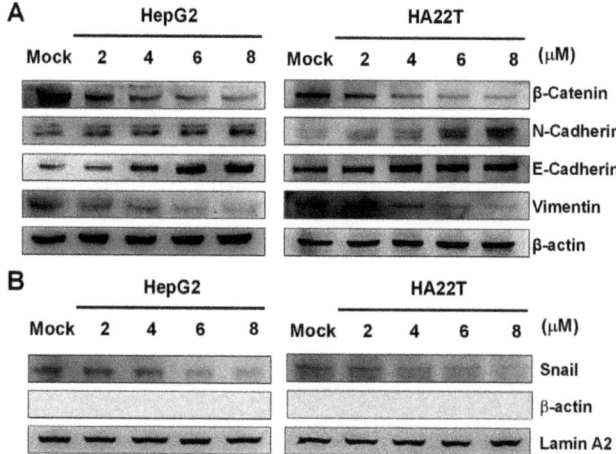

Figure 6. Effects of flaccidoxide-13-acetate at different concentrations on the epithelial-to-mesenchymal transition (EMT) in HA22T and HepG2 cells. (**A**) Protein expression levels of β-catenin, N-cadherin, E-cadherin, and vimentin in cytosol. β-actin: loading control. Mock: DMSO as the vehicle control. (**B**) Protein expression levels of Snail in the nucleus. Internal controls: β-actin for cytosol and lamin A2 for the nucleus.

3. Discussion

Metastases contribute to the majority of cancer deaths, rather than orthotopic tumors. Therefore, the inhibition of tumor metastasis is generally recognized as a key approach for intervention [15,16]. Previous studies of human bladder cancer cells showed that flaccidoxide-13-acetate reduced apoptosis, which is mediated by p38/JNK activation, mitochondrial dysfunction, and endoplasmic reticulum stress [14]; it was also found to inhibit human bladder cancer cell migration and invasion by reduction in the activation of the FAK/PI3K/AKT/mTOR signaling pathway [17]. In this study, we investigated the therapeutic effects of flaccidoxide-13-acetate on tumor metastasis in human HCC. A HA22T cell line was established from a specimen obtained from a 56-year-old Chinese male HCC patient [18], while a HepG2 cell line was obtained from an HCC sample from a 15-year-old Caucasian male [19]. We analyzed the therapeutic effects of flaccidoxide-13-acetate on tumor metastasis in HA22T and HepG2 cell lines, and thereafter, investigated its possible mechanisms of action. Our results showed that, at certain concentrations, flaccidoxide-13-acetate inhibited metastasis in HA22T and HepG2 cells. Reports published in the literature indicated that MMP-2 can enhance the migration of HCC cells by increasing fibronectin cleavage [20] and that the overexpression of MMP-9 is associated with HCC tumor migration and invasion [21].

MMP-2 and MMP-9 have been found to be involved in the metastasis, invasiveness, and prognosis of HCC. Flaccidoxide-13-acetate inhibited the activation of MMP-2, MMP-9, and uPA, whose physiological activities are significantly correlated with TIMPs and uPA. Research has also suggested that the expression of uPA, a key molecule contributing to the activation of MMPs, is associated with cancer invasion [21–24]. The results of the present study showed that flaccidoxide-13-acetate upregulated proteins TIMP-1 and TIMP-2 and downregulated the expression of the uPA protein in treated HCC cells. We suggest that flaccidoxide-13-acetate upregulates the TIMP-1 and TIMP-2 protein expressions and downregulates the uPA protein expression, resulting in the suppression of MMP-2 and MMP-9 activities in HA22T and HepG2 cells.

Focal adhesion kinase (FAK) plays significant roles in cell survival, motility, and proliferation and is associated with EMT, cancer invasion, and migration [25–27]. FAK has been reported to be associated with PI3K/Akt/mTOR signal transduction [28]. The PI3K/Akt/mTOR signaling pathway is also associated with EMT, cancer invasion, and migration. In this study, we showed that flaccidoxide-13-acetate inhibited FAK protein expression and the phosphorylation of PI3K, Akt, and mTOR. We suggest that flaccidoxide-13-acetate may contribute to the inhibition of FAK and the subsequent suppression of PI3K/Akt/mTOR signaling, interrupting the EMT and the invasion and migration of HCC cells.

Snail facilitates the initiation of the EMT and has been found to downregulate the transcription of E-cadherin, which is known to be important in cell–cell adhesion [29,30]. Therefore, Snail and E-cadherin are key markers of EMT [31–33]. Our data showed that flaccidoxide-13-acetate suppressed the protein expression of Snail in the nucleus and promoted the expression of E-cadherin in the cytosol. We suggest that flaccidoxide-13-acetate may suppress the EMT process, including the downregulation of Snail and upregulation of E-cadherin, leading to the inhibition of cell migration.

4. Methods

4.1. Materials and Chemical Reagents

Flaccidoxide-13-acetate was supplied by Dr. Jui-Hsin Su. Rabbit anti-human Akt, FAK, MMP-2, MMP-9, MMP-13, mTOR, PI3K, TIMP-1, TIMP-2, uPA and phosphorylated Akt, mTOR, and PI3K were purchased from Cell Signaling Technology (Danvers, MA, USA). E-cadherin, N-cadherin, lamin A2, and Snail antibodies were supplied by Epitomics (Burlingame, CA, USA). HRP-conjugated goat anti-rabbit immunoglobulin (IgG) was obtained from Millipore (Bellerica, MA, USA). Thiazolyl blue tetrazolium bromide, streptomycin, penicillin, and DMSO were purchased from Sigma (St. Louis, MO, USA). Goat anti-rabbit and horseradish peroxidase-conjugated immunoglobulin IgG and polyvinylidene difluoride (PVDF) membranes were obtained from Millipore (Bellerica, MA, USA). Fetal bovine serum and DMEM were purchased from Biowest (Nuaillé, France).

4.2. Cell Culture

HA22T and HepG2 cells were procured from the Food Industry Research and Development Institute (Hsinchu, Taiwan). We used DMEM to culture cells and maintained cells in a 37 °C humidified incubator under 5% CO_2. The composition of the DMEM culture medium was as follows: 10% fetal bovine serum and streptomycin/penicillin (100 µg/mL and 100 U/mL, respectively).

4.3. Cell Viability Assay

Flaccidoxide-13-acetate was dissolved in DMSO. For all in vitro experiments, the final concentration of DMSO was 0.1% *v/v*, and the solubility of flaccidoxide-13-acetate in the tissue culture media was good, with no precipitation or turbidity. Cells were first seeded in 24-well culture plates at a density of 1×10^4 per well and treated with flaccidoxide-13-acetate at various concentrations (2–8 µM). A thiazolyl blue tetrazolium bromide (MTT) assay was used to measure the cytotoxicity of flaccidoxide-13-acetate after treatment for 24 h.

4.4. Cell Migration Assay

Cell migration was analyzed by seeding HA22T and HepG2 cells (1×10^5 cells per well) in serum-free medium for 24 h, followed by treatment with flaccidoxide-13-acetate at various concentrations (2, 4, and 6 µM). DMSO (0.1% *v/v*) as the vehicle control. The migrated cells were fixed to the bottom chamber with 100% methanol and then stained with 5% Giemsa (Merck, Darmstadt, Germany) before counting using a light microscope.

4.5. Cell Invasion Assay

Cell invasion analysis was carried out by seeding HA22T and HepG2 cells (1×10^5 cells per well) suspended in serum-free DMEM on the top chamber of Matrigel–coated Transwell inserts. The lower chamber was filled with DMEM containing various concentrations of flaccidoxide-13-acetate (2, 4, and 6 µM). DMSO (0.1% *v/v*) as the vehicle control. After 24 h, the Transwell inserts were fixed with 3.7% formaldehyde, followed by Giemsa staining. The invasive cells were counted using a light microscope.

4.6. Gelatin Zymography Assay

Activities of MMPs were analyzed by seeding HA22T and HepG2 cells in 24-well culture plates at a density of 1×10^5 cells per well in serum-free medium (200 µL), followed by treatment with flaccidoxide-13-acetate at various concentrations (2, 4, 6, and 8 µM). DMSO (0.1% *v/v*) as the vehicle control. To measure the activities of MMPs and uPA generated from HA22T and HepG2 cells, gelatin zymography with 8% gelatin gels was used to analyze the conditioned medium after 24 h. The gel was then shifted to a reaction buffer at 37 °C overnight for enzymatic reaction, followed by staining with Coomassie blue solution and destaining with acetic acid (10% *v/v*) and methanol (20% *v/v*) solution.

4.7. Western Blot Analysis

Following incubation, cells were washed with PBS three times and lysed in 250-µL lysis buffer (5-mM bicine buffer, 4-(2-aminoethyl) benzenesulfonyl fluoride (AEBSF 0.3 mM), leupeptin (10 µg/mL), and aprotonin (2 µg/mL)). Supernatants were obtained after centrifuging (8000 rpm) the cell lysates. Nuclear proteins were extracted to detect Snail using an extraction kit (SK-0001; Signosis, Santa Clara, CA, USA). Cells were collected and rinsed with ice-cold PBS, incubated in working reagent I for 10 min, and then centrifuged (8000 rpm) for 5 min at 4 °C. The supernatant was then collected and stored. The pellet was incubated in working reagent II for 2 h and centrifuged (8000 rpm) for 5 min. The supernatant was then collected for Snail detection. Protein concentrations were determined by the

Bradford protein assay (Bio-Rad, Hercules, CA, USA). The total proteins from cell lysates (25 µg) and nuclear proteins (25 µg) were electrophoresed in a 12.5% SDS-PAGE gel. After protein transfer, the PVDF membranes were blocked with 5% dehydrated skim milk and probed with primary antibodies (anti-human Akt, E-cadherin, FAK, MMP-2, MMP-9, N-cadherin, PI3K, Snail, TIMP-1, TIMP-2, mTOR, uPA, p-PI3K, p-Akt, p-mTOR, and actin antibodies) at 4 °C for 16 h, followed by secondary antibodies for 2 h. ECL reagent was used to detect protein expressions.

4.8. Statistical Analysis

Cell viability assay, cell migration, and invasion assay data were collected from three independent experiments and analyzed using Student's *t*-test (Sigma-Stat 2.0, San Rafael, CA, USA). Results with $p < 0.05$ were considered statistically significant.

5. Conclusions

This study revealed that flaccidoxide-13-acetate, a natural product obtained from marine coral, exhibited multiple capacities to suppress bioactivities of HA22T and HepG2 human HCC cells. First, flaccidoxide-13-acetate suppressed the cell migration, cell invasion, activities of MMP-2/-9 and uPA, and activity of upstream molecule uPA. Second, it disrupted the FAK and PI3K/Akt/mTOR signaling pathways. Third, it impaired the EMT process, including the downregulation of Snail and N-cadherin and upregulation of E-cadherin. The hypothetical mechanism of flaccidoxide-13-acetate in HA22T and HepG2 human HCC cells is illustrated in Figure 7. Taken together, these results suggested that flaccidoxide-13-acetate is a good candidate for further development as an anticancer agent to treat human HCC; however, in vivo research is warranted to confirm its effects.

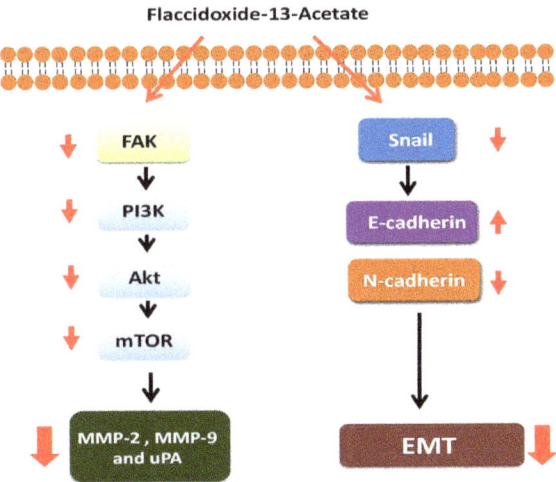

Figure 7. Hypothetical illustration of the flaccidoxide-13-acetate-associated pathway in HA22T and HepG2 human HCC cells.

Author Contributions: Y.-J.W., W.-C.W., and T.-C.T. conceived, designed, and performed the experiments. J.-H.S. isolated and identified the compound. W.-C.W., G.-F.D., J.-H.S., and Y.-H.T. performed the experiments and analyzed the data. T.-C.T. and Y.-J.W. wrote the paper. All authors have read and agreed to the published version of the manuscript.

Funding: This study was supported in part by research grants from the Ministry of Science and Technology (MOST 105-2320-B-276-001-MY3 and MOST 108-2320-B-276-001) to Yu-Jen Wu and research grants from the Antai Medical Care Corporation Antai Tian-Sheng Memorial Hospital to Tsung-Chang Tsai.

Conflicts of Interest: All of the authors declare no conflicts of interest.

References

1. Balogh, J.; Victor, D., III; Asham, E.H.; Burroughs, S.G.; Boktour, M.; Saharia, A.; Li, X.; Ghobrial, R.M.; Monsour, H.P., Jr. Hepatocellular carcinoma: A review. *J. Hepatocell. Carcinoma* **2016**, *3*, 41–53. [CrossRef] [PubMed]
2. McGlynn, K.A.; London, W.T. The global epidemiology of hepatocellular carcinoma: Present and future. *Clin. Liver Dis.* **2011**, *15*, 223–243. [CrossRef] [PubMed]
3. Zhu, R.X.; Seto, W.-K.; Lai, C.-L.; Yuen, M.-F. Epidemiology of Hepatocellular Carcinoma in the Asia-Pacific Region. *Gut Liver* **2016**, *10*, 332–339. [CrossRef] [PubMed]
4. Yuen, M.F.; Hou, J.L.; Chutaputti, A. Hepatocellular carcinoma in the Asia pacific region. *J. Gastroenterol. Hepatol.* **2009**, *24*, 346–353. [CrossRef] [PubMed]
5. Stournaras, E.; Neokosmidis, G.; Stogiannou, D.; Protopapas, A.; Tziomalos, K. Effects of antiviral treatment on the risk of hepatocellular cancer in patients with chronic viral hepatitis. *Eur. J. Gastroenterol. Hepatol.* **2018**, *30*, 1277–1282. [CrossRef]
6. Viveiros, P.; Riaz, A.; Lewandowski, R.J.; Mahalingam, D. Current State of Liver-Directed Therapies and Combinatory Approaches with Systemic Therapy in Hepatocellular Carcinoma (HCC). *Cancers* **2019**, *11*, 1085. [CrossRef]
7. Lurje, I.; Czigany, Z.; Bednarsch, J.; Roderburg, C.; Isfort, P.; Neumann, U.P.; Lurje, G. Treatment Strategies for Hepatocellular Carcinoma (-) a Multidisciplinary Approach. *Int. J. Mol. Sci.* **2019**, *20*, 1465. [CrossRef]
8. Inchingolo, R.; Posa, A.; Mariappan, M.; Spiliopoulos, S. Locoregional treatments for hepatocellular carcinoma: Current evidence and future directions. *World J. Gastroenterol.* **2019**, *25*, 4614–4628. [CrossRef]
9. Malve, H. Exploring the ocean for new drug developments: Marine pharmacology. *J. Pharm. Bioallied. Sci.* **2016**, *8*, 83–91. [CrossRef]
10. Khalifa, S.A.; Elias, N.; Farag, M.A.; Chen, L.; Saeed, A.; Hegazy, M.-E.F.; Moustafa, M.S.; Abd El-Wahed, A.; Al-Mousawi, S.M. Marine Natural Products: A Source of Novel Anticancer Drugs. *Mar. Drugs* **2019**, *17*, 491. [CrossRef]
11. Cragg, G.M.; Pezzuto, J.M. Natural Products as a Vital Source for the Discovery of Cancer Chemotherapeutic and Chemopreventive Agents. *Med. Princ. Pract.* **2016**, *25* (Suppl. 2), 41–59. [CrossRef]
12. Sang, V.T.; Dat, T.T.H.; Vinh, L.B.; Cuong, L.C.V.; Oanh, P.T.T.; Ha, H.; Kim, Y.H.; Anh, H.L.T.; Yang, S.Y. Coral and Coral-Associated Microorganisms: A Prolific Source of Potential Bioactive Natural Products. *Mar. Drugs* **2019**, *17*, 468. [CrossRef] [PubMed]
13. Wei, W.-C.; Sung, P.-J.; Duh, C.-Y.; Chen, B.-W.; Sheu, J.-H.; Yang, N.-S. Anti-inflammatory activities of natural products isolated from soft corals of Taiwan between 2008 and 2012. *Mar. Drugs* **2013**, *11*, 4083–4126. [CrossRef] [PubMed]
14. Wu, Y.-J.; Su, T.-R.; Dai, G.-F.; Su, J.-H.; Liu, C.-I. Flaccidoxide-13-Acetate-Induced Apoptosis in Human Bladder Cancer Cells is through Activation of p38/JNK, Mitochondrial Dysfunction, and Endoplasmic Reticulum Stress Regulated Pathway. *Mar. Drugs* **2019**, *17*, 287. [CrossRef]
15. Plaks, V.; Koopman, C.D.; Werb, Z. Cancer. Circulating tumor cells. *Science* **2013**, *341*, 1186–1188. [CrossRef] [PubMed]
16. Peeters, D.; Van Dam, P.; Van den Eynden, G.; Rutten, A.; Wuyts, H.; Pouillon, L.; Peeters, M.; Pauwels, P.; Van Laere, S.; Van Dam, P. Detection and prognostic significance of circulating tumour cells in patients with metastatic breast cancer according to immunohistochemical subtypes. *Br. J. Cancer* **2014**, *110*, 375–383. [CrossRef] [PubMed]
17. Neoh, C.-A.; Wu, W.-T.; Dai, G.-F.; Su, J.-H.; Liu, C.-I.; Su, T.-R.; Wu, Y.-J. Flaccidoxide-13-Acetate Extracted from the Soft Coral Cladiella kashmani Reduces Human Bladder Cancer Cell Migration and Invasion through Reducing Activation of the FAK/PI3K/AKT/mTOR Signaling Pathway. *Molecules* **2018**, *23*, 58. [CrossRef] [PubMed]
18. Chang, C.; Lin, Y.; O-Lee, T.; Chou, C.; Lee, T.; Liu, T.; P'eng, F.; Chen, T.; Hu, C. Induction of plasma protein secretion in a newly established human hepatoma cell line. *Mol. Cell. Biol.* **1983**, *3*, 1133–1137. [CrossRef] [PubMed]
19. Knowles, B.B.; Howe, C.C.; Aden, D.P. Human hepatocellular carcinoma cell lines secrete the major plasma proteins and hepatitis B surface antigen. *Science* **1980**, *209*, 497–499. [CrossRef] [PubMed]

20. Jiao, Y.; Feng, X.; Zhan, Y.; Wang, R.; Zheng, S.; Liu, W.; Zeng, X. Matrix metalloproteinase-2 promotes alphavbeta3 integrin-mediated adhesion and migration of human melanoma cells by cleaving fibronectin. *PLoS ONE* **2012**, *7*, e41591. [CrossRef] [PubMed]
21. Hofmann, U.B.; Westphal, J.R.; van Muijen, G.N.; Ruiter, D.J. Matrix metalloproteinases in human melanoma. *J. Invest. Dermatol.* **2000**, *115*, 337–344. [CrossRef] [PubMed]
22. Redondo, P.; Lloret, P.; Idoate, M.; Inoges, S. Expression and serum levels of MMP-2 and MMP-9 during human melanoma progression. *Clin. Exp. Dermatol.* **2005**, *30*, 541–545. [CrossRef] [PubMed]
23. Shi, H.; Liu, L.; Liu, L.; Geng, J.; Zhou, Y.; Chen, L. β-Elemene inhibits the metastasis of B16F10 melanoma cells by downregulation of the expression of uPA, uPAR, MMP-2, and MMP-9. *Melanoma Res.* **2014**, *24*, 99–107. [CrossRef] [PubMed]
24. Alpízar-Alpízar, W.; Christensen, I.J.; Santoni-Rugiu, E.; Skarstein, A.; Ovrebo, K.; Illemann, M.; Laerum, O.D. Urokinase plasminogen activator receptor on invasive cancer cells: A prognostic factor in distal gastric adenocarcinoma. *Int. J. Cancer* **2012**, *131*, 329–336.
25. Sonoda, Y.; Hada, N.; Kaneda, T.; Suzuki, T.; Ohshio, T.; Takeda, T.; Kasahara, T. A synthetic glycosphingolipid-induced antiproliferative effect in melanoma cells is associated with suppression of FAK, Akt, and Erk activation. *Biol. Pharm. Bull.* **2008**, *31*, 1279–1283. [CrossRef]
26. Thang, N.D.; Yajima, I.; Kumasaka, M.Y.; Iida, M.; Suzuki, T.; Kato, M. Deltex-3-like (DTX3L) stimulates metastasis of melanoma through FAK/PI3K/AKT but not MEK/ERK pathway. *Oncotarget* **2015**, *6*, 14290–14299. [CrossRef]
27. Zhao, J.; Guan, J.L. Signal transduction by focal adhesion kinase in cancer. *Cancer Metastasis Rev.* **2009**, *28*, 35–49. [CrossRef]
28. Xia, H.; Nho, R.S.; Kahm, J.; Kleidon, J.; Henke, C.A. Focal adhesion kinase is upstream of phosphatidylinositol 3-kinase/Akt in regulating fibroblast survival in response to contraction of type I collagen matrices via a beta 1 integrin viability signaling pathway. *J. Biol. Chem.* **2004**, *279*, 33024–33034. [CrossRef] [PubMed]
29. Hugo, H.; Ackland, M.L.; Blick, T.; Lawrence, M.G.; Clements, J.A.; Williams, E.D.; Thompson, E.W. Epithelial–mesenchymal and mesenchymal–epithelial transitions in carcinoma progression. *J. Cell. Physiol.* **2007**, *213*, 374–383. [CrossRef]
30. Radisky, D.C. Epithelial-mesenchymal transition. *J. Cell. Sci.* **2005**, *118*, 4325–4326. [CrossRef]
31. Batlle, E.; Sancho, E.; Francí, C.; Domínguez, D.; Monfar, M.; Baulida, J.; De Herreros, A.G. The transcription factor snail is a repressor of E-cadherin gene expression in epithelial tumour cells. *Nat. Cell. Biol.* **2000**, *2*, 84–89. [CrossRef] [PubMed]
32. Bolós, V.; Peinado, H.; Pérez-Moreno, M.A.; Fraga, M.F.; Esteller, M.; Cano, A. The transcription factor Slug represses E-cadherin expression and induces epithelial to mesenchymal transitions: A comparison with Snail and E47 repressors. *J. Cell. Sci.* **2003**, *116*, 499–511. [CrossRef] [PubMed]
33. Cano, A.; Pérez-Moreno, M.A.; Rodrigo, I.; Locascio, A.; Blanco, M.J.; del Barrio, M.G.; Portillo, F.; Nieto, M.A. The transcription factor snail controls epithelial-mesenchymal transitions by repressing E-cadherin expression. *Nat. Cell. Biol.* **2000**, *2*, 76–83. [CrossRef] [PubMed]

© 2020 by the authors. Licensee MDPI, Basel, Switzerland. This article is an open access article distributed under the terms and conditions of the Creative Commons Attribution (CC BY) license (http://creativecommons.org/licenses/by/4.0/).

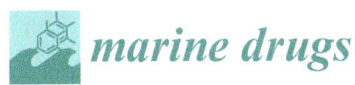

Article

Marine-Derived *Penicillium purpurogenum* Reduces Tumor Size and Ameliorates Inflammation in an Erlich Mice Model

Amanda Mara Teles [1], Leticia Prince Pereira Pontes [2], Sulayne Janayna Araújo Guimarães [2], Ana Luiza Butarelli [2], Gabriel Xavier Silva [1], Flavia Raquel Fernandes do Nascimento [3], Geusa Felipa de Barros Bezerra [4], Carla Junqueira Moragas-Tellis [5], Rui Miguel Gil da Costa [4,6], Marcos Antonio Custódio Neto da Silva [7], Fernando Almeida-Souza [8,9], Kátia da Silva Calabrese [9,*], Ana Paula Silva Azevedo-Santos [2] and Maria do Desterro Soares Brandão Nascimento [4,*]

1. Laboratory for Culture Cell, Postgraduate Program in Biotechnology (RENORBIO), Federal University of Maranhão, São Luís 65080-085, Maranhão, Brazil; damarateles@hotmail.com (A.M.T.); xaviersilva.g@gmail.com (G.X.S.)
2. Laboratory of Applied Cancer Immunology, Biological and Health Sciences Center, Federal University of Maranhão, Avenida dos Portugueses, 1966 Bacanga, São Luis 65080-085, Maranhão, Brazil; leticiaprince22@hotmail.com (L.P.P.P.); sulaynebio@hotmail.com (S.J.A.G.); analuizabutarelli@gmail.com (A.L.B.); apsazevedo@yahoo.com.br (A.P.S.A.-S.)
3. Immunophisiology Laboratory, Biological and Health Sciences Center, Federal University of Maranhão, Avenida dos Portugueses, 1966 Bacanga, São Luís 65080-085, Maranhão, Brazil; nascimentofrf@yahoo.com.br
4. Postgraduate Program in Adult Health (PPGSAD), Federal University of Maranhão, Avenida dos Portugueses, 1966 Bacanga, São Luís 65080-085, Maranhão, Brazil; geusabezerra@gmail.com (G.F.d.B.B.); rmcosta@fe.up.pt (R.M.G.d.C.)
5. Laboratory of Natural Products for Public Health, Institute of Pharmaceutical Techonology, Oswaldo Cruz Foundation, Rio de Janeiro 21041-000, Brazil; carlatellis@far.fiocruz.br
6. Centre for the Research and Technology of Agro-Environmental and Biological Sciences (CITAB), University of Trás-os-Montes and Alto Douro (UTAD), 5001-801 Vila Real, Portugal
7. Post-graduation in Internal Medicine, State University of Campinas, Campinas 13083-887, São Paulo, Brazil; marcos_antonio456@hotmail.com
8. Laboratory of Anamotopathology, Postgraduate Program in Animal Science, State University of Maranhão, São Luis 65055-310, Maranhão, Brazil; fernandoalsouza@gmail.com
9. Laboratory of Immunomodulation and Protozoology, Oswaldo Cruz Institute, Oswaldo Cruz Foundation, Rio de Janeiro 21040-900, Brazil
* Correspondence: calabrese@ioc.fiocruz.br (K.d.S.C.); m.desterro.soares@gmail.com (M.d.D.S.B.N.); Tel.: +55-98-3272-8535 (M.d.D.S.B.N.)

Received: 18 August 2020; Accepted: 4 October 2020; Published: 29 October 2020

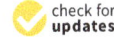

Abstract: Background: This study addresses the antitumoral properties of *Penicillium purpurogenum* isolated from a polluted lagoon in Northeastern Brazil. Methods: Ethyl Acetate Extracellular Extract (EAE) was used. The metabolites were studied using direct infusion mass spectrometry. The solid Ehrlich tumor model was used for antitumor activity. Female Swiss mice were divided into groups (n = 10/group) as follows: The negative control (CTL−), treated with a phosphate buffered solution; the positive control (CTL+), treated with cyclophosphamide (25 mg/kg); extract treatments at doses of 4, 20, and 100 mg/kg; animals without tumors or treatments (Sham); and animals without tumors treated with an intermediate dose (EAE20). All treatments were performed intraperitoneally, daily, for 15 days. Subsequently, the animals were euthanized, and the tumor, lymphoid organs, and serum were used for immunological, histological, and biochemical parameter evaluations. Results: The extract was rich in meroterpenoids. All doses significantly reduced tumor size, and the 20 and 100 mg/kg doses reduced tumor-associated inflammation and tumor necrosis. The extract also reduced the cellular infiltration of lymphoid organs and circulating TNF-α levels. The extract did not induce weight loss or renal and hepatic toxic changes. Conclusions: These results indicate that *P. purpurogenum* exhibits immunomodulatory and antitumor properties in vivo. Thus, fungal fermentation is a valid biotechnological approach to the production of antitumor agents.

Keywords: Ehlich's tumor; *P. purpurogenum*; antitumor; meroterpenoids; inflammation

1. Introduction

Fungi are versatile organisms with promising therapeutic and biotechnological potential that can be found in several habitats and occupy inhospitable ecological niches in all ecosystems on the planet [1]. Several studies show that marine microorganisms are sources of unique natural products, including molecules with potential anticancer uses [2–5].

Penicillium fungi synthesize large amounts of known bioactive secondary metabolites [6,7], including anticarcinogenic drugs and immunosuppressive agents [8,9]. The *P. purpurogenum* species has the ability to synthesize a variety of substances with biotechnological and bioactive potential, but the strains that demonstrate this activity are mutant strains resistant to antibiotics [10,11].

Penicillium purpurogenum MA52 is a strain previously isolated from a polluted marine environment, the Jansen lagoon in the Northeastern Brazilian state of Maranhão [12]. This is a highly polluted environment that receives domestic effluents from the surrounding city of São Luís [12]. However, the specific characteristics of the MA52 strain that allow it to survive in this polluted environment have not yet been described. New drugs are being developed from secondary metabolites to discover less toxic and more effective compounds compared to traditional cancer therapies [13]. Some natural products have also become important nutraceuticals with cancer chemopreventive properties [14,15].

Many in vivo models are used for studying breast cancer, the most common cancer in women worldwide [16]. Breast cancer models include genetically modified animals, xenografted tumors in immune-compromised mice, chemically induced models [17], and syngeneic models like the solid Ehrlich's tumor, which is a spontaneous and highly aggressive murine mammary adenocarcinoma [18]. This syngeneic model is immunocompetent and avoids the use of harmful chemicals, making it particularly useful for tumor and chemotherapy studies [19,20]. Considering the search for bioactive compounds capable of serving as prototypes of new antitumor drugs, the present study aims to describe the in vivo antitumor activity of *P. purpurogenum* extract compounds obtained from the MA52 strain against solid Ehrlich's tumor.

2. Results

2.1. P. purpurogenum Extracellular Extract Contains Meroterpenoids

HPLC-DAD-UV analyses were performed to determine the *P. purpurogenum* extract profile. The obtained chromatogram at 300 nm showed 12 peaks, and all of them presented UV λ_{max} in the range of 258–282 nm, confirming the presence of meroterpenoid compounds (Figure 1 and Table 1).

The mass spectral data obtained by direct infusion in positive mode (ESI-MS/MS), presented in Figure 2, were used to confirm the chemical profile of the *P. purpurogenum* extracellular extract (EAE) and suggested the presence of five meroterpenoidal compounds (**1–5**) commonly produced by fungi [21] by comparing the mass spectral data with those described in the literature.

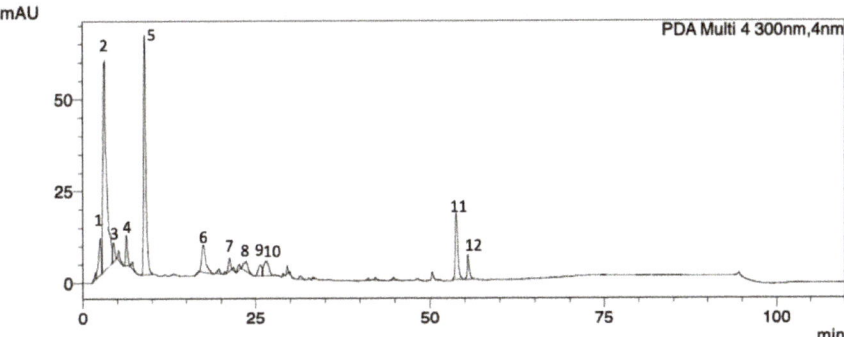

Figure 1. HPLC-DAD-UV chromatogram (300 nm) obtained from the *Penicillium purpurogenum* extract showing 12 peaks of which the UV spectral data (λ max) are characteristic of meroterpenoid compounds.

Table 1. Meroterpenoids of the crude extract of *Penicillium purpurogenum* and their retention times, relative composition, and UV data.

Peak	Rt (min)	Area %	UV (λ_{max}, nm)
1	2.46	4.89	258
2	3.37	37.30	259
3	4.36	2.00	264
4	6.27	2.90	283
5	8.87	26.96	272
6	17.38	5.63	282
7	21.15	1.52	265
8	23.65	2.13	271
9	26.27	2.02	276
10	26.48	3.82	277
11	53.81	8.31	278
12	55.41	2.48	278

Rt: retention time.

Compound **1** (purpurogemutantin) presented an experimental pseudo-molecular ion [M + H]$^+$ at *m/z* 419.1674 compatible with the molecular formula $C_{24}H_{35}O_6$. Compounds **2** (purpurogemutantin) and/or **3** (macrophorin A) showed the same pseudo-molecular ion [M + H]$^+$ at *m/z* 361.1037, corresponding to the molecular formula $C_{22}H_{33}O_4$. These compounds were previously described for *P. purpurogenum* extracts by Fang et al. [22]. Compound **4** (berkeleyacetal C, molecular formula $C_{24}H_{26}O_8$), another meroterpenoid previously described in mutant *P. purpurogenum* by Li et al. [23], presented a pseudo-molecular ion [M + H]$^+$ at *m/z* 443.1696, while compound **5** (rubratoxin B) showed a pseudo-molecular ion [M + H]$^+$ at *m/z* 519.1758 corresponding to the molecular formula $C_{22}H_{33}O_4$. Rubratoxin B is another known meroterpenoid with anticancer activity isolated by *P. purpurogenum* [24].

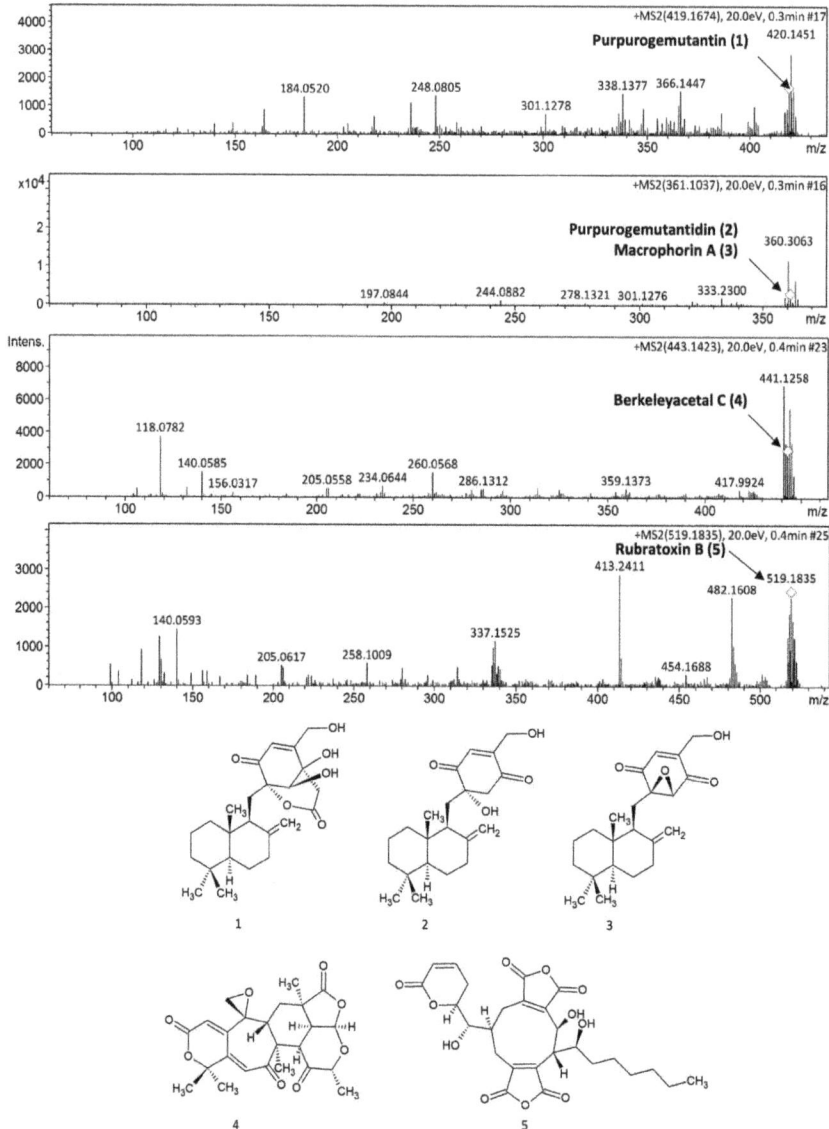

Figure 2. Mass spectra obtained for the tentative identification of meroterpenoids 1–5.

2.2. P. purpurogenum Extract Showed Activity Against Ehrlich's Solid Tumor

In tumor growth kinetics, the results showed that, throughout the experiment, the negative control group presented an upward curve, while those treated with cyclophosphamide and the extract showed linear kinetics. The extract significantly reduced tumor growth from the eighth day compared to CLT−, while cyclophosphamide reduced tumor growth from the tenth day (Figure 3a). The kinetic values of tumor growth agree with the graph of the area under curve (AUC). The extract at doses of 4 mg/kg (422 ± 35.8 mm^2), 20 mg/kg (389.7 ± 49.13 mm^2), and 100 mg/kg (365.5 ± 40.47 mm^2) presented an area smaller than that of the negative control (1240 ± 43.25 mm^2) along with chemotherapy

(599.8 ± 55.51 mm^2) (Figure 3b). At the end of the experimental period, the extract at 4 mg/kg (0.19 ± 0.02 g), 20 mg/kg (0.19 ± 0.05 g), and 100 mg/kg (0.16 ± 0.02 g) showed a low tumor weight when compared to the negative control (0.38 ± 0.07 g) and similar weight to the positive control (0.15 ± 0.05 g) (Figure 3c).

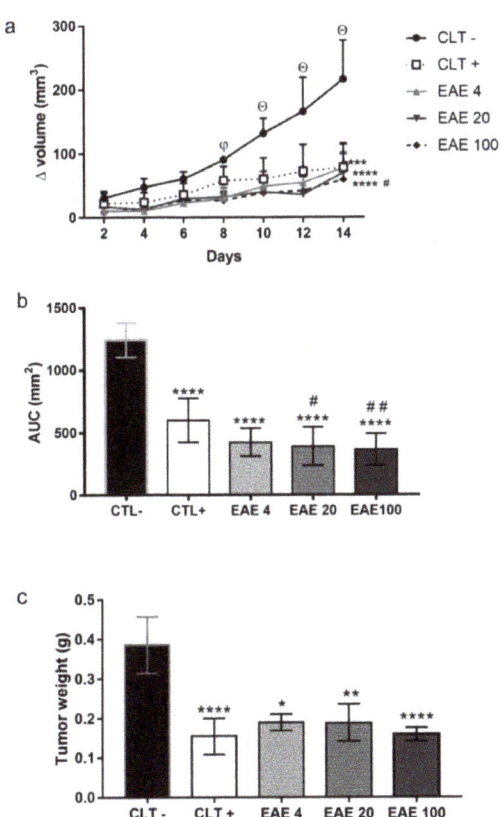

Figure 3. Effect of the *Penicillium purpurogenum* extract on the development of Ehrlich's solid tumor. (**a**) The kinetic of the paw volume inoculated with Ehrlich's tumor followed by intraperitoneal treatment with phosphate buffer solution (CTL−), cyclophosphamide 25 mg/kg (CTL+), and extracts with a concentration of 4 mg/kg (EAE4), 20 mg/kg (EAE20), and 100 mg/kg (EAE10) at 24 h intervals, with the animals being euthanized on day 15. (**b**) The area under the curve (AUC) calculated from the volume growth kinetics. (**c**) The average weight of the paws with a tumor was determined in the groups after treatment. Values are expressed as the mean ± standard error of means (SEM) deviation and analyzed by analysis of variance (one-way or two-way ANOVA) with * $p < 0.05$, ** $p < 0.005$, and **** $p < 0.0001$ relative to the negative control (CTL−); # $p < 0.05$, ## $p < 0.01$ when compared to the positive control (CTL+); and Θ $p < 0.05$ shows a difference in tumor growth for the other groups; φ shows that, on the eighth day, only the extract inhibited tumor growth.

2.3. Histological Results

Histopathological analysis showed the presence of tumor masses in the foot pads of animals from the groups with Ehrlich's solid tumor. The tumor masses exhibited high cellularity and different growth patterns, with central, moderate, or very high pleomorphisms, as well as bizarre nuclear forms, the presence of one or more nucleoli, and heterogeneous chromatin patterns. The cytoplasm was eosinophilic and abundant with poorly defined limits. Occasional multinucleated giant cells (associated with pattern 3 pleomorphism) and up to two mitosis figures per 400× field were identified. Groups with tumor induction presented peritumoral, multifocal, or coalescent lymphohistiocytic inflammatory infiltrates with variable intensity. Areas of multifocal liquefaction necrosis with the accumulation of eosinophilic and amorphous cellular debris associated with neutrophilic infiltrate were also observed. Interestingly, the extract showed an inflammatory process induced by the minor tumors in the groups treated with 20 and 100 mg/kg when compared to the negative control. The extract was also demonstrated to have smaller areas of tumor necrosis, mitotic activity, and invasion compared to the negative control (Figure 4 and Table 2).

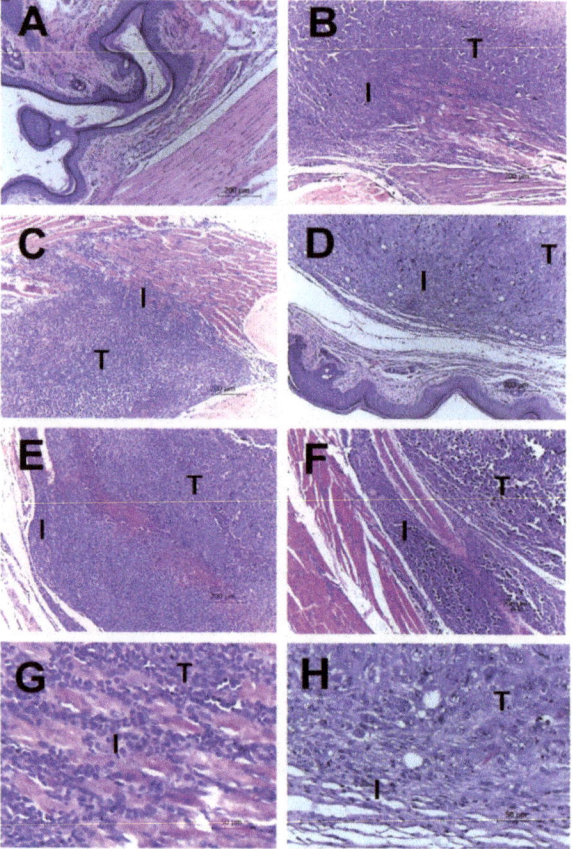

Figure 4. Tumor and leukocyte infiltration in Ehrlich tumors with and without treatments. Leukocyte infiltrates in Ehrlich tumors. Swiss mice were inoculated in the paw with 2×10^6 Ehrlich tumor cells and treated daily with EAE extract intraperitoneally. At the end of the fifteen days of treatment, the animals were euthanized, and their feet were amputated, weighed, and fixed. Histological sections were stained with Hematoxylin–Eosin. In the photos, it is possible to see the tumor cells (indicated by the letter T) and the inflammatory infiltrate (indicated by letter I) present in the paws of the Sham (**A**), CLT− (**B**), and CLT+ (**C**) groups (100× total magnification). The animals treated with the extract showed a decrease in the infiltrate and necrosis are EAE doses of EAE 4 (**D**), EAE 20 (**E**), and EAE 100 (**F**) (100× total magnification). The Sham group is shown in panel **G,** and the animals treated using the extract with a dose of EAE 100 are shown in panel **H** (400× total magnification).

Table 2. Ehrlich tumor histopathological scores (mean ± SD) of groups treated with saline (CTL−), cyclophosphamide (CTL+), or *Penicillium purpurogenum* ethyl acetate extract at 4 mg/kg (EAE4), 20 mg/kg (EAE20), and 100 mg/kg (EAE100).

	Pleomorphism	Necrosis	Mitosis Figures	Inflammation	Invasion
CLT−	2.4 ± 0.511	2.4 ± 0.843	1.0 ± 1.155	2.8 ± 0.421	2.0 ± 0.666
CLT+	0.2 ± 0.421 *	0.2 ± 0.421 *	0.0 ± 0.000 *	1.0 ± 1.333 *	0.6 ± 0.843 *
EAE4	2.2 ± 1.122	1.2 ± 1.033	1.0 ± 1.155	1.4 ± 1.075	1.0 ± 0.667
EAE20	2.0 ± 1.155	0.6 ± 1.265 *	0.2 ± 0.421	0.8 ± 0.788 *	1.0 ± 0.667
EAE100	0.8 ± 1.033 *	0.2 ± 0.421 *	0.0 ± 0.000 *	0.6 ± 0.843 *	0.4 ± 0.843 *

Scores: 0 (absent), 1 (weak), 2 (moderate), and 3 (intense); the result was calculated by the mean of the scores; * $p < 0.05$ relative to the negative control (CLT−). N = 5/group.

2.4. P. purpurogenum Extract Induced Immunomodulatory Effects

Treatment with EAE at doses of 20 and 100 mg/kg presented low number of cells in the popliteal lymph nodes ($9.6 \times 10^4 \pm 1.0$ cells/mL and $4.4 \times 10^4 \pm 0.34$ cells/mL, respectively) compared to the negative control ($326 \times 10^4 \pm 40.83$ cells/mL). Similar results were observed in the cyclophosphamide-treated animals ($8.0 \times 10^4 \pm 1.88$ cells/mL) (Figure 5a). In the spleen cells, the negative control group ($72.7 \times 10^7 \pm 7.06$ cells/mL) showed high cellularity compared to the animals of the Sham group ($1.6 \times 10^7 \pm 0.12$ cells/mL). However, this difference was not observed in animals inoculated with the tumor and treated with cyclophosphamide ($0.7 \times 10^7 \pm 0.02$ cells/mL) or extract doses of 20 mg/kg ($1.6 \times 10^7 \pm 0.14$ cells/mL) and 100 mg/kg ($1.2 \times 10^7 \pm 0.04$ cells/mL) (Figure 5b). The marrow bone cellularity showed that the cyclophosphamide ($12.3 \times 10^5 \pm 3.13$ cells/mL) and the extract treatment ($61.0 \times 10^5 \pm 8.35$ cells/mL, $17.6 \times 10^5 \pm 1.20$ cells/mL and $4.0 \times 10^5 \pm 1.08$ cells/mL, respectively) prevented a high level of cellularity associated with Ehrlich's tumor, since the groups without a tumor (sham: $4.6 \times 10^5 \pm 0.77$ cells/mL and EAE20: $15.44 \times 10^5 \pm 5.04$ cells/mL) had fewer cells than the negative control group ($189.0 \times 10^5 \pm 23.12$ cells/mL) (Figure 5c). The results show that the extract's effect was dose-dependent.

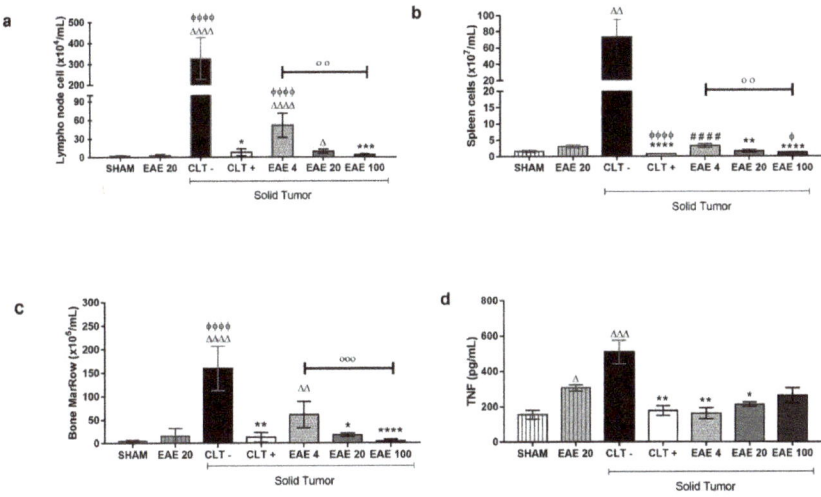

Figure 5. Immunomodulatory effects of *Penicillium purpurogenum* ethyl acetate extract. (**a**–**d**) The results are expressed as the mean ± standard deviation of the total lymph node cell count; bone marrow and splenocytes obtained from the group without tumors treated with saline solution (Sham) from the groups with solid Ehrlich tumors treated intraperitoneally with extracts at doses of 4, 20, and 100 mg/kg,

respectively (EAE4, EAE20, and EAE100); positive and negative control-administered cyclophosphamide (CLT+) and saline solution (CTL−), respectively. Blood serum was used to quantify the tumor necrosis factor (TNF-α). The data were submitted to statistical analyses via Kruskal–Wallis and Dunn multiple comparison tests, with a significance of $\Delta\ p < 0.05$, $\Delta\Delta\ p < 0.005$, $\Delta\Delta\Delta\ p < 0.0005$, and $\Delta\Delta\Delta\Delta\ p < 0.0001$ in relation to the Sham; $\phi\ p < 0.05$, $\phi\phi\phi\phi\ p < 0.0001$ when compared to EA20 without tumor; #### $p < 0.0001$ when compared to CLT+, * $p < 0.05$, ** $p < 0.005$, *** $p < 0.0005$, and **** $p < 0.0001$ when compared to CLT−; and oo $p < 0.0001$ ooo $p < 0.0001$ when comparing the extracts with each other.

Cytokine quantification demonstrated that treatment was able to alter only the TNF levels (Supplementary Information Table S1). The animals with untreated tumors (CTL−) showed an even higher level of TNF-α concentrations (508.8 ± 66.22 pg/mL) compared to the Sham group (156.0 ± 25.14 pg/mL). The cyclophosphamide treatment significantly showed lower TNF-α levels (177.2 ± 27.67 pg/mL) compared to the negative control group. Similarly, the extract at 4, 20, and 100 mg/kg doses also showed low TNF-α concentrations versus the group of CLT− (161.7 ± 30.22, 212.4 ± 12.03 and 261.4 ± 43.16 pg/mL, respectively) in animals with solid tumors. However, the extract treatment in animals without a tumor showed a high level of seric TNF-α concentration (306.9 ± 17.93 pg/mL) compared to normal animals (Figure 5d).

2.5. Toxicity Studies of P. purpurogenum EAE

Daily treatment with *P. purpurogenum* ethyl acetate extract in the solid Ehrlich tumor maintained the body weights of the tumor-inoculated animals (EAE4: 2.38 ± 0.63 g; EAE20: 2.8 ± 0.76 g and EAE100: 0.96 ± 0.67 g) compared with CTL+ (−1.16 ± 0.46 g) and CTL− (−0.24 ± 0.73 g) (Figure 6a). The data show that only the group receiving cyclophosphamide had a body weight reduction compared to the Sham group (1.58 ± 0.96 g). There were no significant differences in the serum AST and ALT levels in any of the groups analyzed, although the CTL− animals showed increased average values compared to the groups treated with the extract in the presence of the tumor (Table 3). Hepatic and renal histological differences were not found between the groups. The survival rate curve showed that the saline (79.12%) and cyclophosphamide (85.72%) groups were statistically different, as expected. Importantly, the tumor-animal groups treated with the extract showed a 100% survival rate under all doses, which is significantly different compared to the controls (Figure 6b).

Table 3. Effect of *Penicillium purpurogenum* ethyl acetate extract on ALT and AST serum levels (mean ± SEM) in all experimental groups.

	ALT (U/L)	AST (U/L)
Sham	125.2 ± 103.5	125.2 ± 103.5
EAE20 *	122.5 ± 101.5	295.3 ± 236.1
CLT−	207.9 ± 181.8	438.3 ± 328.5
CLT+	438.3 ± 328.5	293 ± 131.8
EAE4 + Tumor	50.12 ± 33.38	178.6 ± 95.15
EAE20 + Tumor	68.3 ± 57.5	185.1 ± 111.2
EAE100 + Tumor	48.88 ± 21.68	179.1 ± 61.28

$N = 5$ for each group. The one-way ANOVA showed no statistical differences between the groups. * Tumor free group treated with an extract at a dose of 20 mg/kg. The groups were treated with saline (CTL−), cyclophosphamide (CTL+), and *Penicillium purpurogenum* ethyl acetate extract at 4 mg/kg (EAE4 + Tumor), 20 mg/kg (EAE20 + Tumor), and 100 mg/kg (EAE100 + Tumor).

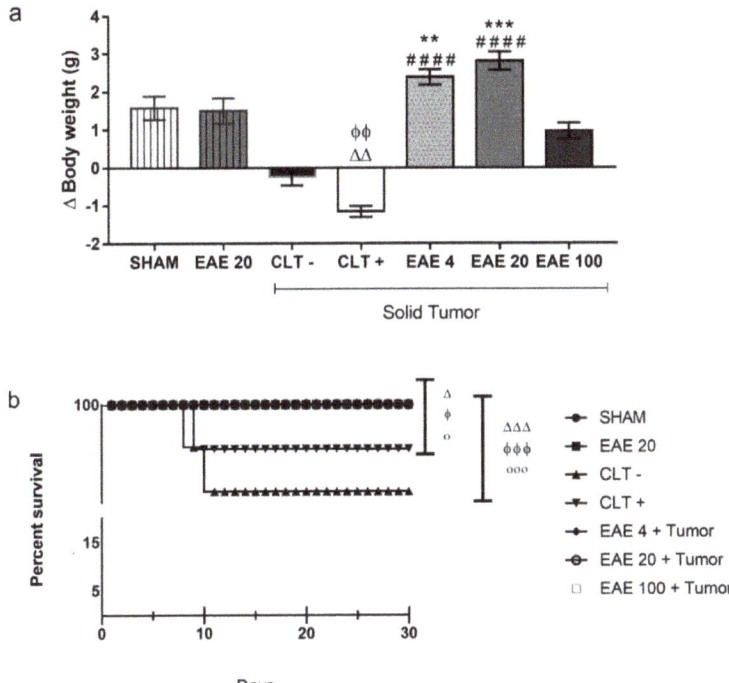

Figure 6. Effect of the toxicity of the extracellular extract of *Penicillium purpurogenum* ethyl acetate extract (EAE). The groups without tumor induction were treated with saline (sham), while the groups with induction received the extract at doses of 4, 20, and 100 mg/kg (EAE4, EAE20, and EAE100), as well as saline (CTL−) and cyclophosphamide (CTL+). The graphs show (**a**) the animals' body weights in the final treatment. (**b**) After the treatment of the animals, the animals remained under observation for thirty days. The data represent the mean ± SEM. The difference was statistically analyzed by a Kruskal–Wallis and Dunn's multiple comparison test, with significance of Δ $p < 0.05$, ΔΔ $p < 0.005$, and ΔΔΔ $p < 0.0005$ in relation to the Sham, ϕ $p < 0.05$ ϕϕ $p < 0.005$, and ϕϕϕ $p < 0.0005$ when compared to EA20 without a tumor, o $p < 0.05$ when compared to CTL+, and ooo $p < 0.0005$ when compared to CTL−, * $p < 0.05$, ** $p < 0.005$, and #### $p < 0.0001$.

2.6. P. purpurogenum Extract Has a Cytotoxic Effect against MCF7 Cells In Vitro

P. purpurogenum isolated from the marine environment exhibited antitumor activity in vitro against MCF7 cells. EAE showed a concentration and time-dependent effect, as observed in the dose–response curve of the viable MCF7 cell percentage in relation to the untreated cells after 24 and 48 h of treatment (Figure 7A). The inhibitory concentration of 50% of cells (IC_{50}) after treatment with EAE was 53.56 ± 1.031 and 27.22 ± 1.029 µg/mL for 24 and 48 h, respectively. The reference drug doxorubicin also presented a concentration and time-dependent effect (Figure 7B) and IC_{50} values of 37.10 ± 1.161 and 19.02 ± 1.223 µg/mL for 24 and 48 h, respectively.

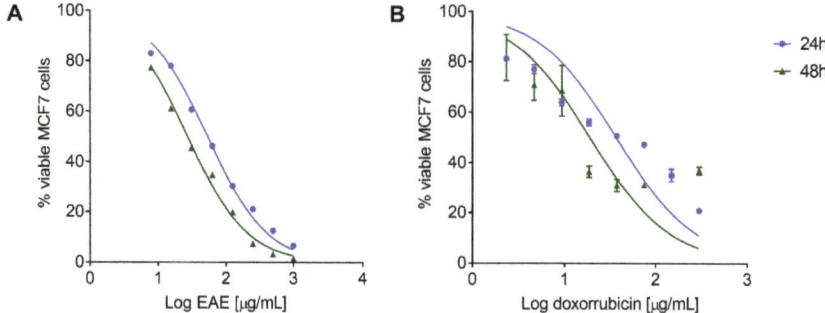

Figure 7. Dose–response curve of *Penicillium purpurogenum* ethyl acetate extract (EAE) for MCF7 cell viability. Data represent the means ± SD of the viable MCF7 cell percentage in relation to the untreated cells after 24 and 48 h of treatment with EAE (**A**) and doxorubicin (**B**).

3. Discussion

P. purpurogenum isolated from a marine environment is capable of secreting secondary bioactive metabolites with anticancer properties. In the present study, the extracellular extract of this fungus revealed the presence of macrophorin A, purpurogemutanthidine, and purpurogemutanthin, corroborating the previous findings by Tang et al. [25], Fang et al. [22], and He et al. [26]. These compounds showed interesting anticancer activities in vitro against cervical cancer, gastric adenocarcinoma, and breast cancer cells, while berkeleyacetal C [27–29] and rubratoxin B [30–32] showed anti-inflammatory and anticancer activity in vitro.

Meroterpenoids, which are formed by the mixed terpenoid–polyketide biosynthetic pathway, are an important class of compounds in the context of the development of new anticancer agents due to their vast structural diversity and broad spectrum of bioactivities [33]. They are known to have activities against cancer through various mechanisms, such as the blocking of cell survival pathways, activity against oxidative stress, and the induction of apoptosis [34]. When checking for the presence of compounds with anticancer activity in vitro, we questioned whether the extract isolated from the marine environment (and not described in the literature to have in vivo activity against Ehrlich's tumor) could be active.

The present study is the first to evaluate the in vivo anticancer effects of *P. purpurogenum* by employing mice inoculated with Ehrlich's tumor cells. The results showed that the extract compounds were able to efficiently reduce the development and weight of Ehrlich's solid tumor.

Ehrlich's tumor exhibits strong inflammatory phenomena, including edema and inflammatory infiltrates, which are believed to play an essential role in tumor growth in various types of cancer [35–39]. However, anti-inflammatory effects were previously reported for meroterpenoids [40] and were also observed in this research, showing that the extract reduces inflammation, thereby reducing the tumor via an indirect route.

We found in our research that the cell line MCF7 is sensitive to the extract. This specificity for MCF-7 cells is possibly due to the cytotoxic effects caused by substances such as meroterpenoids present in the extract [22,27]. However, the research carried out by Chai et al. (2012) [10] to study the strain of the fungus *P. purpurogenum* G59 (originally derived from marine origin) against the K562 strain did not verify a cytotoxic effect or any inhibitory effect at a concentration of 1000 µg/mL. We suggest, based on the research carried out by Darsih et al. (2015) [41] changing the cytotoxic activity in another species of the same genus with the cysteine-targeted Michael acceptor as a possible pharmacophore target for fragment-based drug discovery, bioconjugation, and click reactions [41].

The extract inhibited tumor growth at the same level as the untreated group since the behavior of the animals and the survival of the group treated with the extract were similar to the results in the sham group. Thus, the extract likely acts in tumor cell proliferation, migration, and invasion.

Two factors could inhibit tumor growth: the direct effect on the tumor microenvironment caused by macrophorin A, purpurogutididine, and purpurogemutanthin identified in the extracts to result in smaller tumor size and a reduction in inflammation, thereby decreasing the tumor's size, which may be associated with the presence of Berkeleyacetal C in the extract.

Other meroterpenoids showed the inhibition of tumor activities. Wang et al. [30] studied Guajadial, a natural dialdehyde meroterpenoid able to suppress tumor growth in human xenograft mouse models, with probable proliferation inhibition by blocking the Ras/MAPK pathway.

Wan et al. [42] demonstrated that meroterpenoids have anti-inflammatory and antioxidant activities that can reduce tumor growth. Li et al. [24] found that Berkeleyacetal C significantly inhibits the expression of inducible nitric oxide synthase (iNOS) and the production of nitric oxide by macrophages.

Berkeleyacetal C inhibits the expression and secretion of major pro-inflammatory factors and chemokines, including tumor necrosis factor-α (TNF-α) interleukin-6 (IL-6), interleukin-1β (IL-1β), macrophage inflammatory protein -1α (PImax) -1α), and the monocyte chemotactic protein-1 (MCP-1) [22,28].

Immunosuppression cells can have a pro-tumoral effect. Indeed, higher infiltration by Tregs was observed in tumor tissues, and their depletion augments antitumor immune responses in animal models [37].

There were also systemic effects observed with dose-dependent reduction in the cells of the popliteal lymph node, spleen, and bone marrow compared to the negative control group. This is in line with the low levels of TNF-α, which play an important role in the beginning and apply the activation of adhesion molecules and the expression of inflammatory mediators during inflammatory responses [43]. These pro-inflammatory mediators can cause damage to cells and tissues and also activate macrophages in various diseases associated with inflammation [44].

Increased levels of pro-inflammatory cytokines were previously associated with the development of Ehrlich's tumor [45]. Our data also agree with those of Calixto-Campos et al. [46], Aldubayan et al. [47], and Harun et al. [48], who studied the protective role of fungal extracts against inflammatory events induced by LPS in vitro and found that all the extracts inhibited TNF-α expression. Taken together, these results show that the extracellular extract of *P. purpurogenum* has potent anticancer activity in vivo against Ehrlich's breast adenocarcinoma and that this effect can be mediated, at least in part, by immunomodulatory mechanisms.

Another important set of observations from the present study concerns the safety of the extract. Remarkably, the *P. purpurogenum* extracellular extract was able to improve mouse survival at all doses compared to the negative control and even the cyclophosphamide, providing 100% survival at the end of the study. The extract also preserved the body weight of the animals, preventing the wasting syndrome that is often associated with cancer and intensified by chemotherapy [49–53], as previously reviewed [54,55].

These data suggest that the *P. purpurogenum* extract may have potential clinical use in combination therapies to prevent the loss of body weight in cancer patients. Considering that fungal extracts often display hepatic toxicity, we evaluated the ALT and AST serum levels and hepatic histology. The results did not demonstrate acute hepatic toxicity; instead, the extract did not possess the hepatic histological lesions associated with Ehrlich's tumor and presented low serum levels of hepatic transaminases. In line with these observations, no changes were observed in renal histology. These results support the hypothesis that the extract has a favorable toxicological profile, although these observations should be confirmed and complemented by additional studies.

Thus, the results show that the extract inhibited tumor growth, compared to the negative control, at the same level as standard therapy (cyclophosphamide), even when applied at the lowest dose.

Interestingly, the activity of the extract occurred before that of the cyclophosphamide, suggesting intense antitumor activity in vivo. In addition, these findings correlate with morphological changes of the histological level, showing that *P. purpurogenum* has low mitotic activity and invasive behavior against tumor cells. The extract's antitumor activity is associated with marked immunomodulatory effects.

4. Materials and Methods

4.1. Fermentation and Preparation of Ethyl Acetate Extracellular Extract (EAE)

P. purpurogenum is a marine fungus found in the coastal region (2°29′56″ S 44°17′59″ W) of Maranhão, Brazil. The present strain was isolated by the Mycology Laboratory of the Basic and Applied Immunology Center of the Federal University of Maranhão and deposited into the fungi collection of the Federal University of Maranhão under access code MA52. The fungus strain was grown in Potato Dextrose Agar (BDA) at 28 °C for 7 days until complete growth. After that period, superficial circles of mycelium-containing agar were further cultivated in BDA broth for fermentation at 28 °C for 21 days in a rotary shaker (Quimis, São Paulo, Brazil) at 150 rpm. Afterward, 300 mL of the fermented broth was macerated for 48 h with 600 mL of ethanol to obtain the extracellular extract. Then, the aqueous ethanol solution was filtered and concentrated under reduced pressure to remove the ethanol, and the remaining water was extracted twice with 1:4 (*v/v*) ethyl acetate, resulting in an organic phase that was concentrated and lyophilized to obtain the ethyl acetate extract used for in vivo testing.

4.2. High-Performance Liquid Chromatograph Coupled to Diode-Array UV-Vis Detector (HPLC-DAD-UV)

Chromatographic analyses were performed on a HPLC-DAD-UV using a Shimadzu Nexera XR® liquid chromatograph (Shimadzu, Kyoto, Japan) coupled to a UV detector with an SPDM20A diode array, a CBM20A controller, a DGU20A degasser, an LC20AD binary pump, a CTO20A oven, and an SILA20A auto-injector. Shimadzu LabSolutions Software Version 5.3 (Shimadzu, Kyoto, Japan) was used to analyze the chromatograms. DAD analysis was applied to select the optimized wavelength of the meroterpenoids in this study (300 nm). Combinations of ultrapure water (A) and methanol (HPLC grade, Tedia, Rio de Janeiro, Brazil) (B) were used as the mobile phase (initially 0% B, increasing to 20% in 8.5 min, subsequently rising to 100% of B in 68.5 min, and finally staying at this concentration up to 90 min). The HPLC column was silica-based C18 (250 mm × 4.6 mm i.d. × 5 µm particle size, Shimpack CLC-ODS, Thermo, Waltham, MA, USA). The oven was set to 50 °C, and the injection volume was 10 µL for all analyses.

4.3. Tandem Mass Spectrometry with Electrospray Ionization (ESI-MS/MS)

Ethyl acetate extracellular extract (EAE) was analyzed by direct infusion (ESI-MS/MS) in a Bruker Ion trap amazon SL mass spectrometer (Bruker, Billerica, MA, USA, positive mode (ESI+)). EAE (3 mg) was dissolved in certified HPLC grade methanol containing 0.1% formic acid (*v/v*) using an ultrasonic bath for 20 min. The operating conditions were 1 µL/min infusion, 4.0 kV capillary voltage, 100 °C temperature source, and cone voltage of 20–40 V. The mass spectra were recorded and interpreted by Bruker Compass Data Analysis (Version 4.2, Bruker, Billerica, MA, USA).

4.4. Animals

After approval by the Ethics Committee (CEUA 23115.11239/2017-70), female Swiss mice ($n = 70$), weighing 25–30 g and aged between 3 and 4 months were provided by the Federal University of Maranhão (UFMA). Animals were kept in a room with a controlled temperature of 22 ± 3 °C, with 50 ± 15% relative humidity, a 12 h light/dark photoperiod, and food and water ad libitum. The animal experiments were conducted according to the animal welfare guidelines of the National Council for the Control of Animal Experimentation (CONCEA). Every effort was made to reduce the number of animals used and their discomfort.

4.5. Ehrlich Solid Tumor Model

Animals were anesthetized with ketamine/xylazine (120–150 mg/kg). The Ehrlich ascitic carcinoma was maintained in the mice via intraperitoneal injections of 2×10^6 cells [56]. To induce the solid tumor, transplantable neoplastic cells with 7 days of ascitic evolution were aspirated, and 200 µL of the cell suspension at 2×10^6 cells/mL was injected into the left posterior foot pad. The cells were found to be more than 99% viable by a Trypan blue exclusion method. The experimental treatment began 24 h after the tumor implantation [57].

4.6. Treatment Groups

The animals were separated into two groups: those with tumor inoculation for antitumor activity and those without tumor inoculation used to evaluate the extract toxicity. The tumor inoculation group was subdivided into six subgroups ($n = 10$): the negative control subgroup (CTL−) with tumor induction treated with phosphate buffered solution (PBS); the positive control subgroup (CTL+) treated with cyclophosphamide at a dose of 25 mg/kg; and the subgroups treated with extracts at doses of 4 mg/kg (EAE4 + Tumor), 20 mg/kg (EAE20 + Tumor), and 100 mg/kg (EAE100 + Tumor). To determine the acute toxicity, the two groups without tumor induction were treated with PBS (Sham) or with the extract at a medium dose of 20 mg/kg (EAE20). All treatments were performed intraperitoneally 24 h after tumor inoculation over fifteen days, and the volume administrated was 100 µL. After the treatment, the animals were randomly selected. A portion was euthanized ($n = 5$) for biological analysis, and another portion ($n = 5$) was used for the quality-of-life/survival test. Euthanasia was performed via the intraperitoneal administration of 120 mg/kg ketamine and 150 mg/kg xylazine (2:1 solution) [58] before complete necropsy.

4.7. Tumor Development Assay

The Ehrlich solid tumor model was applied to evaluate antitumoral activity. The paw volume was determined before and after the injection of Ehrlich tumor cells using a digital caliper at 48 h intervals. The volume was calculated by multiplying the thickness, width, and length measurements of the paw with tumor presented as mm^3. After the treatment performed over fifteen days, the animals of each group were randomly chosen ($n = 5$), euthanized, and the paws with tumors were removed and weighed. The area under the curve was calculated from the kinetics graph obtained from the tumor-inoculated paw development data using the GraphPAd Prism software (Version 7.00, GraphPad Software, San Diego, CA, USA).

4.8. Histopathological Analyses

Immediately after euthanasia, the Ehrlich's tumor tissue (and matched normal tissue from the Sham groups), livers, and kidneys were removed and fixed in 10% neutral buffered formalin. The sample sections were stained with hematoxylin and eosin solution and analyzed by a single researcher with expertise, blinded to the experimental groups. For the tumor samples, the following parameters were analyzed: inflammatory infiltrate distribution (focal, multifocal, diffuse, or peripheral); inflammatory infiltrate intensity (scores: absent 0, light 1, moderate 2, and intense 3); necrosis (scores: absent 0, focal 1, focally extensive or multifocal 2, and diffuse 3); mitotic figures (scores: no mitotic figures 0, occasional mitoses 1, single mitotic figure per 400× field 2, and two mitotic figures per 400× field 3); cellular pleomorphism (scores: monomorphic tumor cells 0, minimal intercellular variation 1, variations in nuclear size and shape 2, and major variations with bizarre nuclei 3); and tumor invasion (scores: well-defined borders with no obvious invasion 0, well-defined borders with minimal invasion of adjacent tissues 1, poorly-defined borders with marker invasion 2, and unrecognizable borders with multiple tumor foci 3) [59].

4.9. Lymphoid Organ Cellularity

To obtain and quantify cells in the popliteal lymph node and spleen, these solid organs were removed and macerated in 1 mL PBS. To obtain bone marrow cells, the femur was removed and perfused with 1 mL of PBS. Next, 90 µL of lymph node, spleen, and bone marrow cell suspensions were added to 10 µL violet crystal, and the cells were counted in a Neubauer chamber with the aid of a common light optical microscope (Zeiss, Oberkochen, Germany) [60].

4.10. Blood Samples

Blood samples were obtained by cardiac puncture. The samples were then centrifuged at 5000 rpm for 10 min. The serum was separated and stored in aliquots at −80 °C until needed. Prior to the assay, the samples were thawed at room temperature [59,60].

4.11. Cytokine Quantification

Blood serum was used for the quantification of interleukin-2 (IL-2), interleukin-4 (IL-4), interleukin-6 (IL-6), interferon-γ (IFN-γ), tumor necrosis factor (TNF-α), interleukin 17A (IL-17A), and interleukin-10 (IL-10) by flow cytometry with FACS Calibur equipment (BD Biosciences, San Jose, CA, USA) using the BD™ Cytometric Bead Array (CBA) cytokine kit Mouse Th1/Th2/Th17 (BD Biosciences, San Jose, CA, USA) following the manufacturer's recommendations.

4.12. Extract Toxicity

For the assessment of acute toxicity, we considered the weight of the animals during the treatment (the animals were weighed daily for 15 days). Weight variation was verified before tumor inoculation until the last day of treatment. We also verified the hepatic parameters of the fungus extract. Blood serum was used to perform the biochemical measurement of glutamic-oxalic transaminase (TGO) and glutamic-pyruvic transaminase (TGP) through colorimetric analyses using Labtest kits, following the manufacturer's guidelines. The data were obtained on a visible spectrum plate reader (Lab. Syftemf Multi Skan EX, Version 1.00, Waltham, Ma, USA). Histopathological analysis of the liver and kidney was performed. The parameters analyzed in the liver were the presence of mitotic figures, caryatia (more than 10% hepatocytes with nuclei twice the size of normal hepatocytes), and the presence or absence of necrosis. Hepatitis was classified as mild (hyperplasia of Küpfer cells and/or occasional microabscesses or mild focal periportal leukocytic infiltration) or moderate (multifocal to diffuse leukocytic infiltration in multiple portal spaces or centrilobular veins). Hepatocellular vacuolar degeneration was also classified as mild (restricted to the periportal and/or centrilobular areas) or moderate (extending to the midzonal areas). In the kidney, the presence of tubular degeneration, defined as the swelling of the cells of the outlined proximal or distal tubules, the necrosis of isolated tubular cells, or the loss of cell vesicles in the tubular lumen (bleeding), was evaluated [61]. The quality of life/survival of the animals was verified for 30 days after treatment, following a quality-of-survival protocol in which some of the animals that suffered damage were assessed using a pain scale. Using this scale, if the animal showed three or more potential signs associated with pain or discomfort, they were kept under surveillance for more than 72 h and then euthanized by excess anesthetic [62].

4.13. In Vitro Cytoxicity against MCF7 Cells

The cell line MCF-7 (ATCC® HTB-22™) was kindly donated by the Laboratório de Tecnologia de Anticorpos Monoclonais, Biomanguinhos, Fiocruz-RJ. The cells were grown in a sterile bottle containing modified Dulbecco's Modified Eagle's Medium (DMEM) (Invitrogen, Carlsbad, CA, USA), supplemented with 10% fetal bovine serum with 2 mM glutamine, 100 U/mL penicillin, and 100 µg/mL streptomycin. Then, the cells were incubated at 37 °C in a humid atmosphere containing 5% CO_2. For the experiments, the monolayer cells were trypsinized with a 0.25% (*w/v*) trypsin solution–0.03% (*w/v*) EDTA. The lyophilized extract was dissolved in DMSO 0.1%, and the solution was filtered through a 0.2 µm pore syringe filter and stored at −20 °C until use. The cultured cells were treated with concentrations between 1000 and 7.8 μg/mL, obtained by serial dilution of the extracts (1:2) for 24 and 48 h. In the viability assay, the cells (5×10^4 cells/mL) were grown in 96-well plates in the presence or absence of the extract for 24 and 48 h. In total, 10 μL of 3-(4,5-dimethylthiazol-2-yl)-2,5-diphenyltetrazolium bromide (MTT) at 5 mg/mL was added to each well. The cells were incubated in a CO_2 chamber for 3 h with protection from light. Then, the medium was removed, and 100 μL of DMSO was added to dissolve the formazan crystals. The absorbance at 570 nm was measured with a Biochrom EZ Read 400 spectrophotometer (Biochrom, Cambridge, UK). The data were then normalized, and the inhibitory concentration for 50% of the cells was calculated from the non-linear regression of the percentage of viable cells versus the log of the concentration of the treatment using the GraphPAd Prism software (Version 7.00, GraphPad Software, San Diego, CA, USA) [63].

4.14. Statistical Analysis

The results were expressed as the mean ± standard error of means (SEM or S.D.). The differences were submitted to an analysis of variance (one-way or two-way ANOVA) followed by a Newman–Keuls test and a Student's t-test using the GraphPad Prism software, version 7.0. To evaluate the survival curve, a Kaplan–Meier curve was used, and the statistical analysis was performed by a Log-Rank test. The significance level for rejection of the null hypothesis was 5% ($p < 0.05$).

5. Conclusions

Overall, the present results indicate that the *P. purpurogenum* extract has potent in vivo anticancer activity against Ehrlich's solid tumor, suggesting the presence of immunomodulatory mechanisms. The chemical components present in the extract may serve as lead compounds for the development of new compounds with antitumor effect and immune response modulators. The extract was well-tolerated and improved animal survival compared to cyclophosphamide, suggesting a favorable toxicity profile and potential applications in combination therapies. Further preclinical studies are required to clarify the potential uses of *P. purpurogenum* and better understand the production of bioactive metabolites in fungi for biotechnological applications.

Supplementary Materials: The following are available online at http://www.mdpi.com/1660-3397/18/11/541/s1, Table S1: Cytokine quantification of Swiss mice inoculated with Ehrlich tumor and treated with *Penicillium purpurogenum*.

Author Contributions: Conceptualization, A.M.T., G.F.d.B.B., R.M.G.d.C., M.d.D.S.B.N.; data curation, A.M.T., A.P.S.A.-S., M.d.D.S.B.N.; formal analysis, A.M.T., L.P.P.P., S.J.A.G., A.L.B., G.X.S., F.R.F.d.N., G.F.d.B.B., C.J.M.-T., R.M.G.d.C., M.A.C.N.d.S., K.d.S.C., F.A.-S., A.P.S.A.-S., M.d.D.S.B.N.; funding acquisition, M.d.D.S.B.N. and K.d.S.C.; investigation, F.R.F.d.N. and K.d.S.C.; methodology, A.M.T., L.P.P.P., S.J.A.G., A.L.B., G.X.S., F.R.F.d.N., G.F.d.B.B., C.J.M.-T., K.d.S.C., F.A.-S., A.P.S.A.-S. and M.d.D.S.B.N.; supervision, A.P.S.A.-S., G.F.d.B.B., C.J.M.-T., K.d.S.C., F.A.-S. and M.d.D.S.B.N.; writing—original draft, A.M.T. and F.A.-S.; writing—review and editing, A.M.T., L.P.P.P., S.J.A.G., A.L.B., G.X.S., F.R.F.d.N., G.F.d.B.B., C.J.M.-T., R.M.G.d.C., M.A.C.N.d.S., K.d.S.C., F.A.-S., A.P.S.A.-S., M.d.D.S.B.N. All authors have read and agreed to the published version of the manuscript.

Funding: This research was funded by the Coordenação de Aperfeiçoamento de Pessoal de Nível Superior, Brazil (CAPES) (Finance Code 001) and the Foundation for the Support of Research and Scientific and Technological Development of Maranhão (FAPEMA). Dr. Fernando Almeida-Souza is a postdoctoral researcher fellow of CAPES, grant number 88887.363006/2019-00.

Acknowledgments: We would like to thank Fundação Oswaldo Cruz for providing the in vitro experimental procedures. We would also like to thank the Foundation for the Support of Research and Scientific and Technological Development of Maranhão (FAPEMA) for the financial support.

Conflicts of Interest: The authors declare no conflict of interest.

References

1. Teixeira, T.R.; Santos, G.S.D.; Armstrong, L.; Colepicolo, P.; Debonsi, H.M. Antitumor Potential of Seaweed Derived-Endophytic Fungi. *Antibiotics* **2019**, *8*, 205. [CrossRef] [PubMed]

2. Pejin, B.; Jovanović, K.K.; Mojović, M.; Savić, A.G. New and highly potent antitumor natural products from marine-derived fungi: Covering the period from 2003 to 2012. *Curr. Top. Med. Chem.* **2013**, *13*, 2745–2766. [CrossRef] [PubMed]
3. Rateb, M.E.; Ebel, R. Secondary metabolites of fungi from marine habitats. *Nat. Prod. Rep.* **2011**, *28*, 290–344. [CrossRef] [PubMed]
4. Bhatnagar, I.; Kim, S.K. Immense essence of excellence: Marine microbial bioactive compounds. *Mar. Drugs* **2010**, *8*, 2673–2701. [CrossRef] [PubMed]
5. Newman, D.J.; Cragg, G.M. Marine-sourced anti-cancer and cancer pain control agents in clinical and late preclinical development. *Mar. Drugs* **2014**, *12*, 255–278. [CrossRef] [PubMed]
6. Cafêu, M.C.; Silva, G.H.; Teles, H.L.; Bolzani, V.S.; Araújo, A.R.; Young, M.C.M.; Pfenning, L.H. Substâncias antifúngicas de *Xylaria* sp., um fungo endofítico isolado de *Palicourea marcgravii* (Rubiaceae). *Quim Nov.* **2005**, *28*, 991–995. [CrossRef]
7. Frisvad, J.C.; Smedsgaard, J.; Larsen, T.; Samson, R.A. Mycotoxins, drugs and other extrolites produced by species in *Penicillium* subgenus *Penicillium*. *Stud. Mycol.* **2004**, *49*, 201–241.
8. Baker, C.J.O.; Shaban-Nejad, A.; Su, X.; Haarslev, V.; Butler, G. Semantic Web Infrastructure for Fungal Enzyme Biotechnologists. *J. Web Semant.* **2006**, *4*, 168–180. [CrossRef]
9. Samson, R.A. *Food and Indoor Fungi*; Samson, R.A., Ed.; CBS-KNAW Fungal Biodiversity Centre: Utrecht, The Netherlands, 2010; Volume 2, 390p.
10. Chai, Y.J.; Cui, C.B.; Li, C.W.; Wu, C.J.; Tian, C.K.; Hua, W. Activation of the dormant secondary metabolite production by introducing gentamicin-resistance in a marine-derived *P. purpurogenum* G59. *Mar. Drugs* **2012**, *10*, 559–582. [CrossRef]
11. Wu, C.J.; Yi, L.; Cui, C.B.; Li, C.W.; Wang, N.; Han, X. Activation of the silent secondary metabolite production by introducing neomycin-resistance in a marine-derived *Penicillium purpurogenum* G59. *Mar. Drugs* **2015**, *13*, 2465–2487. [CrossRef]
12. Cutrim, M.V.J.; Ferreira, F.S.; dos Santos, A.K.D.; Cavalcanti, L.F.; de Oliveira Araújo, B.; Gomes de Azevedo-Cutrim, A.C.; Lima Oliveira, A.L. Trophic state of an urban coastal lagoon (northern Brazil), seasonal variation of the phytoplankton community and environmental variables. *Estuar. Coast. Shelf Sci.* **2019**, *217*, 98–109. [CrossRef]
13. Santos, J.M.O.; Moreira-Pais, A.; Neto, T.; Peixoto da Silva, S.; Oliveira, P.A.; Ferreira, R.; Mendes, J.; Bastos, M.M.S.M.; Lopes, C.; Casaca, F.; et al. Dimethylaminoparthenolide reduces the incidence of dysplasia and ameliorates a wasting syndrome in HPV16-transgenic mice. *Drug Dev. Res.* **2019**, *80*, 824–830. [CrossRef] [PubMed]
14. Medeiros-Fonseca, B.; Mestre, V.F.; Colaço, B.; Pires, M.J.; Martins, T.; Gil da Costa, R.M.; Neuparth, M.J.; Medeiros, R.; Moutinho, M.S.S.; Dias, M.I.; et al. *Laurus nobilis* (laurel) aqueous leaf extract's toxicological and anti-tumor activities in HPV16-transgenic mice. *Food Funct.* **2018**, *9*, 4419–4428. [CrossRef] [PubMed]
15. Santos, S.; Ferreira, T.; Almeida, J.; Pires, M.J.; Colaço, A.; Lemos, S.; Gil da Costa, R.M.; Medeiros, R.; Bastos, M.M.S.M.; Neuparth, M.J.; et al. Dietary supplementation with the red seaweed *Porphyra umbilicalis* protects against DNA damage and pre-malignant dysplastic skin lesions in HPV-transgenic mice. *Mar. Drugs* **2019**, *17*, 615. [CrossRef] [PubMed]
16. Bray, F.; Ferlay, J.; Soerjomataram, I.; Siegel, R.L.; Torre, L.A.; Jemal, A. Global cancer statistics 2018: GLOBOCAN estimates of incidence and mortality worldwide for 36 cancers in 185 coutries. *CA Cancer J. Clin.* **2018**, *68*, 394–424. [CrossRef]
17. Faustino-Rocha, A.I.; Silva, A.; Gabriel, J.; Gil da Costa, R.; Gama, A.; Ferreira, R.; Oliveira, P.A.; Ginja, M. Ultrasonographic, thermographic and histologic evaluation of MNU-induced mammary tumors in female Sprague-Dawley rats. *Biomed. Pharmacother.* **2013**, *67*, 771–776. [CrossRef]
18. Faustino-Rocha, A.I.; Colaço, B.; Oliveira, P.A. Experimental mammarycarcinogenesis—Rat models. *Life Sci.* **2017**, *173*, 116–134.
19. Segura, J.A.; Barbero, L.G.; Márquez, J. Ehrlich ascites tumour unbalances splenic cell populations and reduces responsiveness of T cells to *Staphylococcus aureus* enterotoxin B stimulation. *Immunol. Lett.* **2000**, *74*, 111–115. [CrossRef]
20. Ali, A.D.; Badr El-Din, K.N.; Abou-El-Magd, F.R. Antioxidant and hepatoprotective activities of grape seeds and skin against Ehrlich solid tumor induced oxidative stress in mice. *Egypt. J. Basic Appl. Sci.* **2015**, *2*, 98–109. [CrossRef]

21. Geris, R.; Simpson, T.J. Meroterpenoids produced by fungi. *Nat. Prod. Rep.* **2009**, *26*, 1063–1094. [CrossRef]
22. Fang, S.M.; Cui, C.B.; Li, C.W.; Wu, C.J.; Zhang, Z.J.; Li, L.; Huang, X.J.; Ye, W.C. Purpurogemutantin and purpurogemutantidin, new drimenyl cyclohexenone derivatives produced by a mutant obtained by diethyl sulfate mutagenesis of a marine-derived *Penicillium purpurogenum* G59. *Mar. Drugs* **2012**, *10*, 1266–1287. [CrossRef] [PubMed]
23. Natori, S.; Sakaki, S.; Kurata, H.; Udagawa, S.I.; Ichinoe, M. Production of rubratoxin B by *Penicillium purpurogenum* Stoll. *Appl Microbiol.* **1970**, *19*, 613–617. [CrossRef]
24. Li, S.S.; Li, J.; Sun, J.; Guo, R.; Yu, L.Z.; Zhao, Y.F.; Zhu, Z.X.; Tu, P.F. Berkeleyacetal C, a meroterpenoid isolated from the fungus *Penicillium purpurogenum* MHZ 111, exerts anti-inflammatory effects via inhibiting NF-κB, ERK1/2 and IRF3 signaling pathways. *Eur. J. Pharmacol.* **2017**, *814*, 283–293. [CrossRef] [PubMed]
25. Tang, M.C.; Cui, X.; He, X.; Ding, Z.; Zhu, T.; Tang, Y.; Li, D. Late-stage terpene cyclization by an integral membrane cyclase in the biosynthesis of isoprenoid epoxycyclohexenone natural products. *Org. Lett.* **2017**, *19*, 5376–5379. [CrossRef] [PubMed]
26. He, W.J.; Zhou, X.J.; Qin, X.C.; Mai, Y.X.; Lin, X.P.; Liao, S.R.; Yang, B.; Zhang, T.; Tu, Z.C.; Wang, J.F.; et al. Quinone/hydroquinone meroterpenoids with antitubercular and cytotoxic activities produced by the sponge-derived fungus *Gliomastix* sp. ZSDS1-F7. *Nat. Prod. Res.* **2017**, *31*, 604–609. [CrossRef] [PubMed]
27. Stierle, D.B.; Stierle, A.A.; Patacini, B. The berkeleyacetals, three meroterpenes from a deep water acid mine waste *Penicillium*. *J. Nat. Prod.* **2007**, *70*, 1820–1823. [CrossRef] [PubMed]
28. Etoh, T.; Kin, Y.P.; Tanaka, H.; Hayashi, M. Anti-inflammatory effect of berkeleyacetal C through the inhibition of interleukin-1 receptor-associated kinase-4 activity. *Eur. J. Pharmacol.* **2013**, *698*, 435–443. [CrossRef]
29. Nagashima, H.; Goto, T. Calcium channel blockers verapamil and diltiazem impaired rubratoxin B-caused toxicity in HL60 cells. *Toxicol. Lett.* **2000**, *118*, 47–51. [CrossRef]
30. Wang, T.; Zhang, Y.; Wang, Y.; Pei, Y. Anti-tumor effects of Rubratoxin B on cell toxicity, inhibition of cell proliferation, cytotoxic activity and matrix metalloproteinase-2,9. *Toxicol. In Vitro* **2007**, *21*, 646–650. [CrossRef]
31. Nagashima, H. Rubratoxin-B-induced secretion of chemokine ligands of cysteine–cysteine motif chemokine receptor 5 (CCR5) and its dependence on heat shock protein 90 in HL60 cells. *Environm. Toxicol. Pharmacol.* **2015**, *40*, 997–1000. [CrossRef]
32. Qin, X.J.; Yu, Q.; Yan, H.; Khan, A.; Feng, M.Y.; Li, P.P.; Hao, X.J.; An, L.K.; Liu, H.Y. Meroterpenoids with Antitumor Activities from Guava (*Psidium guajava*). *J. Agric. Food Chem.* **2017**, *65*, 4993–4999. [CrossRef]
33. Sharma, S.H.; Thulasingam, S.; Nagarajan, S. Terpenoids as anti-colon cancer agents—A comprehensive review on its mechanistic perspectives. *Eur. J. Pharmacol.* **2017**, *795*, 169–178. [CrossRef]
34. Qin, F.Y.; Yan, Y.M.; Tu, Z.C.; Cheng, Y.X. Meroterpenoid dimers from *Ganoderma cochlear* and their cytotoxic and COX-2 inhibitory activities. *Fitoterapia* **2018**, *129*, 167–172. [CrossRef] [PubMed]
35. Silva, I.P.; Brissow, E.; Kellner Filho, L.C.; Senabio, J.; Siqueira, K.A.; Vandresen Filho, S.; Damasceno, J.L.; Mendes, S.A.; Tavares, D.C.; Magalhaes, L.G.; et al. Bioactive compounds of *Aspergillus terreus*—F7, an endophytic fungus from *Hyptis suaveolens* (L.) Poit. *World J. Microbiol. Biotechnol.* **2017**, *33*, 62. [CrossRef] [PubMed]
36. Santos, O.J.; Sauaia Filho, E.N.; Nascimento, F.R.F.; Silva Júnior, F.C.; Fialho, E.D.S.; Santos, R.H.P.; Santos, R.A.P.; Bogea Serra, I.C.P. Use of raw *Euphorbia tirucalli* extract for inhibition of ascitic Ehrlich tumor. *Rev. Col. Bras. Cir.* **2016**, *43*, 18–21. [CrossRef]
37. Bianchi-Frias, D.; Damodarasamy, M.; Hernandez, S.A.; Gil da Costa, R.M.; Vakar-Lopez, F.; Coleman, I.; Reed, M.J.; Nelson, P.S. The aged microenvironment influences the tumorigenic potential of malignant prostate epithelial cells. *Mol. Cancer Res.* **2019**, *17*, 321–331. [CrossRef] [PubMed]
38. Da Costa, R.M.G.; Bastos, M.M.S.M.; Medeiros, R.; Oliveira, P.A. The NFkB signalling pathway in papillomavirus-induced lesions: Friend or foe? *Anticancer Res.* **2016**, *36*, 2073–2083.
39. Gupta, I.; Burney, I.; Al-Moundhri, M.S.; Tamimi, Y. Molecular genetics complexity impeding research progress in breast and ovarian cancers. *Mol. Clin. Onc.* **2017**, *7*, 3–14. [CrossRef]
40. Zbakh, H.; Zubía, E.; de Los Reyes, C.; Calderón-Montaño, J.M.; López-Lázaro, M.; Motilva, V. Meroterpenoids from the Brown Alga *Cystoseira usneoides* as Potential Anti-Inflammatory and Lung Anticancer Agents. *Mar. Drugs* **2020**, *18*, 207. [CrossRef]

41. Darsih, C.; Prachyawarakorn, V.; Wiyakrutta, S.; Mahidol, C.; Ruchirawat, S.; Kittakoop, P. Cytotoxic metabolites from the endophytic fungus *Penicillium chermesinum*: Discovery of a cysteine-targeted Michael acceptor as a pharmacophore for fragment-based drug discovery, bioconjugation and click reactions. *RSC Adv.* **2015**, *5*, 70595–70603. [CrossRef]
42. Wan, H.; Li, J.; Zhang, K.; Zou, X.; Ge, L.; Zhu, F.; Zhou, H.; Gong, M.; Wang, T.; Chen, D.; et al. A new meroterpenoid functions as an anti-tumor agent in hepatoma cells by downregulating mTOR activation and inhibiting EMT. *Sci. Rep.* **2018**, *8*, 13152. [CrossRef]
43. McCoy, M.K.; Ruhn, K.A.; Blesch, A.; Tansey, M.G. TNF: A Key Neuroinflammatory Mediator of Neurotoxicity and Neurodegeneration in Models of Parkinson's Disease. *Adv. Exp. Med. Biol.* **2011**, *691*, 539–540.
44. Yoon, W.J.; Ham, Y.M.; Kim, S.S.; Yoo, B.S.; Moon, J.Y.; Baik, J.S.; Lee, N.H.; Hyun, C.G. Supressão de citocinas pró-inflamatórias, iNOS e expressão de COX-2 por algas marrons *Sargassum micracanthum* em macrófagos RAW264.7. *Eurásia J. Biosci.* **2009**, *3*, 130–143. [CrossRef]
45. Schefer, F.A.; Ricardo, S.; Blind, C.L.Z.; de Oliveira Souza, B.L.; Filippin, M.F.B.; Weber, B.M.; Orofino, K.M.R. Antitumoral activity of sesquiterpene lactone diacethylpiptocarphol in mice. *J. Ethnopharmacol.* **2017**, *198*, 262–267. [CrossRef] [PubMed]
46. Calixto-Campos, C.; Corrêa, M.P.; Carvalho, T.T.; Zarpelon, A.C.; Hohmann, M.S.N.; Rossaneis, A.C.; Ceolho-Silva, L.; Pavanelli, W.R.; Pinge-Filho, P.; Crespigio, J.; et al. Quercetin reduces Ehrlich tumor-induced cancer pain in mice. *Anal. Cell. Pathol.* **2015**, *2015*, 285708. [CrossRef]
47. Aldubayan, M.A.; Elgharabawy, R.M.; Ahmed, A.S.; Tousson, E. Antineoplastic Activity and Curative Role of Avenanthramides against the Growth of Ehrlich Solid Tumors in Mice. *Oxid. Med. Cell. Longev.* **2019**. [CrossRef]
48. Harun, A.; Vidyadaran, S.; Meng, L.S.; Cole, A.L.J.; Ramasamy, K. Malaysian endophytic fungal extracts-induced anti-inflammation in lipopolysaccharide-activated BV-2 microglia is associated with attenuation of NO production and, IL-6 and TNF-α expression. *BMC Compl. Alt. Med.* **2015**, *15*, 166. [CrossRef] [PubMed]
49. Murphy, R.A.; Mourtzakis, M.; Chu, Q.S.C.; Baracos, V.E.; Reiman, T.; Mazurak, V.C. Nutritional intervention with fish oil provides a benefit over standard of care for weight and skeletal muscle mass in patients with nonsmall cell lung cancer receiving chemotherapy. *Cancer* **2011**, *117*, 1775–1782. [CrossRef] [PubMed]
50. Lordick, F.; Hacker, U. Gewichtsverlust aus Onkologischer Sicht. *Dtsch. Med. Wochenschr* **2016**, *141*, 247–252. [CrossRef]
51. Lau, S.K.M.; Iyengar, P. Implications of weight loss for cancer patients receiving radiotherapy. *Curr. Opin. Support. Palliat. Care* **2017**, *11*, 261–265. [CrossRef] [PubMed]
52. Iyengar, N.M.; Gucalp, A.; Dannenberg, A.J.; Hudis, C.A. Obesity and Cancer Mechanisms: Tumor Microenvironment and Inflammation. *J. Clin. Oncol.* **2016**, *34*, 4270–4276. [CrossRef]
53. Hess, L.M.; Barakat, R.; Tian, C.; Ozols, R.F.; Alberts, D.S. Weight change during chemotherapy as a potential prognostic factor for stage III epithelial ovarian carcinoma: A Gynecologic Oncology Group study. *Gynecol. Oncol.* **2007**, *107*, 260–265. [CrossRef]
54. Moreira-Pais, A.; Ferreira, R.; da Costa, R.M.G. Platinum-induced muscle wasting in cancer chemotherapy: Mechanisms and potential targets for therapeutic intervention. *Life Sci.* **2018**, *208*, 1–9. [CrossRef]
55. Peixoto da Silva, S.; Santos, J.M.O.; Costa e Silva, M.P.; Gil da Costa, R.M.; Medeiros, R. Cancer cachexia and its pathophysiology: Links with sarcopenia, anorexia and asthenia. *J. Cachexia Sarcopenia Muscle* **2020**, *11*, 619–635. [CrossRef]
56. Dagli, M.L.Z.; Guerra, J.L.; Saldiva, P.H.N. An experimental study on the lymphatic dissemination of the solid Ehrlich tumor in mice. *Braz. J. Vet. Res. An. Sci.* **1992**, *29*, 97–103. [CrossRef]
57. Fortes, T.S.; Fialho, S.E.M.; Reis, A.S.; Assunção, A.K.M.; Azevedo, A.P.S.; Barroqueiro, E.S.B.; Guerra, R.N.M.; Nascimento, F.R.F. Desenvolvimento do tumor de Ehrlich em camundongos após tratamento in vitro com mesocarpo de babaçu Mart. *Rev. Ciências Saúde* **2009**, *11*, 101–105.
58. Machado, J.L.; Assunção, A.K.; da Silva, M.C.; Dos Reis, A.S.; Costa, G.C.; de Sousa Arruda, D.; Rocha, B.A.; de Oliveira Lima Leite Vaz, M.M.; de Andrade Paes, A.M.; Guerra, R.N.M.; et al. Brazilian Green Propolis: Anti-Inflammatory Property by an Immunomodulatory Activity. *Evid. Based Complement. Alternat. Med.* **2012**, *2012*, 157652. [CrossRef]

59. Nascimento, F.R.; Cruz, G.V.; Pereira, P.V.; Maciel, M.C.; Silva, L.A.; Azevedo, A.P.S.; Barroqueiro, E.S.B.; Guerra, R.N.M. Ascitic and solid Ehrlich tumor inhibition by *Chenopodium ambrosioides* L. treatment. *Life Sci.* **2006**, *78*, 2650–2653. [CrossRef]
60. Fialho, S.E.M.; Maciel, M.C.G.; Silva, A.C.B.; Reis, A.A.; Assuncao, A.K.M.; Fortes, T.S.; Silva, L.A.; Guerra, R.N.M.; Kwasniewski, F.H.; Nascimento, F.R.F. Immune cells recruitment and activation by *Tityus serrulatus* scorpion venom. *Toxicon* **2011**, *1*, 1–6. [CrossRef]
61. Bancroft, J.D.; Cook, H.C. *Manual of Histological Techniques and Their Diagnostic Application*; Churchill Livingstone: Edinburgh, UK, 1994; Volume 2, 457p.
62. Conselho Nacional de Controle de Experimentação Animal. Available online: http://www.sbcal.org.br/conteudo/view?ID_CONTEUDO=41 (accessed on 18 August 2020).
63. Teles, A.M.; Rosa, T.D.D.S.; Mouchrek, A.N.; Abreu-Silva, A.L.; Calabrese, K.D.S.; Almeida-Souza, F. *Cinnamomum zeylanicum*, *Origanum vulgare*, and *Curcuma longa* Essential Oils: Chemical Composition, Antimicrobial and Antileishmanial Activity. *Evid. Based Complement. Alternat. Med.* **2019**. [CrossRef]

Publisher's Note: MDPI stays neutral with regard to jurisdictional claims in published maps and institutional affiliations.

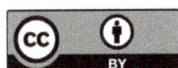

© 2020 by the authors. Licensee MDPI, Basel, Switzerland. This article is an open access article distributed under the terms and conditions of the Creative Commons Attribution (CC BY) license (http://creativecommons.org/licenses/by/4.0/).

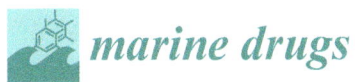

Article

Cytotoxic Secondary Metabolites Isolated from the Marine Alga-Associated Fungus *Penicillium chrysogenum* LD-201810

Lin-Lin Jiang [1,2,3,†], Jin-Xiu Tang [1,†], Yong-Heng Bo [2], You-Zhi Li [2], Tao Feng [2], Hong-Wei Zhu [1,2,3], Xin Yu [1,2,3], Xing-Xiao Zhang [1,3,*], Jian-Long Zhang [1,2,3,*] and Weiyi Wang [4,*]

1. School of Life Sciences, Ludong University, Yantai 264025, China; linlinjiang1986@163.com (L.-L.J.); TJX19950209@163.com (J.-X.T.); hngwzhu@outlook.com (H.-W.Z.); yuxinzghn@163.com (X.Y.)
2. Shandong Provincial Key Laboratory of Quality Safty Monitoring and Risk Assessment for Animal Products, Ji'nan 250022, China; yongheng1980@163.com (Y.-H.B.); liyouzhi2009@126.com (Y.-Z.L.); fengtaojn2019@163.com (T.F.)
3. Yantai Key Laboratory of Animal Pathogenetic Microbiology and Immunology, Yantai 264025, China
4. Key Laboratory of Marine Biogenetic Resources, Third Institute of Oceanography, Ministry of Natural Resources, Xiamen 361005, China
* Correspondence: zhangxingxiao@ldu.edu.cn (X.-X.Z.); zhangjianlong@ldu.edu.cn (J.-L.Z.); wywang@tio.org.cn (W.W.); Tel.: +86-535-6673485 (X.-X.Z.); +86-535-6681162 (J.-L.Z.); +86-592-219-5518 (W.W.)
† These authors contributed equally to this work.

Received: 6 May 2020; Accepted: 20 May 2020; Published: 22 May 2020

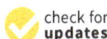

Abstract: A new pentaketide derivative, penilactonol A (**1**), and two new hydroxyphenylacetic acid derivatives, (2′R)-stachyline B (**2**) and (2′R)-westerdijkin A (**3**), together with five known metabolites, bisabolane-type sesquiterpenoids **4**–**6** and meroterpenoids **7** and **8**, were isolated from the solid culture of a marine alga-associated fungus *Penicillium chrysogenum* LD-201810. Their structures were elucidated based on extensive spectroscopic analyses, including 1D/2D NMR and high resolution electrospray ionization mass spectra (HRESIMS). The absolute configurations of the stereogenic carbons in **1** were determined by the $(Mo_2(OAc)_4)$-induced circular dichroism (CD) and comparison of the calculated and experimental electronic circular dichroism (ECD) spectra, while the absolute configuration of the stereogenic carbon in **2** was established using single-crystal X-ray diffraction analysis. Compounds **2** and **3** adapt the 2′R-configuration as compared to known hydroxyphenylacetic acid-derived and O-prenylated natural products. The cytotoxicity of **1**–**8** against human carcinoma cell lines (A549, BT-549, HeLa, HepG2, MCF-7, and THP-1) was evaluated. Compound **3** exhibited cytotoxicity to the HepG2 cell line with an IC_{50} value of 22.0 µM. Furthermore, **5** showed considerable activities against A549 and THP-1 cell lines with IC_{50} values of 21.2 and 18.2 µM, respectively.

Keywords: alga; marine-derived fungus; *Penicillium chrysogenum*; polyketide; hydroxyphenylacetic acid; cytotoxicity

1. Introduction

Microorganisms belonging to marine ecosystems are diverse both taxonomically and biologically [1–3]. These microorganisms developed unique metabolic pathways to overcome the extreme temperature, nutrient scarcity, high salinity, and ultraviolet radiation [4,5]. As one of the most prevalent biocenoses in marine ecosystems, marine-derived filamentous fungi represent an extraordinarily diverse biotic population. They distribute in almost all marine habitats, including marine plants, marine invertebrates and vertebrates, and marine sediments [2,6–8]. Among them, marine alga-associated fungi have drawn considerable attention because they can synthesize valuable secondary metabolites with potential pharmacological properties [6,7].

As part of our ongoing search for bioactive secondary metabolites from marine-derived fungi, the fungus *Penicillium chrysogenum* LD-201810 was isolated from the marine red alga *Grateloupia turuturu*. Subsequent chemical investigation of an EtOAc extract of the culture of this fungal strain led to the isolation of a new pentaketide derivative, penilactonol A (**1**), and two previously unreported hydroxyphenylacetic acid derivatives, (2′R)-stachyline B (**2**) and (2′R)-westerdijkin A (**3**), together with five known metabolites, bisabolane-type sesquiterpenoids **4–6** and meroterpenoids **7** and **8** (Figure 1). The structures and absolute configurations of the stereogenic carbons were unequivocally determined using extensive spectroscopic analyses, (Mo$_2$(OAc)$_4$)-induced circular dichroism (ICD), time-dependent density-functional theory (TDDFT) electronic circular dichroism (ECD) calculations, and single-crystal X-ray diffraction analyses. To the best of our knowledge, **2** and **3** adapt the 2′R-configuration as compared to known hydroxyphenylacetic acid-derived and O-prenylated natural products. Details of the isolation, structure elucidation, and biological activities of the isolated compounds are presented herein.

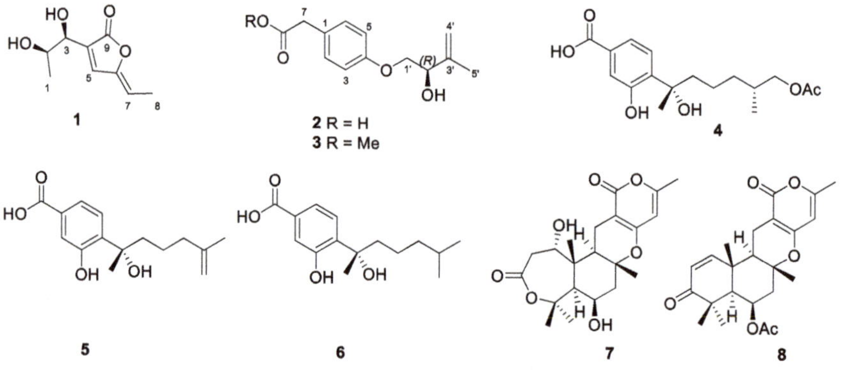

Figure 1. Chemical structures of **1–8**.

2. Results and Discussion

2.1. Structure Elucidation

Compound **1** was obtained as a colorless oil with a molecular formula of C$_9$H$_{12}$O$_4$, established by (+)-HRESIMS *m/z* 185.0803 [M + H]$^+$, corresponding to four degrees of unsaturation. The ^{1}H NMR spectrum (Table 1) showed two methyl doublets at δ$_H$ 1.39 (d, *J* = 6.6 Hz, H$_3$-1) and 1.88 (d, *J* = 7.4 Hz, H$_3$-8), one doublet at δ$_H$ 4.47 (d, *J* = 5.4 Hz, H-3), and a multiplet at δ$_H$ 4.36 (m, H-2), and one singlet at δ$_H$ 7.67 (s, H-5) and one quartet at δ$_H$ 5.60 (q, *J* = 7.4 Hz, H-7) attributable to two olefinic protons. The ^{13}C NMR spectrum, along with distortionless enhancement by polarization transfer (DEPT) and HSQC data, demonstrated the presence of two methyls at δ$_C$ 19.7 (C-1) and 11.7 (C-8); four methines, including two oxygenated sp^3 at δ$_C$ 59.3 (C-2) and 69.1 (C-3) and two sp^2 at δ$_C$ 140.4 (C-5) and 112.2 (C-7); and three quaternary carbons, including two sp^2 carbons at δ$_C$ 132.1 (C-4) and 148.6 (C-6) and one carbonyl carbon at δ$_C$ 168.4 (C-9). The COSY correlations (Figure 2A) from H$_3$-1 to H-2 and from H-2 to H-3, combined with the downfield chemical shifts of C-2 (δ$_C$ 59.3) and C-3 (δ$_C$ 69.1), revealed a presence of a *vic*-diols moiety. The key HMBC correlations from H-2 to C-4, H-3 to C-5, H-5 to C-3 and C-7, H$_3$-8 to C-6, and the COSY correlation of H-7 and H$_3$-8 extended the fragment to C-4–C-8. The HMBC correlations from H-3 and H-5 to C-9 located the carbonyl carbon C-9 linked to C-4. To satisfy the molecular formula and a degree of unsaturation, C-9 should connect to C-6 by an ester linkage to form the α,β-unsaturated γ-lactone ring. Hence, the planar structure of **1** was assigned. The key NOE correlation (Supplementary Materials, Figure S6) between H-5 and H-7 assigned the *Z* configuration of the double bond between C-6 and C-7. According to the literature, the coupling constant between the H-2 and H-3 is larger than 4 Hz in *erythro* isomers but smaller than 2 Hz in *threo* isomers in the α,β-unsaturated γ-lactones [9]. Therefore, the coupling constant of 5.4 Hz between H-2 and H-3 indicated the *erythro* relative configuration of 2,3-diol in **1** [10]. The absolute configuration of the *erythro*-2,3-diol in **1** was determined by the dimolybdenum-induced circular dichroism (ICD) analysis [11]. In the ICD analyses using Snatzke's method with dimolybdenum tetraacetate [Mo$_2$(OAc)$_4$] in MeOH, the Mo$_2$-complex of **1** gave a negative CD Cotton effect near 400 nm (Figure 2B). Using Snatzke's helicity rule [11–13], the sign of the O–C–C–O torsional angle in the favored conformation of the chiral Mo$_2$-complex determines the sign of the CD Cotton effect near 400 nm, and the conformation with an antiperiplanar orientation of the OH and the methyl group, O–C–C–CH$_3$, is a favored conformation of the Mo$_2$-complex in the *erythro*-diols closely resembling **1**, as shown in Figure 2B. Furthermore, the TDDFT method was employed at the CAM-B3LYP-SCRF/def2-SVP//B3LYP/6-31G(d) level to obtain the calculated ECD spectra of **1**. The experimental ECD spectrum of **1** was in good agreement with that of the calculated for (2*R*, 3*S*)-**1** at this level (Figure 3). Hence, the absolute configurations at C-2 and C-3 in **1** were finally determined to be 2*R*, 3*S*, respectively.

Table 1. ^{1}H (500 MHz) and ^{13}C NMR (125 MHz) data of compounds **1-3** in DMSO-d_6.

	Compound 1			Compound 2		Compound 3	
No.	δ$_H$ (Mult, *J* in Hz)	δ$_C$, Type	No.	δ$_H$ (Mult, *J* in Hz)	δ$_C$, Type	δ$_H$ (Mult, *J* in Hz)	δ$_C$, Type
1	1.39 (d, 6.6)	19.7, CH$_3$	1		127.4, C		126.3, C
2	4.36 (m)	59.3, CH	2/6	7.14 (d, 8.3)	130.8, CH	7.15 (d, 8.6)	130.4, CH
3	4.47 (d, 5.4)	69.1, CH	3/5	6.86 (d, 8.3)	114.8, CH	6.88 (d, 8.6)	114.5, CH
4		132.1, C	4		157.8, C		157.6, C
5	7.67 (s)	140.4, CH	7	3.46 (br s)	40.2, CH$_2$	3.58 (d, 5.3)	39.3, CH$_2$
6		148.6, C	8		173.4, C		171.9, C
7	5.60 (q, 7.4)	112.2, CH	1'	3.92 (dd, 9.9, 4.4) 3.84 (m)	71.3, CH$_2$	3.93 (dd, 9.9, 4.5) 3.86 (dd, 9.9, 6.9)	70.9, CH$_2$
8	1.88 (d, 7.4)	11.7, CH$_3$	2'	4.24 (t, 5.3)	72.7, CH	4.25 (m)	72.3, CH
9		168.4, C	3'		145.8, C		145.4, C
			4'	4.86 (br s) 5.02 (br s)	112.1, CH$_2$	4.87 (br s) 5.03 (br s)	111.7, CH$_2$
			5'	1.72 (s)	18.9, CH$_3$	1.73 (s)	18.5, CH$_3$
			8-OMe			3.58 (s)	51.6, CH$_3$
			2'-OH			5.23 (br s)	

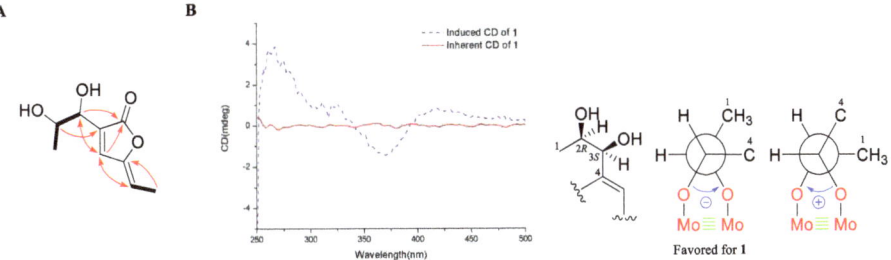

Figure 2. (**A**) COSY and key HMBC correlations in **1**; (**B**) induced circular dichroism (ICD) spectra from the Mo$_2$-complex and inherent CD of **1**.

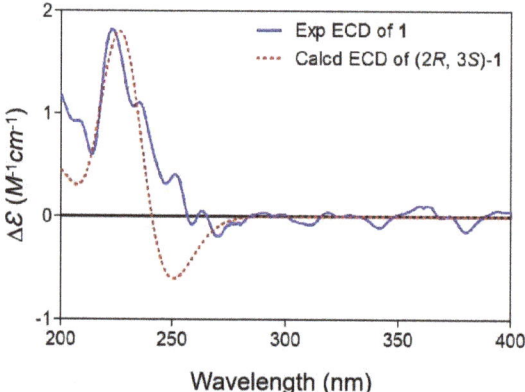

Figure 3. Experimental electronic circular dichroism (ECD) spectrum of **1** (blue solid); calculated ECD spectrum of (2*R*, 3*S*)-**1** (UV correction = −19 nm, red dash) at the CAM-B3LYP-SCRF/def2-SVP//B3LYP/6-31G(d) level of theory in MeOH with IEFPCM solvent model (Polarized Continuum Model using the Intergral Equation Formalism).

Compound **2** was acquired as colorless needles. The molecular formula $C_{13}H_{16}O_4$ was established on the basis of (+)-HRESIMS data at *m/z* 254.1389 ([M + NH$_4$]$^+$) and 259.0942 ([M + Na]$^+$). The ^{1}H and ^{13}C NMR data (Table 1), in combination with the HSQC spectrum, displayed signals that were attributed to one methyl at δ_H 1.72 (s, H-5′) and δ_C 18.9 (C-5′); three methylenes, including one oxygenated sp^3 at δ_H 3.92 (dd, *J* = 9.9, 4.4 Hz, H-1′α), 3.84 (m, H-1′β), and δ_C 71.3 (C-1′), one sp^3 at δ_H 3.46 (br s, H-7) and δ_C 40.2 (C-7), and one exocyclic sp^2 at δ_H 4.86 (br s, H-4′α), 5.02 (br s, H-4′β) and δ_C 112.1 (C-4′); five methines, including four sp^2 at δ_H 7.14 (d, *J* = 8.3 Hz, H-2/6), 6.86 (d, *J* = 8.4 Hz, H-3/5), δ_C 130.8 (C-2/6), 114.8 (C-3/5), and one sp^3 at δ_H 4.24 (t, *J* = 5.3 Hz, H-2′) and δ_C 72.7 (C-2′); three non-protonated sp^2 carbons at δ_C 127.4 (C-1), 157.8 (C-4), 145.8 (C-3′), and one carbonyl carbon at δ_C 173.4 (C-8). The above-mentioned spectroscopic features as well as the COSY correlation between H-2/6 and H-3/5 (Figure 4A) were interpreted as characteristic for a *para*-substituted aromatic ring. Besides, H$_2$-1′ and H-2′ were coupled as evidenced by the COSY correlation (Figure 4A). The key HMBC correlations from H$_3$-5′ to C-2′, C-3′, and C-4′, from H$_2$-1′ to C-3′, and from H-2′ to C-4′ and C-5′ delineated an unsaturated and hydroxylated isoprene unit, (2-hydroxy-3-methylbut-3-en-1-yl)oxy (Figure 4A). Additional HMBC correlation from H$_2$-1′ to C-4 showed that the isoprene unit was connected to the *para*-substituted aromatic ring via an oxygen atom. Furthermore, the interactive HMBC correlations from H$_2$-7 to C-2, C-6, and C-8 constructed the other group (C7-C8) linked to the aromatic ring. The planar structure of **2** was therefore determined. A literature search revealed that it possessed the same planar structure as stachyline B, a secondary metabolite previously isolated from the sponge-derived fungus *Stachylidium* sp. [14]. The configuration at C-2′ of stachyline B was determined as *S* by Mosher's method [14]. Since **2** possessed the opposite sign of the optical rotation when compared to that of stachyline B (+16.1 in **2** vs −12 in stachyline B), the *R* configuration was proposed for C-2′ of **2**. X-ray diffraction crystallographic analysis enabled us to undoubtedly confirm its absolute configuration (Figure 4B).

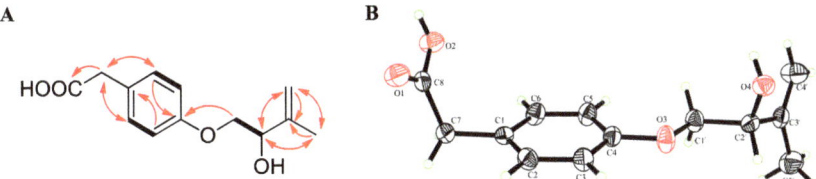

Figure 4. (**A**) COSY and key HMBC correlations of **2**; (**B**) ORTEP (Oak Ridge Thermal-Ellipsoid Plot Program) diagram for the single-crystal X-ray structure of **2**.

Compound **3** was obtained as a white amorphous powder and possessed a molecular formula of $C_{14}H_{18}O_4$ by (+)-HRESIMS data m/z 268.1548 [M + NH$_4$]$^+$ and 273.1095 [M + Na]$^+$. With compound **2** in hand, the structure elucidation of **3** was quite straightforward. The ^{1}H and ^{13}C NMR spectra of **3** (Table 1) closely resembled those of **2**, except that **3** had one methyl group ($\delta_{H/C}$ 3.58/51.6, 8-OMe) more than **2**. Accordingly, **3** was elucidated as a methyl ester of **2**. Because **3** is dextrorotatory, it was concluded that **3** also has R-configuration at C-2'.

In addition, another five previously reported metabolites including bisabolane-type sesquiterpenoids **4–6** and meroterpenoids **7** and **8** were also isolated in this study. They were identified as (7S,11S)-(+)-12-acetoxysydonic acid (**4**) [15], (S)-(+)-11-dehydrosydonic acid (**5**) [15], sydonic acid (**6**) [16], asperdemin (**7**) [17], and asperversin G (**8**) [18], respectively, by comparing their NMR data with those from the literature.

2.2. Cytotoxicity of Compounds **1–8**

The isolated compounds **1–8** were submitted to Cell Counting Kit-8 (CCK-8) colorimetric assays toward six human carcinoma cell lines (human lung adenocarcinoma epithelial cell line A549, human breast cancer cell line BT-549, human cervix carcinoma cell line HeLa, human liver carcinoma cell line HepG2, human breast adenocarcinoma cell line MCF-7, and human monocytic cell line THP-1) to estimate their cytotoxicities. Compound **3** exhibited cytotoxicity to the HepG2 cell line with an IC$_{50}$ value of 22.0 µM. Furthermore, **5** also showed considerable activities against the A549 and THP-1 cell lines with IC$_{50}$ values of 21.2 and 18.2 µM, respectively (Table 2). To determine whether the compounds could induce apoptosis, 4',6-diamidino-2-phenylindole (DAPI) staining was conducted using a confocal laser scanning microscope. We found that many cells had typical apoptotic features, such as fragmented/condensed nucleus and apoptotic body formation (Figure 5). All staining results indicated that **3** and **5** had apoptosis-inducing activity against the HepG2, A549, and THP-1 cell lines, respectively.

Table 2. Cytotoxicity of **1–8** (IC$_{50}$, µM, mean ± SD, n = 3).

Compound	A549	BT-549	HeLa	HepG2	MCF-7	THP-1
1	>100	>100	>100	>100	>100	>100
2	>100	87.3 ± 3.5	96.6 ± 1.5	>100	>100	>100
3	70.0 ± 1.2	>100	>100	22.0 ± 1.2	>100	>100
4	63.6 ± 2.6	>100	78.7 ± 2.9	>100	>100	78.7 ± 1.9
5	21.2 ± 2.3	>100	61.7 ± 2.2	>100	>100	18.2 ± 1.2
6	>100	>100	>100	>100	>100	>100
7	>100	>100	>100	>100	>100	>100
8	>100	>100	>100	>100	>100	>100
Epirubicin [a]	6.6 ± 0.5	4.4 ± 0.2	2.2 ± 0.3	3.7 ± 0.2	3.9 ± 0.1	4.8 ± 0.2

[a] Positive control.

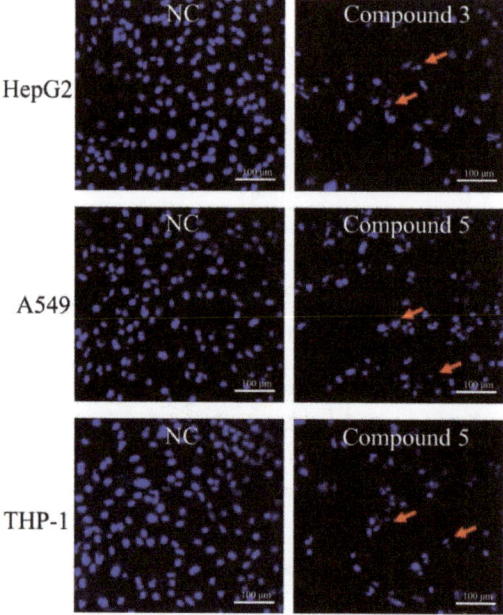

Figure 5. Apoptosis-related morphological changes were detected by staining cells with 4′,6-diamidino-2-phenylindole (DAPI). Apoptotic cells were defined as those with blue-stained cells that exhibited a fragmented/condensed nucleus and apoptotic body (red arrow).

3. Materials and Methods

3.1. General Experimental Procedures

The UV spectra were measured using a Shimadzu UV-2700 spectrometer (Shimadzu Co., Ltd., Kyoto, Japan). The optical rotations were measured using a Jasco P-1020 automatic polarimeter (JASCO, Tokyo, Japan). The NMR spectra were recorded on an Agilent DD2 500 MHz NMR spectrometer (Agilent Technologies, Waldbronn, Germany) with tetramethylsilane (TMS) as an internal standard. The HRESIMS data were obtained in the positive ion mode on a Waters Xevo G2-XS QTof mass spectrometer (Waters, Milford, MA, USA). Commercially available silica gel (100–200 and 200–300 mesh, Qingdao Marine Chemical Inc., Qingdao, China), Lobar LiChroprep RP-18 (40-60 μm, Merck, Darmstadt, Germany), and Sephadex LH-20 (Merck) were used for open column chromatography.

3.2. Fungal Material

The fungal strain LD-201810 was previously isolated from the marine red alga *Grateloupia turuturu* collected in August 2016 from Qingdao, China. This strain was identified as *P. chrysogenum* according to its morphological characteristics and sequencing of the ITS region (GenBank no. MT075873). The strain was deposited in the Key Laboratory of Marine Biotechnology at the Universities of Shandong (Ludong University), School of Life Sciences, Ludong University, Yantai, China.

3.3. Fermentation, Extraction, and Isolation

The fermentation was performed statically on sterilized solid rice medium (70 g of rice, 0.1 g of corn flour, 0.3 g of peptone, 0.1 g of monosodium glutamate, and 100 mL of filtered seawater in each 1 L Erlenmeyer flask) at room temperature. After incubation for 30 days, a total of 50 flasks of cultured mycelium were exhaustively extracted with EtOAc (3 × 10 L). Then, the organic phase was filtered and evaporated under reduced pressure to afford 40.6 g of EtOAc crude extract. Chromatographic fractionation of the EtOAc crude extract was performed using an open silica gel vacuum liquid chromatography (VLC) gradient system (bed 10 × 60 cm, silica gel 300 g, 100–200 mesh); the column was eluted with mixtures of petroleum ether (PE)–EtOAc (from 5:1 to 1:1, v/v, collected 1 L for each fraction) and dichloromethane (DCM)–methanol (MeOH) (from 20:1 to 5:1, v/v, collected 1 L for each fraction). A total of eight fractions, i.e., fractions A (11.2 g), B (2.6 g), C (5.8 g), D (5.2 g), E (2.6 g), F (6.0 g), G (2.1 g), and H (1.9 g), were obtained and concentrated under reduced pressure. Fraction A (11.2 g), eluted with PE–EtOAc (5:1, v/v, collected 2 L eluent), was re-fractionated by a silica gel column (bed 8 × 80 cm, silica gel 200 g, 200–300 mesh; PE–EtOAc gradient, from 10:1 to 1:1, v/v) to yield subfractions A1 and A2. Fraction A1 (4.5 g, eluted with PE–EtOAc 5:1, v/v, collected 1 L eluent) was subjected to a Sephadex LH-20 column (MeOH, bed 1.5 × 135 cm) to obtain **7** (23.6 mg). Fraction A2 (3.2 g, eluted with PE–EtOAc 1:1, v/v, collected 1 L eluent) was purified using preparative thin layer chromatography (PTLC, plate: 20 × 20 cm; developing solvents: DCM–MeOH, 20:1, v/v, 160 mL) to obtain **8** (42.3 mg). Fraction C (5.8 g), eluted with PE–EtOAc (1:1, v/v, collected 1 L eluent), was further re-fractionated by a silica gel column (bed 8 × 80 cm, silica gel 200 g, 200–300 mesh; DCM–MeOH, from 20:1 to 10:1, v/v) to yield subfractions C1 and C2. Fraction C1 (1.2 g, eluted with DCM–MeOH 20:1, v/v, collected 500 mL eluent) was purified by a Sephadex LH-20 column (MeOH, bed 1.5 × 135 cm) to obtain **1** (10.5 mg). Fraction E (2.6 g) was subjected to reversed-phase column chromatography (bed 2 × 5 cm) over Lobar LiChroprep RP-18 with a MeOH–H$_2$O gradient system (from 1:9 to 10:0, v/v, collected 1.2 L for each fraction) to afford five subfractions (Fr.E1–E5). Fr.E1 (123 mg, eluted with MeOH–H$_2$O 3:7, v/v) was purified using prep-HPLC (SunFire® C18, 250 mm × 10 mm, 5 μm; mobile phase: 50% MeOH–H$_2$O; flow rate: 2 mL/min; UV detection: 235 nm) to afford **2** (8.5 mg, t_R 12.6 min). Fr.E2 (89 mg, eluted with MeOH–H$_2$O 2:3, v/v) was subjected to PTLC (plate: 20 × 20 cm; developing solvents: DCM–acetone–acetic acid, 10:1:0.05, v/v, 80 mL) to afford **6** (9.5 mg). Fr.E3 (120 mg, eluted with MeOH–H$_2$O 1:1, v/v) was chromatographed on a prep-HPLC column (SunFire® C18, 250 mm × 10 mm, 5 μm; mobile phase: 60% MeOH–H$_2$O; flow rate: 2 mL/min; UV detection: 235 nm) to obtain **3** (12.3 mg, t_R 15.0 min). Fr.E4 (200 mg, eluted with MeOH–H$_2$O 3:2, v/v) was subjected to PTLC (plate: 20 × 20 cm; developing solvents: DCM–MeOH–CH$_3$CO$_2$H, 10:1:0.05, v/v, 4 × 40 mL) to afford **4** (11.3 mg) and **5** (26.3 mg).

Penilactonol A (**1**): colorless oil; $[\alpha]^{25}_D$ +7.3° (c 0.20, MeOH); UV (MeOH) λ_{max} (log ε) 207 (0.22) nm; ECD (0.20 mg/mL, MeOH) λ_{max} ($\Delta\varepsilon$) 224 (+1.80) nm; ^{1}H and ^{13}C NMR data, Table 1; (+)-HRESIMS m/z 185.0803 [M + H]$^+$ (calcd for C$_9$H$_{13}$O$_4$, 185.0808).

(2'R)-Stachyline B (**2**): colorless needles; mp 188–190 °C; $[\alpha]^{25}_D$ +16.1° (c 0.25, MeOH); UV (MeOH) λ_{max} (log ε) 203 (3.37), 228 (3.81), 278 (3.12), 285 (2.79) nm; ^{1}H and ^{13}C NMR data, Table 1; (+)-HRESIMS m/z 254.1389 [M + NH$_4$]$^+$ (calcd for C$_{13}$H$_{20}$NO$_4$, 254.1387) and 259.0942 [M + Na]$^+$ (calcd for C$_{13}$H$_{16}$O$_4$Na, 259.0941).

(2'R)-Westerdijkin A (**3**): white amorphous powder; $[\alpha]^{25}_D$ +70.3° (c 0.30, MeOH); UV (MeOH) λ_{max} (log ε) 201 (3.33), 226 (3.79), 277 (3.06), 283 (2.80) nm; ^{1}H and ^{13}C NMR data, Table 1; (+)-HRESIMS m/z 268.1548 [M + NH$_4$]$^+$ (calcd for C$_{14}$H$_{22}$NO$_4$, 268.1543) and 273.1095 [M + Na]$^+$ (calcd for C$_{14}$H$_{18}$O$_4$Na, 273.1097).

*3.4. Measurement of ICD Spectrum of **1** Using Mo$_2$(OAc)$_4$*

The ICD spectrum was measured using spectroscopy-grade anhydrous MeOH. A mixture of the ligand (**1**) and Mo$_2$(OAc)$_4$ in MeOH in an approximate 1:2 molar ratio was subjected to ICD measurement. The first CD spectrum was recorded immediately after mixing, and its time evolution was monitored until stationary ICD was reached about 10 min after mixing. After the inherent CD data of the compound were subtracted, the ICD spectrum was normalized to a molar concentration of **1** and was presented as the $\Delta\varepsilon'$ values. The observed signs of the Cotton effect near 400 nm in the ICD were correlated to the absolute configuration of the 1,2-diol moiety [11].

3.5. Computational Section

The conformational search was conducted via the conformer–rotamer ensemble sampling tool (CREST) [19,20]. Density-functional theory (DFT) calculations were carried out using the Gaussian 16 program [21]. The conformers within an energy window of 4 kcal/mol were optimized with DFT calculations at the B3LYP/6-31G(d) level of theory with Grimme's D3 dispersion correction. Next, energies of all optimized conformations were evaluated by M06-2X/6-311+g(2d,p) with D3 dispersion correction. Those conformers accounting for over 98% of the population were subjected to TDDFT ECD calculations at the CAM-B3LYP/def2-SVP level of theory in MeOH with the IEFPCM solvent model, respectively. For each conformer, 30 excited states were calculated [22]. The calculated ECD curves were generated using Multiwfn 3.6 software with a full width at half maximum (FWHM) for each peak set to 0.4 eV [23].

3.6. X-ray Crystallographic Analysis of **2**

Single-crystal X-ray diffraction data of **2** were obtained on an Agilent Xcalibur Eos Gemini Charge Couple Device (CCD) plate diffractometer using graphite monochromatized Cu/Kα radiation (λ = 1.54178 Å). The structures were solved by direct methods with the SHELXTL software package [24]. All non-hydrogen atoms were refined anisotropically. The H atoms were located using geometrical calculations, and their positions and thermal parameters were fixed during the structure refinement. The structure was refined using full-matrix least-squares techniques [25]. Crystallographic data of **2** have been deposited in the Cambridge Crystallographic Data Centre (CCDC) with the CCDC number of 1999572. The data can be obtained free of charge via CCDC, 12 Union Road, Cambridge CB21EZ, UK (e-mail: deposit@ccdc.cam.ac.uk).

Crystal data for compound **2**: $C_{13}H_{16}O_4$, F.W. = 236.26, monoclinic space group P2(1), unit cell dimensions a = 5.8770(7) Å, b = 7.7029(13) Å, c = 27.763(4) Å, V = 1256.8(3) Å^3, $\alpha = \beta = \gamma$ = 90°, Z = 4, d_{calcd} = 1.249 mg/m^3, crystal dimensions 0.36 × 0.22 × 0.12 mm, μ = 0.762 mm^{-1}, F(000) = 504. The 1774 measurements yielded 1500 independent reflections after equivalent data were averaged, and Lorentz and polarization corrections were applied. The final refinement gave R_1 = 0.0379 and wR_2 = 0.1050 [$I > 2\sigma(I)$]. The Flack parameter was −0.2(3) in the final refinement for all 1774 reflections with 157 Friedel pairs.

3.7. Cytotoxic Assays

The CCK-8 colorimetric method and DAPI staining were used to determine the cytotoxicities of compounds **1–8** against six human carcinoma cell lines (A549, BT-549, HeLa, HepG2, MCF-7, and THP-1) [26]. For the DAPI staining, HepG2, A549, and THP-1 cells were initially incubated for 24 h and then exposed to compounds for 48 h. Then, the cells were fixed with 70% ethanol. Subsequently, the cells were stained with 4 ng/mL DAPI at 4 °C for 5–10 min. Stained cells in each group were observed using a confocal laser scanning microscope.

3.8. Statistical Analysis

In this study, experiments were performed in triplicate and in parallel. For data analysis, the SPSS 21.0 software package (Chicago, IL, USA) was used to detect the half-maximal inhibitory concentration (IC_{50}) value.

4. Conclusions

Secondary metabolites produced by marine-derived fungi have gained remarkable attention due to their intriguing structures and potential pharmacological applications. In this study, a new pentaketide derivative, penilactonol A (**1**), and two previously unreported hydroxyphenylacetic acid derivatives, (2′R)-stachyline B (**2**) and (2′R)-westerdijkin A (**3**), together with five known metabolites including bisabolane-type sesquiterpenoids **4–6** and meroterpenoids **7** and **8**, were isolated from the solid culture of marine alga-associated fungus *P. chrysogenum* LD-201810. It should be pointed out that **2** and **3** adapt the 2′*R*-configuration as compared to known hydroxyphenylacetic acid-derived and *O*-prenylated natural products. The cytotoxicities of the isolated compounds were evaluated. Compound **3** exhibited cytotoxicity to the HepG2 cell line with an IC$_{50}$ value of 22.0 μM, whereas **5** showed considerable activities against A549 and THP-1 cell lines with IC$_{50}$ values of 21.2 and 18.2 μM, respectively. Moreover, DAPI staining indicated that **3** and **5** had apoptosis-inducing activity. The present study may provide further proof that marine natural products are promising candidates for the discovery of new lead compounds of antitumor drugs.

Supplementary Materials: The following are available online at http://www.mdpi.com/1660-3397/18/5/276/s1. Figures S1–S19: ^{1}H NMR, ^{13}C NMR, HSQC, ^{1}H-^{1}H COSY, HMBC, NOESY, and HRESIMS spectra of compounds **1–3**; Figures S20–S28: Cytotoxicity of **1–8** and epirubicin; Tables S1–S19: Gibbs free energies and equilibrium populations of the calculated conformers.

Author Contributions: Conceptualization, J.-X.T. and Y.-H.B.; writing—original draft preparation, L.-L.J.; writing—review and editing, Y.-Z.L., T.F., H.-W.Z., and X.Y.; funding acquisition, X.-X.Z., W.W., and J.-L.Z. All authors have read and approved the final manuscript.

Funding: This research was supported by the National Key Research and Development Program of China (Grant No. 2016YFD0501010, 2017YFD0500806 and 2018YFD0501402), the Major Agricultural Applied Technological Innovation Projects of Shandong Province (to X.X.Z.), the Key Research and Development Plan of Yantai (No. 2018XSCC045), the Foundation of Third Institute of Oceanography SOA (2018021 and 2017001), and the Natural Science Foundation of Fujian Province (2018J01064).

Conflicts of Interest: The authors declare no conflict of interest.

References

1. Hou, X.-M.; Xu, R.-F.; Gu, Y.-C.; Wang, C.; Shao, C.-L. Biological and Chemical Diversity of Coral-Derived Microorganisms. *Curr. Med. Chem.* **2015**, *22*, 3707–3762. [CrossRef] [PubMed]
2. Carroll, A.R.; Copp, B.R.; Davis, R.A.; Keyzers, R.A.; Prinsep, M.R. Marine natural products. *Nat. Prod. Rep.* **2019**, *36*, 122–173. [CrossRef] [PubMed]
3. Shah, M.; Sun, C.; Sun, Z.; Zhang, G.; Che, Q.; Gu, Q.; Zhu, T.; Li, D. Sun Antibacterial Polyketides from Antarctica Sponge-Derived Fungus *Penicillium* sp. HDN151272. *Mar. Drugs* **2020**, *18*, 71. [CrossRef] [PubMed]
4. Xu, K.; Yuan, X.-L.; Li, C.; Li, X.-D. Recent Discovery of Heterocyclic Alkaloids from Marine-Derived *Aspergillus* Species. *Mar. Drugs* **2020**, *18*, 54. [CrossRef]
5. Rateb, M.E.M.; Ebel, R. Secondary metabolites of fungi from marine habitats. *Nat. Prod. Rep.* **2011**, *28*, 290. [CrossRef]
6. Ji, N.-Y.; Wang, B.-G. Mycochemistry of marine algicolous fungi. *Fungal Divers.* **2016**, *80*, 301–342. [CrossRef]
7. Zhang, P.; Li, X.; Wang, B.-G. Secondary Metabolites from the Marine Algal-Derived Endophytic Fungi: Chemical Diversity and Biological Activity. *Planta Medica* **2016**, *82*, 832–842. [CrossRef]
8. Soldatou, S.; Baker, B.J. Cold-water marine natural products, 2006 to 2016. *Nat. Prod. Rep.* **2017**, *34*, 585–626. [CrossRef]
9. Chen, X.-W.; Li, C.-W.; Cui, C.-B.; Hua, W.; Zhu, T.-J.; Gu, Q.-Q. Nine New and Five Known Polyketides Derived from a Deep Sea-Sourced *Aspergillus* sp. 16-02-1. *Mar. Drugs* **2014**, *12*, 3116–3137. [CrossRef]
10. Huang, L.; Ding, L.; Li, X.; Wang, N.; Yan, Y.; Yang, M.; Cui, W.; Naman, C.B.; Cheng, K.; Zhang, W.; et al. A new lateral root growth inhibitor from the sponge-derived fungus *Aspergillus* sp. LS45. *Bioorg. Med. Chem. Lett.* **2019**, *29*, 1593–1596. [CrossRef]
11. Di Bari, L.; Pescitelli, G.; Pratelli, C.; Pini, D.; Salvadori, P. Determination of absolute configuration of acyclic 1,2-diols with Mo2(OAc)4. 1. Snatzke's method revisited. *J. Org. Chem.* **2001**, *66*, 4819–4825. [CrossRef] [PubMed]
12. Frelek, J.; Ruskowska, P.; Suszczynska, A.; Szewczyk, K.; Osuch, A.; Jarosz, S.; Jagodzinski, J. Configurational assignment of sugar erythro-1,2-diols from their electronic circular dichroism spectra with dimolybdenum tetraacetate. *Tetrahedron: Asymmetry* **2008**, *19*, 1709–1713. [CrossRef]

13. Xia, M.-W.; Cheng-Bin, C.; Li, C.-W.; Wu, C.-J. Three New and Eleven Known Unusual C25 Steroids: Activated Production of Silent Metabolites in a Marine-Derived Fungus by Chemical Mutagenesis Strategy using Diethyl Sulphate. *Mar. Drugs* **2014**, *12*, 1545–1568. [CrossRef] [PubMed]
14. Almeida, C.; Part, N.; Bouhired, S.; Kehraus, S.; König, G.M. Stachylines A–D from the Sponge-Derived Fungus *Stachylidium* sp. *J. Nat. Prod.* **2011**, *74*, 21–25. [CrossRef]
15. Lu, Z.; Zhu, H.; Fu, P.; Wang, Y.; Zhang, Z.; Lin, H.; Liu, P.; Zhuang, Y.; Hong, K.; Zhu, W. Cytotoxic Polyphenols from the Marine-Derived Fungus *Penicillium expansum*. *J. Nat. Prod.* **2010**, *73*, 911–914. [CrossRef]
16. Hamasaki, T.; Nagayama, K.; Hatsuda, Y. Two new metabolites, sydonic acid and hydroxysydonic acid from *Aspergillus sydowi*. *Agric. Biol. Chem.* **1978**, *42*, 37–40. [CrossRef]
17. Yurchenko, A.N.; Smetanina, O.F.; Kalinovsky, A.I.; Pivkin, M.V.; Dmitrenok, P.S.; Kuznetsova, T.A. A new meroterpenoid from the marine fungus *Aspergillus versicolor* (Vuill.) Tirab. *Russ. Chem. Bull.* **2010**, *59*, 852–856. [CrossRef]
18. Li, H.; Sun, W.; Deng, M.; Qi, C.; Chen, C.; Zhu, H.; Luo, Z.; Wang, J.; Xue, Y.; Zhang, Y. Asperversins A and B, two novel meroterpenoids with an unusual 5/6/6/6 ring from the marine-derived fungus *Aspergillus versicolor*. *Mar. Drugs* **2018**, *16*, 177. [CrossRef]
19. Pracht, P.; Bohle, F.; Grimme, S. Automated exploration of the low-energy chemical space with fast quantum chemical methods. *Phys. Chem. Chem. Phys.* **2020**, *22*, 7169–7192. [CrossRef]
20. Grimme, S. Exploration of Chemical Compound, Conformer, and Reaction Space with Meta-Dynamics Simulations Based on Tight-Binding Quantum Chemical Calculations. *J. Chem. Theory Comput.* **2019**, *15*, 2847–2862. [CrossRef]
21. Frisch, M.J.; Trucks, G.W.; Schlegel, H.B.; Scuseria, G.E.; Robb, M.A.; Cheeseman, J.R.; Scalmani, G.; Barone, V.; Petersson, G.A.; Nakatsuji, H.; et al. *Gaussian 16 Rev. C.01*; Gaussian, Inc.: Wallingford, CT, USA, 2016.
22. Pescitelli, G.; Bruhn, T. Good Computational Practice in the Assignment of Absolute Configurations by TDDFT Calculations of ECD Spectra. *Chirality* **2016**, *28*, 466–474. [CrossRef] [PubMed]
23. Lu, T.; Chen, F. Multiwfn: A multifunctional wavefunction analyzer. *J. Comput. Chem.* **2011**, *33*, 580–592. [CrossRef] [PubMed]
24. Sheldrick, G.M. *SHELXTL, Structure Determination Software Programs*; Bruker Analytical X-ray System Inc.: Madison, WI, USA, 1997.
25. Sheldrick, G.M. *SHELXL-97 and SHELXS-97, Program for X-ray Crystal Structure Solution and Refinement*; University of Göttingen: Göttingen, Germany, 1997.
26. Yuan, X.-L.; Zhang, P.; Liu, X.-M.; Du, Y.-M.; Hou, X.-D.; Cheng, S.; Zhang, Z.-F. Cytological Assessments and Transcriptome Profiling Demonstrate that Evodiamine Inhibits Growth and Induces Apoptosis in a Renal Carcinoma Cell Line. *Sci. Rep.* **2017**, *7*, 12572. [CrossRef] [PubMed]

© 2020 by the authors. Licensee MDPI, Basel, Switzerland. This article is an open access article distributed under the terms and conditions of the Creative Commons Attribution (CC BY) license (http://creativecommons.org/licenses/by/4.0/).

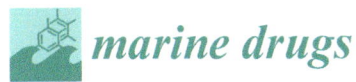

Article

New Biscembranoids Sardigitolides A–D and Known Cembranoid-Related Compounds from *Sarcophyton digitatum*: Isolation, Structure Elucidation, and Bioactivities

Tzu-Yin Huang [1], Chiung-Yao Huang [2], Chih-Hua Chao [3,4], Chi-Chien Lin [5,6], Chang-Feng Dai [7], Jui-Hsin Su [8], Ping-Jyun Sung [8], Shih-Hsiung Wu [9] and Jyh-Horng Sheu [1,2,6,10,*]

1. Doctoral Degree Program in Marine Biotechnology, National Sun Yat-sen University, Kaohsiung 804, Taiwan; slime112229@gmail.com
2. Department of Marine Biotechnology and Resources, National Sun Yat-sen University, Kaohsiung 804, Taiwan; huangcy@mail.nsysu.edu.tw
3. School of Pharmacy, China Medical University, Taichung 404, Taiwan; chchao@mail.cmu.edu.tw
4. Chinese Medicine Research and Development Center, China Medical University Hospital, Taichung 404, Taiwan
5. Institute of Biomedical Science, National Chung-Hsing University, Taichung 402, Taiwan; lincc@dragon.nchu.edu.tw
6. Department of Medical Research, China Medical University Hospital, China Medical University, Taichung 404, Taiwan
7. Institute of Oceanography, National Taiwan University, Taipei 112, Taiwan; corallab@ntu.edu.tw
8. National Museum of Marine Biology and Aquarium, Pingtung 944, Taiwan; x2219@nmmba.gov.tw (J.-H.S.); pjsung@nmmba.gov.tw (P.-J.S.)
9. Institute of Biological Chemistry and Chemical Biology and Molecular Biophysics Program, Taiwan International Graduate Program, Academia Sinica, Taipei 112, Taiwan; shwu@gate.sinica.edu.tw
10. Graduate Institute of Natural Products, Kaohsiung Medical University, Kaohsiung 807, Taiwan
* Correspondence: sheu@mail.nsysu.edu.tw; Tel.: +886-7-5252000 (ext. 5030); Fax: +886-7-5255020

Received: 7 July 2020; Accepted: 27 August 2020; Published: 29 August 2020

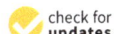

Abstract: Chemical examination from the cultured soft coral *Sarcophyton digitatum* resulted in the isolation and structural identification of four new biscembranoidal metabolites, sardigitolides A–D (**1**–**4**), along with three previously isolated biscembranoids, sarcophytolide L (**5**), glaucumolide A (**6**), glaucumolide B (**7**), and two known cembranoids (**8** and **9**). The chemical structures of all isolates were elucidated on the basis of 1D and 2D NMR spectroscopic analyses. Additionally, in order to discover bioactivity of marine natural products, **1**–**8** were examined in terms of their inhibitory potential against the upregulation of inflammatory factor production in lipopolysaccharide (LPS)-stimulated murine macrophage J774A.1 cells and their cytotoxicities against a limited panel of cancer cells. The anti-inflammatory results showed that at a concentration of 10 µg/mL, **6** and **8** inhibited the production of IL-1β to 68 ± 1 and 56 ± 1%, respectively, in LPS-stimulated murine macrophages J774A.1. Furthermore, sardigitolide B (**2**) displayed cytotoxicities toward MCF-7 and MDA-MB-231 cancer cell lines with the IC_{50} values of 9.6 ± 3.0 and 14.8 ± 4.0 µg/mL, respectively.

Keywords: *Sarcophyton digitatum*; biscembranoid-type metabolites; cytotoxicity; inflammatory factor production; LPS-stimulated murine macrophage

1. Introduction

Cembrane diterpenoids and their derivatives are an abundant and structurally diverse group of secondary metabolites of soft corals and gorgonians. The 14-membered ring structures of cembranoids are biosynthetically formed by cyclization of a geranylgeranyl pyrophosphate precursor between carbons 1 and 14 [1]. These compounds possess a defense mechanism against their natural predators and protect corals against viral infections [2]. Cembranoids exhibit various useful biological properties, such as antitumor [3–8] and anti-inflammatory activities [7,9–12].

Previous studies indicated that species of *Sarcophyton* are rich sources of compounds, such as cembranoids [13–16], biscembranoids [17–21], and steroids [22]. Until now, more than 500 marine natural objects have been found from the soft corals of the genus *Sarcophyton* [23]. It is worth mentioning that biscembranoid-type metabolites are mainly biosynthetically rationalized by a Diels–Alder reaction of two monocembranoidal members, a 1,3-diene cembranoid unit, and a dienophile cembranoid unit. The diene unit forms new trisubstituted conjugated double bonds at C-34/C-35. Normally, most biscembranoids are biosynthesized by the endo-type cyclization of a Diels–Alder reaction [21]. Although many specimens of *Sarcophyton* genus have been chemically studied, there is only one chemical investigation of the soft coral *Sarcophyton digitatum* that has been reported by Zeng et al. in 2000, which led to the isolation of a polyhydroxylated sterol, sardisterol, from this species [24]. Due to the structure diversity and attracting bioactivities of natural products from soft corals, it is well worth further investigating for the discovery of new metabolites from *S. digitatum*. As part of our continuing investigations of discovering bioactive compounds from soft corals, herein is reported the chemical examination of a cultured *S. digitatum*, which resulted in the isolation and structure identification of four new biscembranoidal metabolites, sardigitolides A–D (**1**–**4**), along with five known compounds, sarcophytolide L (**5**) [25], glaucumolide A (**6**) [18], glaucumolide B (**7**) [18], isosarcophytonolide D (**8**) [26], and (4Z,8S,9S,12Z,14E)-9-hydroxy-1-isopropyl-8,12-dimethyloxabicyclo [9.3.2]-hexadeca-4,12,14-trien-18-one (**9**) [27]. Lipopolysaccharide (LPS), a known endotoxin, is the main component of the outer membrane of gram-negative bacteria, which could induce an inflammatory response in mammalian tissues. In most cases, the inflammatory response helps the organism to clear the LPS or pathogen. However, the violent inflammation caused by overproduced LPS could lead to tissue damage [28]. In the present study, the inhibitory effect of isolates **1**–**8** against the enhanced production of inflammatory factors in LPS-treated murine macrophage J774A.1 cells was examined. Furthermore, the in vitro cytotoxicities toward MCF-7, MDA-MB-231, HepG2, and HeLa cells of compounds **1**–**8** were investigated.

2. Results and Discussion

Soft coral *Sarcophyton digitatum* was cultured in the National Museum of Marine Biology & Aquarium. A frozen sample was initially extracted with *n*-hexane and subsequently by ethyl acetate. The ethyl acetate layer was concentrated and repeatedly chromatographed to isolate compounds **1**–**9** (Figure 1), and structure of new compounds **1**–**4** were established based on spectroscopic analyses (Supplementary Materials S1–S40).

Sardigitolide A (**1**) was isolated as a white amorphous powder. High-resolution electron spray ionization mass spectroscopy (HRESIMS) showed a molecular ion peak at *m/z* 721.4287 [M + Na]$^+$ corresponding to the molecular formula $C_{41}H_{62}O_9$ and implying 11 degrees of unsaturation. In the IR spectrum, a characteristic absorption at 3433 cm^{-1} indicated the presence of a hydroxy group. The ^{13}C spectrum (Table 1) showed 41 carbon signals, including 9 methyl groups, 11 methylene, 10 methines, and 11 quaternary carbons. Its ^{1}H (Table 2) and ^{13}C NMR spectra revealed signals of three olefinic methyl groups (δ_H 1.89, s; 1.86, s; 1.70, s and δ_C 26.6; 19.3; 17.9, respectively), two methyl groups linked to oxygen-bearing quaternary carbons (δ_H 1.16, s; 1.13, s and δ_C 23.7; 25.3, respectively), one methoxy group (δ_H 3.55, s; δ_C 51.3), an isopropyl group (δ_H 2.19, m; 0.95, d, *J* = 6.8 Hz; 0.76, d, *J* = 6.8 Hz and δ_C 29.1, CH; 21.1, CH$_3$; 18.3, CH$_3$, respectively), two trisubstituted double bond (δ_H 6.44, s; δ_C 126.0, CH; 160.9, C and δ_H 5.06, d, *J* = 10.0 Hz; 125.2, CH; 138.4, C, respectively), one tetrasubstituted double bond (δ_C 131.7, C and 130.6, C), three oxygen-bearing methines (δ_H 4.86, t, J = 6.4 Hz; 3.49, m; 3.44, dd, J = 4.0, 12.0 Hz and δ_C 67.8, CH; 81.7, CH; 73.8, CH, respectively), two oxygen-bearing quaternary carbons (δ_C 73.8, C and 70.4, C), and four carbonyl carbons (δ_C 214.2, C; 210.0, C; 202.5, C; and 174.9, C). All of the above evidence suggested that **1** contained a biscembranoid skeleton. The planar structure of **1** was further determined. The correlations spectroscopy (COSY) signals revealed eight different structural units from H-2 to H$_2$-36; H$_2$-6 via H$_2$-7 and H$_2$-8; H-9 to H$_3$-18; isopropyl protons H$_3$-16 and H$_3$-17 via H-15, H-12, and H-11; H-21 to H-22; H$_2$-24 via H$_2$-25 and H$_2$-26; H$_2$-28 via H$_2$-29 and H-30; and H$_2$-32 to H-33. These units were assembled by heteronuclear multiple bond correlations (HMBCs) of H$_3$-16 to C-12, C-15, and C-17; H$_3$-18 to C-8, C-9, and C-10; H$_3$-19 to C-4, C-5, and C-6; H$_3$-37 to C-34, C-35, and C-36; H$_3$-38 to C-22, C-23, and C-24; H$_3$-39 to C-27, C-28, and C-29; H$_3$-40 to C-30, C-31, and C-32; H-2 to C-1, C-3, and C-14; H$_2$-11 to C-10; H-12 to C-13; H$_2$-14 to C-1 and C-20; and H-33 to C-34 and C-35. Accordingly, compound **1** had an additional degree of unsaturation, which was suggested to be of an ether ring between C-26 and C-30 established via an HMBC from H-26 to C-30. The gross structure of **1** was thus confirmed as shown in Figure 2 which possesses a biscembranoid skeleton similar to ximaolides E and F [29].

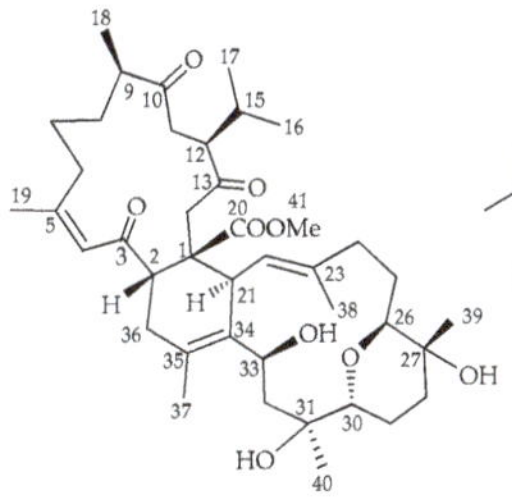

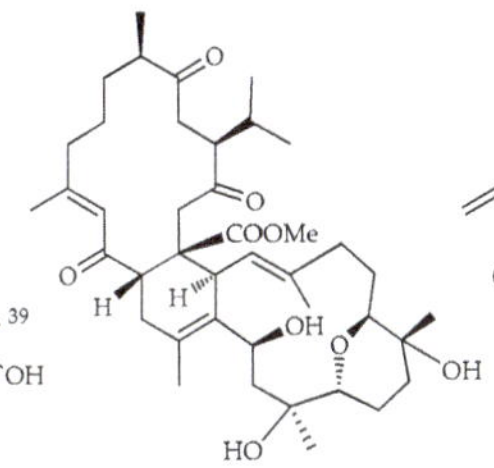

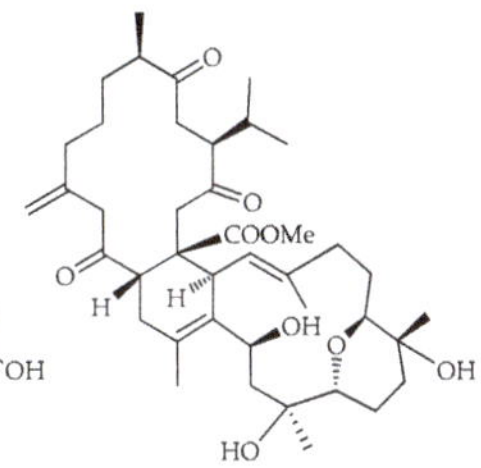

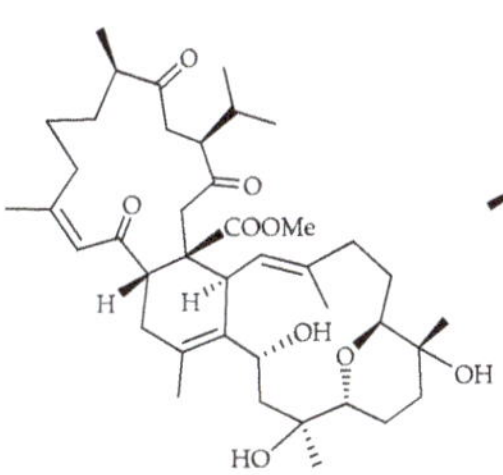

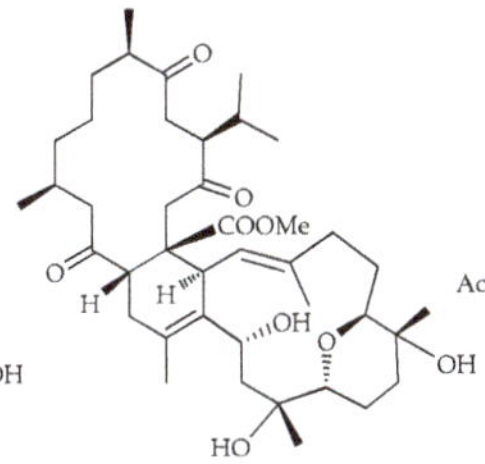

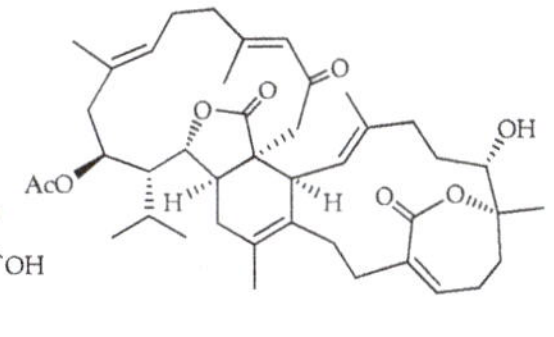

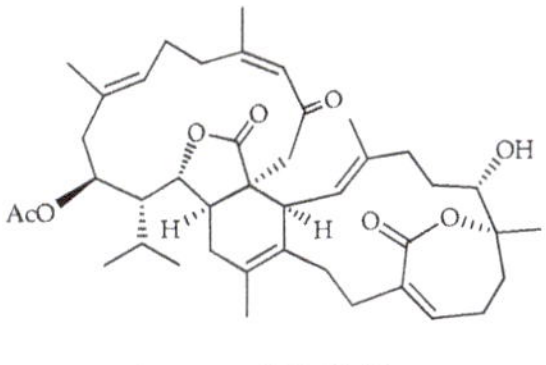

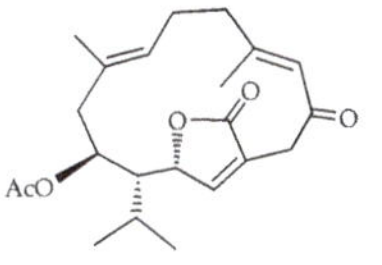

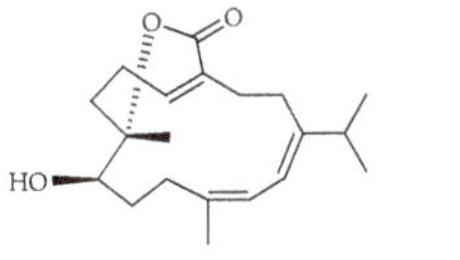

Figure 1. Structures of compounds **1–9**.

Table 1. ^{13}C NMR spectroscopic data of 1–4.

Position	1 [a]	2	3	4 [b]
1	50.2 (C)	48.7 (C)	49.8 (C)	49.4 (C)
2	46.0 (CH) [c]	47.3 (CH)	45.8 (CH)	44.0 (CH)
3	202.5 (C)	203.8 (C)	210.3 (C)	201.5 (C)
4	126.0 (CH)	126.0 (CH)	51.0 (CH$_2$)	124.7 (CH)
5	160.9 (C)	159.8 (C)	143.2 (C)	159.4 (C)
6	32.3 (CH$_2$)	39.8 (CH$_2$)	36.5 (CH$_2$)	34.0 (CH$_2$)
7	24.7 (CH$_2$)	24.1 (CH$_2$)	25.7 (CH$_2$)	25.2 (CH$_2$)
8	31.0 (CH$_2$)	31.1 (CH$_2$)	33.8 (CH$_2$)	33.6 (CH$_2$)
9	44.6 (CH)	45.7 (CH)	47.7 (CH)	44.7 (CH)
10	214.2 (C)	213.3 (C)	213.6 (C)	213.6 (C)
11	34.7 (CH$_2$)	35.1 (CH$_2$)	34.2 (CH$_2$)	37.1 (CH$_2$)
12	52.6 (CH)	52.1 (CH)	51.1 (CH)	52.3 (CH)
13	210.0 (C)	211.2 (C)	211.6 (C)	207.6 (C)
14	46.6 (CH$_2$)	47.7 (CH$_2$)	46.8 (CH$_2$)	45.2 (CH$_2$)
15	29.1 (CH)	29.4 (CH)	29.2 (CH)	28.3 (CH)
16	18.3 (CH$_3$)	17.9 (CH$_3$)	18.4 (CH$_3$)	17.3 (CH$_3$)
17	21.1 (CH$_3$)	20.8 (CH$_3$)	21.0 (CH$_3$)	21.0 (CH$_3$)
18	17.2 (CH$_3$)	16.3 (CH$_3$)	17.6 (CH$_3$)	18.3 (CH$_3$)
19	26.6 (CH$_3$)	20.3 (CH$_3$)	114.9 (CH$_2$)	26.4 (CH$_3$)
20	174.9 (C)	174.4 (C)	175.0 (C)	174.1 (C)
21	42.9 (CH)	40.8 (CH)	42.5 (CH)	41.7 (CH)
22	125.2 (CH)	124.0 (CH)	124.5 (CH)	126.8 (CH)
23	138.4 (C)	140.2 (C)	139.3 (C)	134.9 (C)
24	36.7 (CH$_2$)	38.5 (CH$_2$)	37.6 (CH$_2$)	34.9 (CH$_2$)
25	25.8 (CH$_2$)	26.8 (CH$_2$)	26.3 (CH$_2$)	24.4 (CH$_2$)
26	81.7 (CH)	84.8 (CH)	82.7 (CH)	79.8 (CH)
27	70.4 (C)	70.1 (C)	70.4 (C)	69.0 (C)
28	33.6 (CH$_2$)	32.0 (CH$_2$)	33.2 (CH$_2$)	33.6 (CH$_2$)
29	19.5 (CH$_2$)	19.8 (CH$_2$)	19.9 (CH$_2$)	19.2 (CH$_2$)
30	73.8 (CH)	74.0 (CH)	73.9 (CH)	72.8 (CH)
31	73.8 (C)	74.0 (C)	73.9 (C)	72.8 (C)
32	40.2 (CH$_2$)	41.2 (CH$_2$)	40.6 (CH$_2$)	39.8 (CH$_2$)
33	67.8 (CH)	69.9 (CH)	68.5 (CH)	64.9 (CH)
34	131.7 (C)	131.5 (C)	132.8 (C)	132.7 (C)
35	130.6 (C)	130.2 (C)	130.1 (C)	125.2 (C)
36	34.0 (CH$_2$)	34.0 (CH$_2$)	34.2 (CH$_2$)	32.9 (CH$_2$)
37	19.3 (CH$_3$)	19.8 (CH$_3$)	19.6 (CH$_3$)	16.8 (CH$_3$)
38	17.9 (CH$_3$)	18.9 (CH$_3$)	18.5 (CH$_3$)	17.2 (CH$_3$)
39	25.3 (CH$_3$)	25.4 (CH$_3$)	25.4 (CH$_3$)	26.2 (CH$_3$)
40	23.7 (CH$_3$)	22.9 (CH$_3$)	23.4 (CH$_3$)	24.7 (CH$_3$)
41	51.3 (CH$_3$)	51.6 (CH$_3$)	51.3 (CH$_3$)	50.6 (CH$_3$)

[a] Spectroscopic data of 1–3 were recorded at 100 MHz in CDCl$_3$. [b] Spectroscopic data of 4 was recorded at 125 MHz in DMSO-d_6. [c] Attached protons were deduced by DEPT experiments.

The relative configuration of **1** was determined by the analysis of correlations recorded by nuclear Overhauser effect spectroscopy (NOESY). As shown in Figure 3, the NOE correlations of H-4 (δ_H 6.44, s) with H$_3$-19 (δ_H 1.89, s), together with the obviously downfield-shifted methyl group at C-19 (δ_C 26.6, CH$_3$), suggested a *cis* geometry of C-4/C-5 trisubstituted double bond. Assuming the β-orientations of H$_3$-41 as previously reported [30], NOE correlations of H$_3$-41 with both of H$_3$-16 (δ_H 0.76, d, J = 6.8 Hz) and H$_3$-17 (δ_H 0.95, d, J = 6.8 Hz), and all of H$_3$-16, H$_3$-17 and H$_3$-18 (δ_H 1.08, d, J = 7.2 Hz) with H-11 (δ_H 2.13, m) suggested the β-orientations of H$_3$-18 and C-1 carbomethoxy groups, on the basis that metabolites of this type with absolute configurations determined previously all possessed 1*S* and 2*S* configurations [30]. Furthermore, the correlations of H-2 with H-22 (δ_H 5.06, d, J = 10.0 Hz); H-22 with H-24β (δ_H 2.43, m); and H-24β with H-25β (δ_H 1.84, m); H-25β with H$_3$-39 (δ_H 1.13, s); H$_3$-39 with H-28β (δ_H 1.52, m); H-28β with H-30 (δ_H 3.44, dd, J = 4.0, 12.0 Hz) reflected the β-orientation of H-30 and H$_3$-39. In contrast, the α-orientations of H-9 and H-12 were confirmed by the NOE correlations of H-11α (δ$_H$ 2.76, m) with both H-9 (δ$_H$ 2.71, m) and H-12 (δ$_H$ 2.97, m). The α-orientation of H-26 was determined by the NOE correlations of H-21 (δ$_H$ 3.37, m) with H$_3$-38 (δ$_H$ 1.70, s); H$_3$-38 with H-24α (δ$_H$ 1.98, m); H-24α with H-25α (δ$_H$ 1.64, m); H-25α with H-26 (δ$_H$ 3.49, m). Also, the α-orientations of H-33 and H$_3$-40 were determined by the NOE correlations of H-33 (δ$_H$ 4.86, t, J = 6.4 Hz) with both H$_3$-37 (δ$_H$ 1.86, s) and H$_3$-40 (δ$_H$ 1.16, s). Moreover, the ^{13}C NMR signals of C-37 (δ$_C$ 19.3, CH$_3$) and C-38 (δ$_C$ 17.9, CH$_3$) indicated the E geometry of the trisubstituted C-22/C-23 and tetrasubstituted C-34/C-35 double bonds. According to the above described evidence, and since compounds of this type are likely biosynthesized from the same or similar precursors and pathway, the absolute configuration of **1** was proposed as 1S,2S,9R,12S,21S,26S,27R,30R,31S,33S.

The pseudomolecular ion peak of sardigitolide B (**2**) [M + Na]$^+$ at m/z = 721.4283 indicated the same molecular formula of **2**, C$_{41}$H$_{62}$O$_9$, as that of **1**. The ^{13}C NMR spectrum of **2** showed similar signals to those of **1**. Also, it displayed carbon signals of 9 methyls, 11 methylenes, 10 methines, and 11 quaternary carbons. By detailed analysis of the 2D NMR spectral data of **2**, a similar gross structure to that of **1** was deduced. However, it was found that **2** possesses a remarkably upfield-shifted signal of H-4 (δ$_H$ 5.85, s), while **1** displayed a downfield-shifted resonance for H-4 (δ$_H$ 6.44, s). Also, the ^{13}C NMR spectroscopy data were found to be quite similar to those of **1**, with the exception of CH$_3$-19 at δ$_C$ 26.6 in **1** and δ$_C$ 20.3 in **2**, suggesting the presence of a *trans* geometry of 4,5-double bond.

Table 2. ^{1}H NMR spectroscopic data of **1**–**4**.

Position	1 [α]	2	3	4 [b]
2	3.59, m	3.73, m	3.74, t (7.6) [c]	3.37, m
4	6.44, s	5.85, s	3.20, m; 3.64 m	6.30, s
6	1.68, m; 3.30, m	1.99, m; 2.21, m	1.80, m; 2.16 m	2.11, m
7	1.34, m; 1.52, m	1.51, m; 1.60, m	1.27, m	1.10, m; 1.30, m
8	1.34, m; 1.64, m	1.49, m	1.52, m; 1.63 m	1.23, m; 1.54, m
9	2.71, m	2.24, m	2.43, m	2.73, m
11	2.13, m; 2.76, m	2.09, m; 2.98, m	2.04, m; 3.0, m	2.05, m; 3.01, m
12	2.97, m	2.82, m	3.05, m	2.99, m
14	2.84, m; 3.11, m	2.58, m; 3.23, m	3.10, m	2.58, m; 2.82, m
15	2.19, m	2.07, m	2.03, m	2.03, m
16	0.76, d (6.8)	0.77, d (6.8)	0.79, d (6.8)	0.59, d (7.0)
17	0.95, d (6.8)	0.94, d (6.8)	0.95, d (6.4)	0.90, d (6.5)
18	1.08, d (7.2)	1.13, d (6.8)	1.13, d (7.2)	0.96, (7.0)
19	1.89, s	2.12, s	4.72, 4.88, brs	1.84, s
21	3.37, m	3.73, d (10.8)	3.50, m	3.36, m
22	5.06, d (10.0)	5.25, d (10.8)	5.17, d (10.4)	4.99, d (10.5)
24	1.98, m; 2.43, m	1.94, m; 2.52, m	1.94, m; 2.50 m	1.82, m; 2.24, m
25	1.64, m; 1.84, m	1.61, m; 1.99, m	1.63, m; 1.94 m	1.58, m; 1.64, m
26	3.49, m	3.60, m	3.54, m (9.6)	3.28, d (10.5)
28	1.52, m; 1.72, m	1.52, m; 1.71, m	1.58, m; 1.72 m	1.62, m; 2.16, m
29	1.57, m; 1.70, m	1.70, m;	1.63, m; 1.71, m	1.29, m; 1.64, m
30	3.44, dd (4.0; 12.0)	3.63, m	3.52, m	3.15, dd (4.0; 12.0)
32	1.55, m; 2.19 m	1.71, m; 1.92, m	1.60, m; 2.03 m	2.19, m
33	4.86, t (6.4)	4.80, t (6.4)	4.83, t (6.4)	4.78, d (10.5)
36	2.26, m	2.26 m; 2.56 m	2.15, m; 2.40, m	1.92, m
37	1.86, s	1.91, s	1.89, s	1.66, s
38	1.70, s	1.77, s	1.75, s	1.57, s
39	1.13, s	1.13, s	1.14, s	0.96, s
40	1.16, s	1.14, s	1.15, s	1.01, s
41	3.55, s	3.58, s	3.58, s	3.40, s

[α] Spectroscopic data of **1**–**3** were recorded at 400 MHz in CDCl$_3$. [b] Spectroscopic data of **4** was recorded at 500 MHz in DMSO-d_6. [c] J values (in Hz) in parentheses.

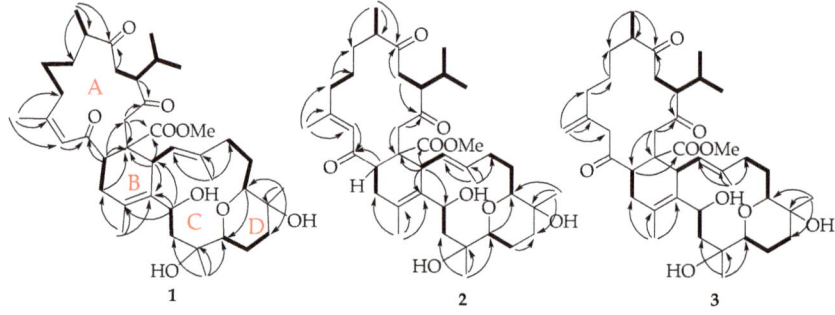

Figure 2. Selected COSY and HMBC correlations of **1**–**3**.

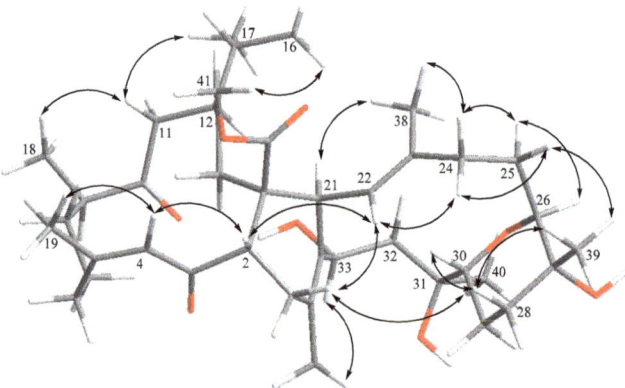

Figure 3. Key NOE correlations of compound **1**.

The relative configurations of the stereogenic centers in **2** were determined from the NOESY spectrum, which also showed similar NOE correlations to those of **1**. In contrast, H-4 (δ_H 5.85, s) showed an NOE correlation with H-2 (δ_H 3.73, m), but not with H$_3$-19 (δ_H 2.12, s), confirming the E geometry of the double bond at C-4 and C-5 again. These results determined **2** to be the 4E isomer of **1**.

Sardigitolide C (**3**) exhibited a protonated molecular peak at m/z 721.4281 [M + Na]$^+$ in the HR-ESI-MS spectrum, establishing the same molecular formula, $C_{41}H_{62}O_9$, and 11 degrees of unsaturation as those of **1** and **2**. The ^{13}C NMR spectroscopy data also showed 41 carbon signals, including 8 methyl groups, 13 methylene, 9 methines, and 11 quaternary carbons. Analyzing the 2D NMR spectral data of **3** in detail showed a similar gross structure of **3** to that of **1**, except that the chemical shifts of CH$_2$-19 (δ_H 4.72, 4.88, brs; δ_C 114.9) in **3** indicated the presence of 1,1-disubstituted double bond at C-5/C-19. The relative configuration of **3** was also determined from NOESY spectrum, which showed similar NOE correlations among the corresponding protons to those of **1**. This is the first ximaolide-type compound containing a disubstituted double bond at C-5.

Sardigitolide D (**4**) was isolated as a white amorphous solid. The HR-ESI-MS of **4** showed a pseudomolecular ion peak at 721.4268 [M + Na]$^+$, indicating the molecular formula $C_{41}H_{62}O_9$ and implying 11 degrees of unsaturation. In the ^{13}C and DEPT-135 spectra, **4** showed 41 carbon signals resembling those of **1** including 9 methyls, 11 methylenes, 10 methines, and 11 quaternary carbons. Also, **4** had the same gross structure as **1** according to the detailed analyses of 1D and 2D NMR (COSY and HMBC) spectra. However, it was found that H-33 of **4** showed a different coupling constant

(J = 10.5 Hz) to that of H-33 (J = 6.4 Hz) in **1**. Furthermore, **4** did not show NOE correlation between H-22 (δ_H 4.99, d, J = 10.5 Hz) and H-33 (δ_H 4.78, d, J = 10.5 Hz), while **1**–**3** exhibited NOE interactions between H-22 and H-33, revealing the 33R configuration. On the basis of the above findings, the molecular structure of **4** was determined unambiguously to be the 33-epimer of **1**.

It is known that IL-1β, the cytokine family member of interleukin-1 produced by activated macrophages, can lead to a strong immune response, and many studies have shown that IL-1β is related to various diseases, such as rheumatoid arthritis [31,32], neuropathic pain [33], and cardiovascular disease [34]. Furthermore, IL-1β has been suggested as a therapeutic target for the treatment of diabetic retinopathy [35,36]. In this study, we also attempted to screen the bioactivity of isolates with potential anti-inflammatory and cytotoxic abilities. Therefore, **1**–**8** were screened for their inhibitory potential against the upregulation of proinflammatory cytokine IL-1β in LPS-stimulated murine macrophage J774A.1 cells. The results showed that, at a concentration of 10 µg/mL, **6** and **8** potently inhibited LPS-induced IL-1β production to 68 ± 1 and 56 ± 1%, respectively, with IC$_{50}$ values of 10.7 ± 2.7 and 14.9 ± 5.1 µg/mL, respectively. In addition, compounds **1**–**8** were assayed for their cytotoxicities toward MCF-7, MDA-MB-231, HepG2, and HeLa carcinoma cell lines. The results (Table 3) showed that sardigitolide B (**2**) exhibited inhibitory activity toward MCF-7 and MDA-MB-231 cells with IC$_{50}$ values of 9.6 ± 3.0 and 14.8 ± 4.0 µg/mL, respectively, and glacumolide A (**6**) showed cytotoxicity toward MCF-7, HepG2, and HeLa cell lines with IC$_{50}$ values of 10.1 ± 3.3, 14.9 ± 3.5, and 17.1 ± 4.5 µg/mL, respectively. Glacumolide B (**7**) also was found to display cytotoxicity toward MCF-7, MDA-MB-231, and HepG2 cell lines, with IC$_{50}$ values of 9.4 ± 3.0, 17.8 ± 4.5, and 14.9 ± 4.2 µg/mL, respectively. The monocembranoid **8** (molecular weight 374) showed cytotoxicity against the growth of MCF-7 cancer cell line with IC$_{50}$ value of 10.9 ± 4.3 µg/mL (29.1 ± 11.4 µM). The remaining compounds did not show any effective cytotoxic and anti-inflammatory activities.

Table 3. Cytotoxicities of compounds **1**–**8**. IC$_{50}$ (µg/mL) values are the mean ± SEM (n = 3).

Compound	MCF-7	MDA-MB-231	HepG2	HeLa
1	–[a]	–	–	–
2	9.6 ± 3.0	14.8 ± 4.0	–	–
3	–	–	–	–
4	–	–	–	–
5	–	–	–	–
6	10.1 ± 3.3	–	14.9 ± 3.5	17.1 ± 4.5
7	9.4 ± 3.0	17.8 ± 4.5	14.9 ± 4.2	–
8	10.9 ± 4.3	–	–	–
Doxorubicin	0.7 ± 0.1	1.3 ± 0.2	1.2 ± 0.4	0.4 ± 0.1

[a] —> 20 µg/mL.

Methyl tortuosoate, also called methyl tetrahydrosarcoate (**10**) (Figure 4), has been frequently discovered to be the dienophile monomeric cembranoid in the Diels–Alder reaction to biosynthesize relevant biscembranoid, while methyl sarcoate (**11**) has been found to be the dienophile part of this series biscembranoids for only one time [37]. Biscembranoids **1** and **4** are the Diels–Alder reaction products using (7Z,8)-dehydromethyl tortuosoate (**12**), **2** using (7E,8)-dehydromethyl tortuosoate (**13**), and **3** using (7,19)-dehydromethyl tortuosoate (**14**), respectively, as the dienophiles in the biscembranoids biosynthesis. Cembranoids **12**–**14** are waiting for discovery in future investigations.

Our previous investigation of secondary metabolites from the soft coral *Sarcophyton glacum* led to the discovery of two biscembranoid-type compounds, glaucumolide A (**6**) and glaucumolide B (**7**) [19]. The absolute configurations of **6**, **7**, and analogs have been confirmed in 2019 by Wen et al. from the X-ray single crystal diffraction of the same compound **6**, isolated from the soft coral *S. trocheliophorum* [20].

Recently, with the development of molecular phylogenetic analysis technology, McFadden et al. suggested that *S. glacum* contained more than seven genetically distinct clades which might be the reason for the continuous discovery of high chemical diversity of secondary metabolites of the soft coral *S. glacum* [38]. For the same reason, it is possible that the corals of *Sarcophyton* genus could generate similar structure biscembranoids as our present study.

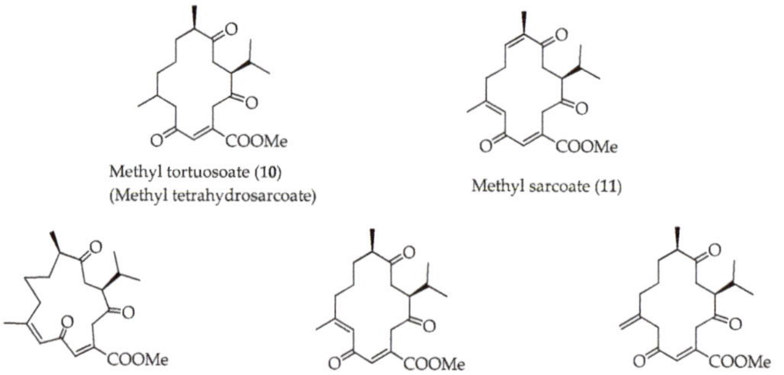

Methyl tortuosoate (**10**)
(Methyl tetrahydrosarcoate)

Methyl sarcoate (**11**)

(7Z,8)-dehydromethyl tortuosoate (**12**)   (7E,8)-dehydromethyl tortuosoate (**13**)   (7,19)-dehydromethyl tortuosoate (**14**)

Figure 4. Structures of dienophiles **10–14**.

3. Materials and Methods

3.1. General Experimental Procedures

Optical rotations and IR spectra were recorded on a JASCO P-1020 polarimeter and FR/IR-4100 infrared spectrophotometer (Jasco Corporation, Tokyo, Japan), respectively. NMR spectra were acquired on a Varian Unity Inova 500 FT-NMR (Varian Inc., Palo Alto, CA, USA) at 500 and 125 MHz for ^{1}H and ^{13}C, respectively; or on Varian 400 MR FT-NMR instrument at 400 MHz and 100 MHz for ^{1}H and ^{13}C, respectively. The data of low-resolution electron spray ionization mass spectroscopy (LRESIMS) were measured by Bruker APEX II mass spectrometer. The data of HRESIMS were obtained by Bruker Apex-Qe 9.4T mass spectrometer. Silica gel 60 and reverse-phased silica gel (RP-18; 230–400 mesh) were used for normal-phase and reverse-phased column chromatography. Precoated silica gel plates (Kieselgel 60 F254, 0.2 mm) (Merck, Darmstadt, Germany) were used for analytical TLC. High-performance liquid chromatography was performed on a Hitachi L-2455 HPLC apparatus with a Supelco C18 column (ODS-3, 5 μm, 250 × 20 mm; Sciences Inc., Tokyo, Japan).

3.2. Soft Coral Material

The cultured soft coral *Sarcophyton digitatum* of this study was originally collected from the wild in an 80-ton cultivation tank (height 1.6 m) located in the National Museum of Marine Biology and Aquarium, Taiwan. The tank was designed to simulate the fringing reefs in southern Taiwan [39]. The bottom of the tank was covered by a 3–5 cm layer of coral sand, and artificial rocks were distributed on the sand. Sand-filtered seawater pumped directly from the adjacent reef coast and added to the tank at an exchange rate of 10% per day of the total volume. The tank was a semiclosed recirculating aquaculture system and did not require deliberate feeding [40]. The water temperatures were maintained between 24 and 27 °C via a heat-exchanger cooling system. The soft coral *S. digitatum* was harvested in the National Museum of Marine Biology & Aquarium, Pingtung, in 2014. The coral was identified by one of the authors of this study (C.-F.D.). The animal sample was stored at the Department of Marine Biotechnology and Marine Resources, National Sun Yat-Sen University.

3.3. Extraction and Isolation

A sample of S. digitatum (0.9 kg) was sliced and exhaustively extracted with ethyl acetate (1 L × 5), and the solvent-free residue was sequentially partitioned between water and n-hexane, ethyl acetate, and n-butanol to yield three samples from the above solvents. The resulted EtOAc extract (1.098 g) was purified over silica gel by column chromatography and eluted with acetone in n-hexane (10–100%, stepwise), and then with methanol in acetone (0–100%, stepwise) to yield 13 fractions. Fraction 2 was eluted with the solvent system of acetone–n-hexane (6:1) to obtain 4 subfractions (A–D). Subfraction 2-B was purified by RP-HPLC using MeOH/H$_2$O (3:1) at a flow rate of 5 mL/min to afford **8** (2.1 mg). Fraction 3 was eluted with acetone–n-hexane (1:5) followed by isolation over a silica gel column to yield 5 subfractions (A–E). Subfraction 3-D was also purified by RP-HPLC with the solvent system of MeOH/H$_2$O (4:1) at a flow rate of 5 mL/min to obtain **9** (3.4 mg). Fraction 10 was eluted with acetone–n-hexane (1:3) and rechromatographed over RP-18 gel to obtain 6 subfractions (A–F). Subfraction 10-F was exhaustively purified by RP-HPLC using MeOH/H$_2$O (2:1) at a flow rate of 5 mL/min to yield **6** (20.2 mg) and **7** (13.5 mg). Fraction 11, eluting with acetone–n-hexane (1:2), was carefully isolated by a reverse-phase silica gel column to yield 6 subfractions (A–F). Subfraction 11-C was further purified by RP-HPLC using MeOH/H$_2$O (2:1) at a flow rate of 5 mL/min to obtain **1** (8.6 mg), **2** (4.0 mg), **3** (2.5 mg), **4** (2.0 mg), and **5** (23.3 mg).

Compound **1**: white powder; $[\alpha]_D^{25}$ = +48 (c 1.3, CHCl$_3$), IR (KBr) v_{max} 3433, 2958, 1705, 1603, 1436, 1373, 1205, 1135, 1061, 1029 cm^{-1}, ^{13}C and ^{1}H NMR data, Tables 1 and 2; ESIMS m/z 721 [M + Na]$^+$; HRESIMS m/z 721.4287 [M + Na]$^+$ (calcd for C$_{41}$H$_{62}$O$_9$Na, 721.4292)

Compound **2**: white powder; $[\alpha]_D^{25}$ = +88 (c 0.1, CHCl$_3$), IR (KBr) v_{max} 3398, 2927, 1704, 1607, 1372, 1204, 1135, 1070 cm^{-1}, ^{13}C and ^{1}H NMR data, Tables 1 and 2; ESIMS m/z 721 [M + Na]$^+$; HRESIMS m/z 721.4283 [M + Na]$^+$ (calcd for C$_{41}$H$_{62}$O$_9$Na, 721.4292)

Compound **3**: white powder; $[\alpha]_D^{25}$ = +39 (c 0.8, CHCl$_3$), IR (KBr) v_{max} 3445, 2959, 1703, 1435, 1372, 1206, 1061 cm^{-1}, ^{13}C and ^{1}H NMR data, Tables 1 and 2; ESIMS m/z 721 [M + Na]$^+$; HRESIMS m/z 721.4281 [M + Na]$^+$ (calcd for C$_{41}$H$_{62}$O$_9$Na, 721.4292)

Compound **4**: white powder; $[\alpha]_D^{25}$ = +76 (c 0.5, CHCl$_3$), IR (KBr) v_{max} 3446, 2957, 2925, 1706, 1603, 1435, 1375, 1206, 1061 cm^{-1}, ^{13}C and ^{1}H NMR data, Tables 1 and 2; ESIMS m/z 721 [M + Na]$^+$; HRESIMS m/z 721.4268 [M + Na]$^+$ (calcd for C$_{41}$H$_{62}$O$_9$Na, 721.4292)

3.4. Cytotoxicity Assay

Cell lines were purchased from the American Type Culture Collection (Rockville, MD). Cytotoxicity assays were carried out using the MTT assays [41]. MCF-7, MDA-MB-231, and HepG2, and HeLa cell lines were cultured and then exposed to various concentrations of **1–8** in dimethyl sulfoxide (DMSO) for 72 h to screen cytotoxicity. Doxorubicin, the positive control of the MTT assay, showed cytotoxicity towards MCF-7, MDA-MB-231, HepG2, and HeLa cancer cell lines, with IC$_{50}$ values of, 0.7 ± 0.1, 1.3 ± 0.2, 1.2 ± 0.4, and 0.4 ± 0.1 (μg/mL), respectively.

3.5. Anti-Inflammatory Assay

Murine macrophage cell line J774A.1 was purchased from the American Type Culture Collection (Rockville, MD). J774A.1 cells were cultured in 96-well plates at a concentration of 5 × 10^4 cells/mL and allowed to grow overnight. The cell cultures were added to the DMSO as control or different concentrations of compounds **1–8**, followed by treatment with LPS 1 μg/mL for 24 h. Determination of the cytokine concentration was performed by ELISA according to the manufacturer's protocol and previously reported method [42].

4. Conclusions

Investigation of *Sarcophyton digitatum* led to the purification of four new biscembranoids **1–4**, along with five known compounds **5–9**. With regards to biological activities, compounds **2**, **6**, and **7** displayed inhibitory activities against the proliferation of a limited panel of cancer cell lines in a cytotoxic assay. Furthermore, compounds **6** and **8** showed anti-inflammatory activity, which inhibited LPS-induced enhanced IL-1β production. The soft coral *Sarcophyton* sp. has been shown to produce various biscembranoid metabolites. Up to date, more than 60 biscembranoids biosynthesized via Diels–Alder reaction were isolated. Interestingly, these biscembranoids and their biosynthetic monocembranoid precursors are often found in *Sarcophyton* species [17–21,30,43–46]. The results of this study suggest that aquaculture of *Sarcophyton* species might produce structurally diversified bioactive compounds that could be beneficial for future drug development. Furthermore, the three dienophiles **12–14** are waiting for discovery as new cembranoids in future studies.

Supplementary Materials: The following are available online at http://www.mdpi.com/1660-3397/18/9/452/s1, IR, HRESIMS, ^{1}H, ^{13}C, distortionless enhancement by polarization transfer (DEPT), heteronuclear single quantum coherence spectroscopy (HSQC), COSY, HMBC, and NOESY spectra of new Compounds **1–4** are available online at http://www.mdpi.com/1660-3397/18/9/452/s1, Figure S1: IR spectrum of **1**, Figure S2: ESIMS spectrum of **1**, Figure S3: HRESIMS spectrum of **1**, Figure S4: ^{1}H NMR spectrum of **1** in CDCl$_3$ at 400 MHz, **Figure S5**: ^{13}C NMR spectrum of **1** in CDCl$_3$ at 100 MHz, Figure S6: DEPT spectrum of **1**, **Figure S7**: HSQC spectrum of **1**, **Figure S8**: COSY spectrum of **1**, Figure S9: HMBC spectrum of **1**, Figure S10: NOESY spectrum of **1**, **Figure S11**: IR spectrum of **2**, Figure S12: ESIMS spectrum of **2**, Figure S13: HRESIMS spectrum of **2**, Figure S14: ^{1}H NMR spectrum of **2** in CDCl$_3$ at 400 MHz, **Figure S15**: ^{13}C NMR spectrum of **2** in CDCl$_3$ at 100 MHz, Figure S16: DEPT spectrum of **2**, **Figure S17**: HSQC spectrum of **2**, **Figure S18**: COSY spectrum of **2**, Figure S19: HMBC spectrum of **2**, Figure S20: NOESY spectrum of **2**, Figure S21: IR spectrum of **3**, Figure S22: ESIMS spectrum of **3**, Figure S23: HRESIMS spectrum of **3**, Figure S24: ^{1}H NMR spectrum of **3** in CDCl$_3$ at 400 MHz, **Figure S25**: ^{13}C NMR spectrum of **3** in CDCl$_3$ at 100 MHz, **Figure S26**: DEPT spectrum of **2**, Figure S27: HSQC spectrum of **3**, **Figure S28**: COSY spectrum of **3**, Figure S29: HMBC spectrum of **3**, Figure S30: NOESY spectrum of **3**, Figure S31: IR spectrum of **4**, Figure S32. ESIMS spectrum of **3**, Figure S33: HRESIMS spectrum of **4**, Figure S34: ^{1}H NMR spectrum of **4** in DMSO-d_6 at 500 MHz, **Figure S35**: ^{13}C NMR spectrum of **4** in DMSO-d_6 at 125 MHz, Figure S36: DEPT spectrum of **4**, **Figure S37**: HSQC spectrum of **4**, Figure S38: COSY spectrum of **4**, Figure S39: HMBC spectrum of **4**, Figure S40: NOESY spectrum of **4**. Figure S41: ESIMS spectrum of **5**, **Figure S42**: ^{1}H NMR spectrum of **5** in CDCl$_3$ at 400 MHz, Figure S43: ^{13}C NMR spectrum of **5** in CDCl$_3$ at 100 MHz, Figure S44: ESIMS spectrum of **6**, Figure S45: ^{1}H NMR spectrum of **6** in CDCl$_3$ at 400 MHz, Figure S46: ^{13}C NMR spectrum of **6** in CDCl$_3$ at 100 MHz, Figure S47: ESIMS spectrum of **7**, Figure S48: ^{1}H NMR spectrum of **7** in CDCl$_3$ at 400 MHz, Figure S49: ^{13}C NMR spectrum of **7** in CDCl$_3$ at 100 MHz, Figure S50: ESIMS spectrum of **8**, Figure S51: ^{1}H NMR spectrum of **8** in CDCl$_3$ at 500 MHz, Figure S52: ^{13}C NMR spectrum of **8** in CDCl$_3$ at 125 MHz.

Author Contributions: Conceptualization, J.-H.S. (Jyh-Horng Sheu); investigation, T.-Y.H., C.-Y.H., C.-C.L., C.-F.D., J.-H.S. (Jui-Hsin Su), P.-J.S., and J.-H.S. (Jyh-Horng Sheu); writing-original draft, T.-Y.H., C.-Y.H., C.-H.C., and S.-H.W.; writing-review and editing, T.-Y.H., C.-H.C., S.-H.W., and J.-H.S. (Jyh-Horng Sheu); material resources, C.-C.L., C.-F.D., J.-H.S. (Jui-Hsin Su), and P.-J.S. All authors have read and agreed to the published version of the manuscript.

Funding: This research was mainly funded by the Ministry of Science and Technology of Taiwan (MOST 104-2113-M-110-006, 104-2320-B-110-001-MY2, and 107-2320-B-110-001-MY3).

Acknowledgments: Financial support of this work from the Ministry of Science and Technology of Taiwan (MOST 104-2113-M-110-006, 104-2320-B-110-001-MY2, and 107-2320-B-110-001-MY3) to J.-H.S. is gratefully acknowledged.

Conflicts of Interest: The authors declare no conflict of interest.

References

1. Rodríguez, A.D.; Li, Y.; Dhasmana, H. New marine cembrane diterpenoids isolated from the Caribbean gorgonian *Eunicea mammosa*. *J. Nat. Prod.* **1993**, *7*, 1101–1113. [CrossRef]
2. Katsuyama, I.; Fahmy, H.; Zjawiony, J.K.; Khalifa, S.I.; Kilada, R.W.; Konoshima, T.; Takasaki, M.; Tokuda, H. Semisynthesis of new sarcophine derivatives with chemopreventive activity. *J. Nat. Prod.* **2002**, *65*, 1809–1814. [CrossRef]

3. Hegazy, M.E.F.; Elshamy, A.I.; Mohamed, T.A.; Hamed, A.R.; Ibrahim, M.A.A.; Ohta, S.; Paré, P.W. Cembrene diterpenoids with ether linkages from *Sarcophyton ehrenbergi*: An anti-proliferation and molecular-docking assessment. *Mar. Drugs* **2017**, *15*, 192. [CrossRef]
4. Tang, G.H.; Sun, Z.H.; Zou, Y.H.; Yin, S. New cembrane-type diterpenoids from the South China Sea soft coral *Sarcophyton ehrenbergi*. *Molecules* **2016**, *21*, 587. [CrossRef]
5. Hegazy, M.E.F.; Mohamed, T.A.; Elshamy, A.I.; Hamed, A.R.; Ibrahim, M.A.A.; Ohta, S.; Umeyama, A.; Paré, P.W.; Efferth, T. Sarcoehrenbergilides D–F: Cytotoxic cembrene diterpenoids from the soft coral *Sarcophyton ehrenbergi*. *RSC Adv.* **2019**, *9*, 27183–27189. [CrossRef]
6. Hassan, H.M.; Rateb, M.E.; Hassan, M.H.; Sayed, A.M.; Shabana, S.; Raslan, M.; Amin, E.; Behery, F.A.; Ahmed, O.M.; Bin Muhsinah, A.; et al. New antiproliferative cembrane diterpenes from the Red Sea *Sarcophyton* species. *Mar. Drugs* **2019**, *17*, 411. [CrossRef] [PubMed]
7. Li, S.W.; Ye, F.; Zhu, Z.D.; Huang, H.; Mao, S.C.; Guo, Y.W. Cembrane-type diterpenoids from the South China Sea soft coral *Sarcophyton mililatensis*. *Acta Pharm. Sin. B* **2018**, *8*, 944–955. [CrossRef] [PubMed]
8. Sala, G.D.; Agriesti, F.; Mazzoccoli, C.; Tataranni, T.; Costantino, V.; Piccoli, C. Clogging the ubiquitin-proteasome machinery with marine natural products: Last decade update. *Mar. Drugs* **2018**, *16*, 467. [CrossRef] [PubMed]
9. Li, G.; Li, H.; Zhang, Q.; Yang, M.; Gu, Y.C.; Liang, L.F.; Tang, W.; Guo, Y.W. Rare cembranoids from Chinese soft coral *Sarcophyton ehrenbergi*: Structural and stereochemical studies. *J. Org. Chem.* **2019**, *84*, 5091–5098. [CrossRef] [PubMed]
10. Peng, C.C.; Huang, C.Y.; Ahmed, A.F.; Hwang, T.L.; Dai, C.F.; Sheu, J.H. New cembranoids and a biscembranoid peroxide from the soft coral *Sarcophyton cherbonnieri*. *Mar. Drugs* **2018**, *16*, 276. [CrossRef]
11. Ahmed, A.F.; Chen, Y.W.; Huang, C.Y.; Tseng, Y.J.; Lin, C.C.; Dai, C.F.; Wu, Y.C.; Sheu, J.H. Isolation and structure elucidation of cembranoids from a Dongsha Atoll soft coral *Sarcophyton stellatum*. *Mar. Drugs* **2018**, *16*, 210. [CrossRef]
12. Kamada, T.; Kang, M.C.; Phan, C.S.; Zanil, I.I.; Jeon, Y.J.; Vairappan, C.S. Bioactive cembranoids from the soft coral genus *Sinularia* sp. in Borneo. *Mar. Drugs* **2018**, *16*, 99. [CrossRef] [PubMed]
13. Lin, W.Y.; Chen, B.W.; Huang, C.Y.; Wen, Z.H.; Sung, P.J.; Su, J.H.; Dai, C.F.; Sheu, J.H. Bioactive cembranoids, sarcocrassocolides P–R, from the Dongsha Atoll soft coral *Sarcophyton crassocaule*. *Mar. Drugs* **2014**, *12*, 840–850. [CrossRef] [PubMed]
14. Lin, W.Y.; Su, J.H.; Wen, Z.H.; Kuo, Y.H.; Sheu, J.H. Cytotoxic and anti-inflammatory cembranoids from the Dongsha Atoll soft coral *Sarcophyton crassocaule*. *Bioorganic Med. Chem.* **2010**, *18*, 1936–1941. [CrossRef] [PubMed]
15. Huang, H.C.; Ahmed, A.F.; Su, J.H.; Chao, C.H.; Wu, Y.C.; Chiang, M.Y.; Sheu, J.H. Crassocolides A–F, Cembranoids with a *trans*-Fused Lactone from the Soft Coral *Sarcophyton crassocaule*. *J. Nat. Prod.* **2006**, *69*, 1554–1559. [CrossRef] [PubMed]
16. Chao, C.H.; Li, W.L.; Huang, C.Y.; Ahmed, A.F.; Dai, C.F.; Wu, Y.C.; Lu, M.C.; Liaw, C.C.; Sheu, J.H. Isoprenoids from the soft coral *Sarcophyton glaucum*. *Mar. Drugs* **2017**, *15*, 202. [CrossRef]
17. Jia, R.; Kurtán, T.; Mándi, A.; Yan, X.H.; Zhang, W.; Guo, Y.W. Biscembranoids formed from an α,β-unsaturated γ-lactone ring as a dienophile: Structure revision and establishment of their absolute configurations using theoretical calculations of electronic circular dichroism spectra. *J. Org. Chem.* **2013**, *78*, 3113–3119. [CrossRef] [PubMed]
18. Huang, C.Y.; Sung, P.J.; Uvarani, C.; Su, J.H.; Lu, M.C.; Hwang, T.L.; Dai, C.F.; Sheu, J.H. Glaucumolides A and B, biscembranoids with new structural type from a cultured soft coral *Sarcophyton glaucum*. *Sci. Rep.* **2015**, *5*, 15624. [CrossRef] [PubMed]
19. Sun, P.; Yu, Q.; Li, J.; Riccio, R.; Lauro, G.; Bifulco, G.; Kurtán, T.; Mándi, A.; Tang, H.; Li, T.J.; et al. Bissubvilides A and B, cembrane–capnosane heterodimers from the soft coral *Sarcophyton subviride*. *J. Nat. Prod.* **2016**, *79*, 2552–2558. [CrossRef]
20. Sun, P.; Cai, F.Y.; Lauro, G.; Tang, H.; Su, L.; Wang, H.L.; Li, H.H.; Mándi, A.; Kurtán, T.; Riccio, R.; et al. Immunomodulatory biscembranoids and assignment of their relative and absolute configurations: Data set modulation in the density functional theory/nuclear magnetic resonance approach. *J. Nat. Prod.* **2019**, *82*, 1264–1273. [CrossRef]
21. Yan, P.C.; Lv, Y.; van Ofwegen, L.; Proksch, P.; Lin, W.H. Lobophytones A–G, new isobiscembranoids from the soft coral *Lobophytum pauciflorum*. *Org. Lett.* **2010**, *12*, 2484–2487. [CrossRef] [PubMed]

22. Zubair, M.S.; Al-Footy, K.O.; Ayyed, S.-E.N.; Al-Lihaibi, S.S.; Alarif, W.M. A review of steroids from *Sarcophyton* species. *Nat. Prod. Res.* **2016**, *30*, 869–879. [CrossRef] [PubMed]
23. Elkhawas, Y.A.; Elissawy, A.M.; Elnaggar, M.S.; Mostafa, N.M.; Al-Sayed, E.; Bishr, M.M.; Singab, A.N.B.; Salama, O.M. Chemical diversity in species belonging to soft coral genus *Sacrophyton* and its impact on biological activity: A review. *Mar. Drugs* **2020**, *18*, 41. [CrossRef] [PubMed]
24. Su, J.Y.; Yang, R.L.; Zeng, L.M. Sardisterol, a new polyhydroxylated sterol from the soft coral *Sarcophyton digitatum* moser. *Chin. J. Chem.* **2001**, *19*, 515–517. [CrossRef]
25. Xi, Z.F.; Bie, W.; Chen, W.; Liu, D.; van Ofwegen, L.; Proksch, P.; Lin, W.H. Sarcophytolides G–L, new biscembranoids from the soft coral *Sarcophyton elegans*. *Helv. Chim. Acta.* **2013**, *96*, 2218–2227. [CrossRef]
26. Yan, X.H.; Gavagnin, M.; Cimino, G.; Guo, Y.W. Two new biscembranes with unprecedented carbon skeleton and their probable biogenetic precursor from the Hainan soft coral *Sarcophyton latum*. *Tetrahedron Lett.* **2007**, *48*, 5313–5316. [CrossRef]
27. Gross, H.; Wright, A.D.; Beli, W.; König, G.M. Two new bicyclic cembranolides from a new *Sarcophyton* species and determination of the absolute configuration of sarcoglaucol-16-one. *Org. Biomol. Chem.* **2004**, *2*, 1133–1138. [CrossRef] [PubMed]
28. Fang, H.; Liu, A.; Chen, X.; Cheng, W.; Dirsch, O.; Dahmen, U. The severity of LPS induced inflammatory injury is negatively associated with the functional liver mass after LPS injection in rat model. *J. Inflamm.* **2018**, *15*, 21. [CrossRef]
29. Jia, R.; Guo, Y.W.; Chen, P.; Yang, Y.M.; Mollo, E.; Gavagnin, M.; Cimino, G. Biscembranoids and their probable biogenetic precursor from the Hainan soft coral *Sarcophyton tortuosum*. *J. Nat. Prod.* **2007**, *70*, 1158–1166. [CrossRef]
30. Kurtán, T.; Jia, R.; Li, Y.; Pescitelli, G.; Guo, Y.W. Absolute configuration of highly flexible natural products by the solid-state ECD/TDDFT method: Ximaolides and sinulaparvalides. *Eur. J. Org. Chem.* **2012**, *34*, 6722–6728. [CrossRef]
31. Dayer, J.M.; Oliviero, F.; Punzi, L. A brief history of IL-1 and IL-1 Ra in rheumatology. *Front. Pharmacol.* **2017**, *8*, 293. [CrossRef] [PubMed]
32. Kay, J.; Calabrese, L. The role of interleukin-1 in the pathogenesis of rheumatoid arthritis. *Rheumatology* **2004**, *43*, iii2–iii9. [CrossRef] [PubMed]
33. Gui, W.S.; Wei, X.; Mai, C.L.; Murugan, M.; Wu, L.J.; Xin, W.J.; Zhou, L.J.; Liu, X.G. Interleukin-1β overproduction is a common cause for neuropathic pain, memory deficit, and depression following peripheral nerve injury in rodents. *Mol. Pain* **2016**, *12*, 1–15. [CrossRef] [PubMed]
34. Szekely, Y.; Arbel, Y. A review of interleukin-1 in heart disease: Where do we stand today? *Cardiol. Ther.* **2018**, *7*, 25–44. [CrossRef] [PubMed]
35. Liu, Y.; Costa, M.B.; Gerhardinger, C. IL-1β is upregulated in the diabetic retina and retinal vessels: Cell-specific effect of high glucose and IL-1β autostimulation. *PLoS ONE* **2012**, *7*, e36949. [CrossRef]
36. Kowluru, R.A.; Odenbach, S. Role of interleukin-1β in the pathogenesis of diabetic retinopathy. *Br. J. Ophthalmol.* **2004**, *88*, 1343–1347. [CrossRef]
37. Ichige, T.; Okano, Y.; Kanoh, N.; Nakata, M. Total synthesis of methyl sarcophytoate, a marine natural biscembranoid. *J. Org. Chem.* **2009**, *74*, 230–243. [CrossRef]
38. Maloney, K.N.; Botts, R.T.; Davis, T.S.; Okada, B.K.; Maloney, E.M.; Leber, C.A.; Alvarado, O.; Brayton, C.; Caraballo-Rodríguez, A.M.; Chari, J.V.; et al. Cryptic species account for the seemingly idiosyncratic secondary metabolism of *Sarcophyton glaucum* specimens collected in Palau. *J. Nat. Prod.* **2020**, *83*, 693–705. [CrossRef]
39. Liu, P.J.; Lin, S.M.; Fan, T.Y.; Meng, P.J.; Shao, K.T.; Lin, H.J. Rates of overgrowth by macroalgae and attack by sea anemones are greater for live coral than dead coral under conditions of nutrient enrichment. *Limnol. Oceanogr.* **2009**, *54*, 1167–1175. [CrossRef]
40. Chou, W.C.; Liu, P.J.; Chen, Y.H.; Huang, W.J. Contrasting changes in diel variation of net community calcification support that carbonate dissolution can be more sensitive to ocean acidification than coral calcification. *Front. Mar. Sci.* **2020**, *7*, 3. [CrossRef]
41. Cole, S.P.C. Rapid chemosensitivity testing of human lung tumor cells using the MTT assay. *Cancer Chemother. Pharmacol.* **1986**, *17*, 259–263. [CrossRef] [PubMed]

42. Chen, L.; Lin, S.X.; Agha-Majzoub, R.; Overbergh, L.; Mathieu, C.; Chan, L.S. CCL27 is a critical factor for the development of atopic dermatitis in the keratin-14 IL-4 transgenic mouse model. *Int. Immunol.* **2006**, *18*, 1233–1242. [CrossRef] [PubMed]
43. Feller, M.; Rudi, A.; Berer, N.; Goldberg, I.; Stein, Z.; Benayahu, Y.; Schleyer, M.; Kashman, Y. Isoprenoids of the soft coral *Sarcophyton glaucum*: nyalolide, a new biscembranoid, and other terpenoids. *J. Nat. Prod.* **2004**, *67*, 1303–1308. [CrossRef] [PubMed]
44. Zeng, L.M.; Lan, W.J.; Su, J.Y.; Zhang, G.W.; Feng, X.L.; Liang, Y.J.; Yang, X.P. Two new cytotoxic tetracyclic tetraterpenoids from the Soft coral *Sarcophyton tortuosum*. *J. Nat. Prod.* **2004**, *67*, 1915–1918. [CrossRef] [PubMed]
45. Yan, P.C.; Deng, Z.W.; van Ofwegen, L.; Proksch, P.; Lin, W.H. Lobophytones O–T, new biscembranoids and cembranoid from soft coral *Lobophytum pauciflorum*. *Mar. Drugs* **2010**, *8*, 2837–2848. [CrossRef] [PubMed]
46. Yan, P.C.; Deng, Z.W.; van Ofwegen, L.; Proksch, P.; Lin, W.H. Lobophytones U–Z_1, biscembranoids from the chinese soft coral *Lobophytum pauciflorum*. *Chem. Biodivers.* **2011**, *8*, 1724–1734. [CrossRef] [PubMed]

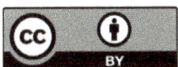

© 2020 by the authors. Licensee MDPI, Basel, Switzerland. This article is an open access article distributed under the terms and conditions of the Creative Commons Attribution (CC BY) license (http://creativecommons.org/licenses/by/4.0/).

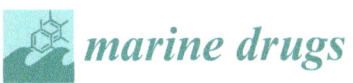

Communication

Optimization of Two Steps in Scale-Up Synthesis of Nannocystin A

Tingrong Zhang, Shaojie Miao, Mingxiao Zhang, Wenjie Liu, Liang Wang * and Yue Chen *

State Key Laboratory of Medicinal Chemical Biology, College of Pharmacy, and Tianjin Key Laboratory of Molecular Drug Research, Nankai University, Tianjin 300350, China; tingrongzhang@mail.nankai.edu.cn (T.Z.); miaoshaojie@mail.nankai.edu.cn (S.M.); mingxiaozhang@mail.nankai.edu.cn (M.Z.); liuwenjie@mail.nankai.edu.cn (W.L.)
* Correspondence: lwang@nankai.edu.cn (L.W.); yuechen@nankai.edu.cn (Y.C.); Tel.: +86-22-85358387 (L.W. & Y.C.)

Abstract: We have accomplished a 10-step (longest linear) total synthesis of nannocystin A on a four hundred milligram scale. The previously reported Kobayashi vinylogous Mukaiyama aldol reaction to connect C4 and C5 was unreproducible during the scaling up process. A more convenient and cost-efficient Keck asymmetric vinylogous aldol reaction was employed to improve this transformation.

Keywords: total synthesis; natural product; nannocystin; anti-cancer; gram-scale

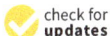

Citation: Zhang, T.; Miao, S.; Zhang, M.; Liu, W.; Wang, L.; Chen, Y. Optimization of Two Steps in Scale-Up Synthesis of Nannocystin A. *Mar. Drugs* 2021, 19, 198. https://doi.org/10.3390/md19040198

Academic Editors: Celso Alves and Marc Diederich

Received: 15 February 2021
Accepted: 29 March 2021
Published: 31 March 2021

Publisher's Note: MDPI stays neutral with regard to jurisdictional claims in published maps and institutional affiliations.

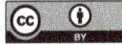

Copyright: © 2021 by the authors. Licensee MDPI, Basel, Switzerland. This article is an open access article distributed under the terms and conditions of the Creative Commons Attribution (CC BY) license (https://creativecommons.org/licenses/by/4.0/).

1. Introduction

Marine myxobacteria are prolific producers of secondary metabolites owning unique structures and exhibiting multiple biological activities ranging from antibiotic to anti-cancer [1,2]. The discovery of epothilones [3] from myxobacteria and their metabolic stable analogue Ixabepilone [4,5] (approved for the treatment of aggressive breast cancer) for clinical use highlight the powerful potential of myxobacteria as resources for drug discovery. More importantly, novel modes of action [6] were also identified during the pharmacological study of these myxobacteria-derived natural products, and hereby proceeded the target-oriented drug discovery.

Nannocystin A (**1**) and its natural congener (**2–6**) (Figure 1) are myxobacterial secondary metabolites isolated by Hoepfner [7] and BrÖnstrup [8] independently from *Nannocystis sp*. They exhibit significant inhibitory activity against a broad variety of human cancer cells at nanomolar concentrations [7,8]. This anti-neoplastic activity is attributed to the binding affinity with elongation factor 1A (eEF1A) [7]. Since this mechanism is shared by plitidepsin [9,10] (isolated from the marine tunicate *Aplidium albicans*, Figure 1) which has recently been approved by the Australia Therapeutic Goods Administration for clinical use against multiple myeloma, it is obvious that nannocystins might be a promising lead for anti-cancer drug discovery.

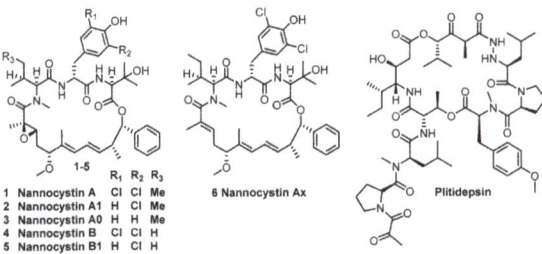

Figure 1. Structure of nannocystins and plitidepsin.

Structurally, nannocystins share a rigid 21-membered macroskeleton bearing nine chiral centers (7 chiral centers for **6**), an N-methyl α,β-epoxy amide (for **1–5**) and two conjugated E-alkenes. Its novel macroskeleton, strong antineoplastic activity and unusual mechanism attracted the interests of the chemical community. Thus far, seven total syntheses [11–20] of **1** and **6** have been finished. For efficiency, all synthetic routes fully utilized the principle of convergency, endowing freedom of structural modification of individual moieties, which help to uncover the preliminary of structure-activity relationship of the macroskeleton [17,21–24]. However, the quantities of nannocystins obtained from previously reported studies are insufficient for multipronged biological testing. Only Liu and Ye reported 75 mg and 20 mg-scaled synthesis of nannocystins, respectively, whereas others (including us) reported it on a milligram scale. This might be an explanation that the biological testing of nannocystin A is stagnant at the in vitro level, and tardily cannot advance to the in vivo level. To address the supply issue for in vivo study, we enlarged the synthetic procedures we previously reported. Herein, we describe the details of our efforts in the optimization of some procedures. The key improvement is that a Keck asymmetric vinylogous Mukaiyanma aldol reaction was employed to construct the carbon bond between C4 and C5. We finally obtained 420 mg of nannocystin A for future biological testing.

2. Results

Chemistry

In our previous paper [13], we provided a concise route in 10 steps (longest linear sequence) featuring an intramolecular Heck cross-coupling for the final macrocyclization. Connections of building blocks (**7–11**, Figure 2) via well-established esterification, amidation and the Mitsunobu reaction succeeded in providing the penultimate linear precursor **19** (Figure 3). Considering that five chiral centers (C2, C3, C5, C10, C11) were built on our own and the other four were innate in commercially available amino acid-derived starting materials, we paid key attention to these five chiral centers during the amplification process.

We first amplified the synthesis of **18** (structure shown in Figure 3). The Mitsunobu reaction between anti-homoallylic alcohol **10** and N-Boc-3-hydroxy-D-valine **9** went smoothly according to a previously reported procedure to give **18** in 70% yield, with 12 g obtained for the current batch.

As for the establishment of the C5 chiral center, all seven reported synthetic routes deployed nucleophilic attack of carbon anions towards carbonyl groups, five of which including us employed an asymmetric vinylous Mukaiyama-type aldol reaction (Figure 4). Kobayashi et al. [25] first developed this type aldol reaction of an aldehyde with vinylketene silyl N,O-acetal, and the enantio-selectivity was controlled by the remote Evans auxiliary. By employing this methodology, we produced **14** (Figure 4) in an acceptable yield with a d.r. value > 10:1, and 8.1 g of product **14** was obtained for the previous batch. However, when we reperformed this reaction, we found it was capricious because upon scale-up to 5 g, the yield dropped considerably to 10%. Strictly following the previous operation, we repeated this reaction several times; the yield can occasionally reach up to 50% but it was unreproducible. In most cases, the yield ranged from 5% to 20%. Then, we carefully checked the details of this reaction such as the purity of reactants and solvent, the equivalents and concentrations of reactants, the reaction time and temperature, the stirring speed, the method of quench, etc., but still failed in furnishing **14** in a stable yield more than 20%. Meanwhile, Liu et al. [20] also reported the fruitlessness during the synthesis of nannocystin Ax utilizing **20** and aldehyde **23** (Figure 4). They found both reactants decomposed rapidly under treatment with Lewis acid such as $TiCl_4$. In addition, considering the potential hazards of $TiCl_4$ in the amplification process, we set out for an alternative method to achieve this transformation.

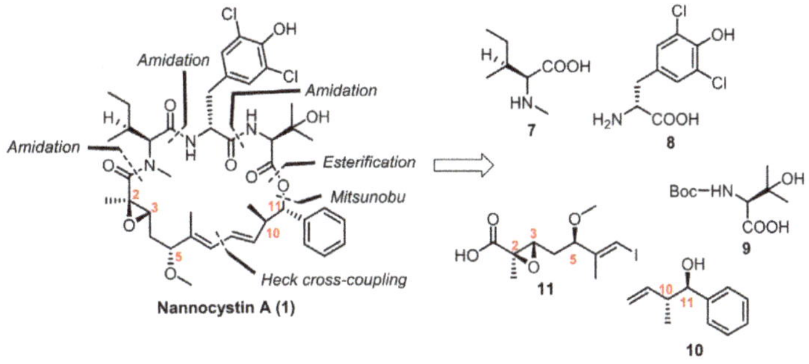

Figure 2. Retrosynthetic analysis of our route.

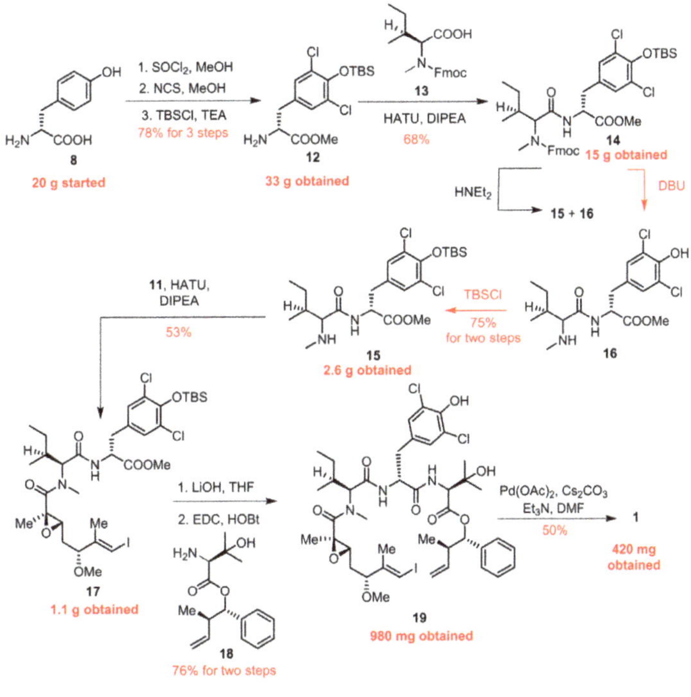

Figure 3. Previously reported synthetic route towards **1**, scaled up synthesis for the current batch was marked red.

Ti(O*i*Pr)$_4$ is a mild reagent compared to TiCl$_4$, and its combination with BINOL can also mediate the asymmetric Mukaiyama-type aldol reaction between aldehyde and vinylketene silyl acetal [26]. By employing the chiral BINOL reagents, this reaction can proceed in an enantio-selective manner with high e.e. value evidenced by our recent synthetic work of ovatodiolide [27]. Besides, the external addition of BINOL can save the installation and removal of auxiliaries on reactants compared to Evans auxiliary methodology, and BINOL can be recovered after the reaction is completed. Then, we chose economical material **24** (Figure 5) to form **25** as the coupling partner on a milligram scale. The reaction between aldehyde **21** and **25** with the addition of Ti(O*i*Pr)$_4$ and (*R*)-BINOL went smoothly to provide **26** in a stable >55% yield with an e.e. value = 85% [13]. The temperature was maintained at −78 °C only for 30 min after the reaction began and was allowed to warm to 0 °C for another 10 h stirring. By far, the biggest batch we preformed was 20 g for compound **21** without any erosion of yield (for a complete comparison between two vinylous Mukaiyama aldol reactions, see Figure 5). Since the two produced enantiomers could not be easily separated, purification was deferred to later steps. Compound **26** was then converted to **27** under treatment with Ag$_2$O and CH$_3$I. The reduction of the methyl ester group with DIBAL-H afforded us 3.6 g of allylic alcohol **28**. With the aid of Sharpless' conditions, epoxidation proceeded stereoselectively and we obtained **29** as a mixture of two diastereomers. Next, building block **11** was obtained via two successive oxidations on a gram scale according to previous procedures. The compound with an undesired configuration at C5 disappeared after condensation with amine **15** according to the ^{1}H-NMR of isolated product **17**.

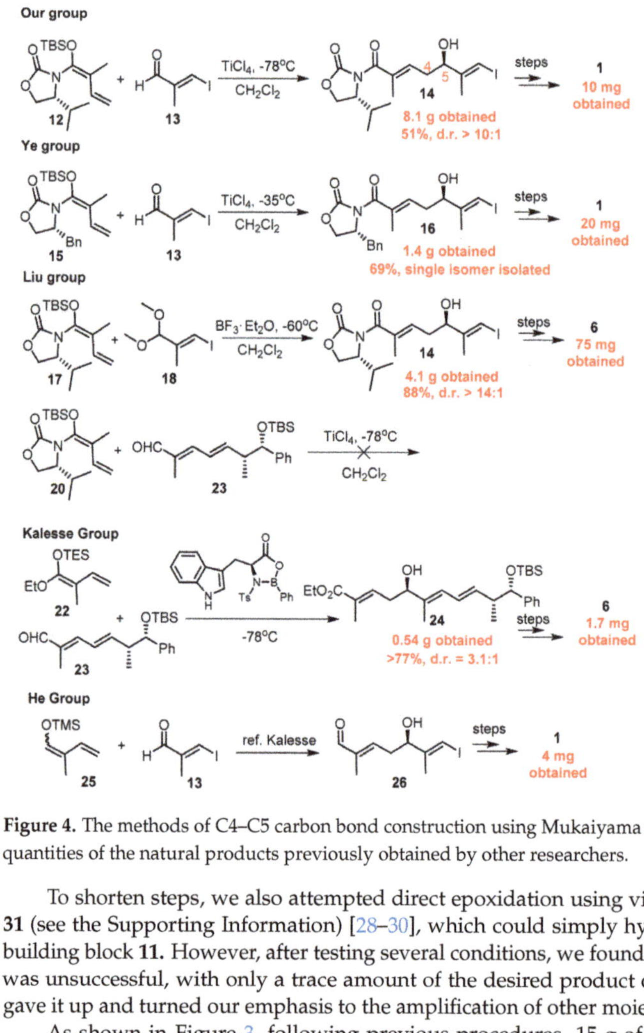

Figure 4. The methods of C4–C5 carbon bond construction using Mukaiyama aldol reaction and the quantities of the natural products previously obtained by other researchers.

To shorten steps, we also attempted direct epoxidation using vinyl ester **27** to give **31** (see the Supporting Information) [28–30], which could simply hydrolyze to provide building block **11**. However, after testing several conditions, we found this transformation was unsuccessful, with only a trace amount of the desired product obtained. Thus, we gave it up and turned our emphasis to the amplification of other moieties.

As shown in Figure 3, following previous procedures, 15 g of compound **14** was obtained unimpededly. However, the removal of the Fmoc group with Et$_2$NH was problematic when scaled up to 1 g. The *t*-butyldimethylsilyl (TBS) group could be simultaneously cleaved partially. We extended the reaction time and increased the equiv. of Et$_2$NH, but still TBS could not be cleaved entirely and two products (**15** and **16**) were detectable through thin-layer chromatography (TLC) analysis. The isolation process was cumbersome because the secondary amine was hard to remove. Therefore, we employed circuitous tactics. First, the treatment of **14** with 1,5-diazabicyclo[4.3.0]non-5-ene (DBU) rapidly delivered us **16**. With the concern that the phenol might make an impact on the following coupling, we unmasked it with a TBS group again to obtain **15**.

The subsequent transformation from **15** to the penultimate linear precursor proceeded smoothly to give rise to 980 mg of **19** for the current batch. By subjecting **19** to the intramolecular Heck macrocyclization, we finally obtained 420 mg of **1** in 50% yield (brsm). It was noteworthy that no cis/trans isomers were detected during this transformation.

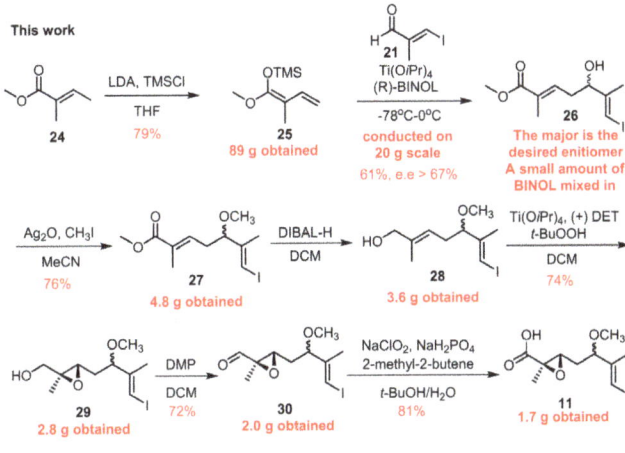

conditions	previous Kobayashi Mukaiyama aldol	Keck Mukaiyama aldol in this work
Lewis acid	TiCl$_4$	Ti(O*i*Pr)$_4$
temperature and time	-78 °C (5 h)	-78 °C (0.5 h), then 0 °C (10 h)
yield	unreproducable up to 1 g, from 5% to 50%	20 g scale, 61%
d.r./ e.r. value	d.r. > 10:1	e.r. = 12.7:1

Addition:
1. All the costs of obtaining compound 28 in this work is about one-fifth of that in the previous work.
2. The operation of Keck Mukaiyama aldol reaction is simpler and easier to scale up, by avoiding usage of TiCl$_4$.
3. The route in this work is one-step shorter.
4. BINOL can be recycled compared to unrecycleable Evans auxiliary.

Figure 5. The optimization of vinylous Mukaiyama aldol reaction.

3. Materials and Methods

3.1. General Information

Reagents were purchased from commercial suppliers and used without purification unless otherwise stated: lithium diisopropylamide (LDA), 1-(3-dimethylaminopropyl)-3-ethylcarbodiimide (EDC), N-chlorosuccinimide (NCS), Nhydroxybenzotrizole (HOBt), 1-(2-hydroxynaphthalen-1-yl)naphthalen-2-ol (BINOL), dichloromethane (DCM), Dess-Martin periodinane (DMP), 1-(bis(dimethylamino)methylene)-1H-1,2,3-triazolo(4,5-b)pyridinium 3-oxid hexafluorophosphate (HATU), and N,N-Diisopropy-lethylamine (DIPEA), *t*-butyldimethylchlorosilane (TBSCl), diisobutyl aluminium hydride (DIBAL-H).

All reactions were carried out under an argon atmosphere with dry solvents under anhydrous conditions, unless otherwise noted. Tetrahydrofuran (THF) was distilled immediately before use from sodium-benzophenone ketyl. Solvents for chromatography were used as supplied by Tianjin Reagents Chemical (Tianjin, China). Reactions were monitored by thin-layer chromatography (TLC) carried out on silica gel plates, using UV light as the visualizing agent and aqueous phosphomolybdic acid or basic aqueous potassium permanganate as the developing agent. A 200–300 mesh silica gel was used for column chromatography.

Optical rotations were recorded on an Insmark IP 120 digital polarimeter (Insmark, Shanghai, China). IR spectra were recorded on a Bruker Tensor 27 instrument (Ettlingen, Germany). Only the strongest and/or most structurally important absorptions of IR spectra were reported in wavenumbers (cm^{-1}). ^{1}H NMR, ^{13}C NMR, and 2D NMR were recorded on Bruker AV 400 and calibrated by using internal references and solvent signals CDCl$_3$ (δ_H = 7.26 ppm, δ_C = 77.16 ppm) and CD$_3$OD (δ_H =3.31 ppm, δ_C = 49.0 ppm), unless otherwise noted. ^{1}H NMR data are reported as follows: chemical shift, multiplicity (s = singlet, d = doublet, t = triplet, q = quartet, p = quintet, br = broad, m = multiplet), coupling constants and integration. High-resolution mass spectra (HRMS) were detected on an IonSpec Fourier transform ion cyclotron resonance mass spectrometer by Varian 7.0T FTMS (Kuala Lumpur, Malaysia).

3.2. Chemistry

Compounds **8**, **12**, **17**, **18**, **19**, **1**, **29**, **30**, and **11** were obtained following the procedure reported previously.

*Methyl-(2R)-3-(3,5-dichloro-4-hydroxyphenyl)-2-((3S)-3-methyl-2-(methylamino)pentanamido) propanoate (**16**)*

To a solution of compound **14** (5.0 g, 6.9 mmol) in dry DCM (100 mL), DBU (5 mL, 33.4 mmol) was added. The reaction mixture was stirred for 30 min at room temperature. The reaction was quenched by silica gel, then purified by column chromatography (DCM:MeOH=50:1) to give the product **16** (2.7 g, crude) as a colorless oil.

*Methyl-(2R)-3-(4-((tert-butyldimethylsilyl)oxy)-3,5-dichlorophenyl)-2-((3S)-3-methyl-2-(methylamino)pentanamido)propanoate (**15**)*

To a solution of **16** (2.7 g, 6.9 mmol) in dry DCM (30 mL), triethylamine (1.9 mL, 13.8 mmol) was added, followed by TBSCl (1.6 g, 10.4 mmol) under ice bath. The reaction was stirred for 2 h at room temperature. Then, the reaction was quenched by water (10 mL), extracted with DCM (15 mL × 3). The combined organic layers were dried over MgSO$_4$, filtered and concentrated to give the crude. The crude was purified by column chromatography (DCM:MeOH, 100:1–70:1) to give the product **15** (2.6 g, 75% for two steps) as a colorless oil. The spectroscopic data are consistent with those reported in the literature.

*(Z)-((1-methoxy-2-methylbuta-1,3-dien-1-yl)oxy)trimethylsilane (**25**)*

To a solution of diisopropylamine (67 g, 0.66 mol) in dry THF (250 mL), n-BuLi (266 mL, 2.5 M in hexane) was added at −78 °C. The reaction mixture was warmed to 0 °C for 30 min, then cooled to −65 °C. Methyl tiglate **24** (68 g, 0.60 mol) in THF (30 mL) was added dropwise. The reaction mixture was stirred for 2 h, and after that, TMSCl (78 g, 0.72 mol) in THF (30 mL) was added dropwise. Then, the reaction was warmed to room temperature at a period of 4 h, diluted by hexane (1000 mL), and then filtered and concentrated to give a crude. The crude was distilled at 80 °C under reduced pressure to give the compound **25** as a light yellow liquid (89 g, 79%), which was directly used in the next step.

*Methyl-(2E,6E)-5-hydroxy-7-iodo-2,6-dimethylhepta-2,6-dienoate (**26**)*

To a solution of R-BINOL (15.2 g, 53 mmol) and CaH$_2$ (2.2 g) in dry THF (200 mL), Ti(OiPr)$_4$ (15.1 g, 53 mmol) was added at room temperature. The mixture turned orange while adding it. Then, the mixture was cooled to −78 °C after stirring at room temperature for 30 min, and then aldehyde **21** (21 g, 107 mmol) in THF (20 mL) was added dropwise, followed by dropwise addition of a solution of **25** (20 g, 107 mmol) in THF (20 mL). The mixture was then stirred at −78 °C for 30 min, and warmed to 0 °C for 10 h of stirring.

Then, the reaction was quenched by saturated aqueous NaHCO$_3$ (20 mL) and Rochelle salt (20 mL), extracted with EtOAc (80 mL × 3). The combined organic layers were dried over Na$_2$SO$_4$, filtered, and concentrated to give a crude. The crude was purified by column chromatography (PE:EA = 10:1), then redissolved by hexane, filtered, and concentrated to give the product **26** (20 g, 61%) as a yellow oil. ^{1}H NMR (400 MHz, CDCl$_3$) δ 6.72 (td, J = 7.2, 1.7 Hz, 1H), 6.31 (s, 1H), 4.29 (t, J = 6.5 Hz, 1H), 3.72 (s, 3H), 3.57 (d, J = 29.5 Hz, 1H), 2.44 (t, J = 6.9 Hz, 2H), 1.83 (d, J = 2.4 Hz, 6H). ^{13}C NMR (101 MHz, CDCl$_3$) δ 168.55, 149.18, 137.84, 129.46, 78.94, 75.11, 51.97, 34.55, 20.03, 12.72. IR(KBr)ν$_{max}$: 3445, 2936, 1699, 1437, 1275, 1084, 795, 661 cm^{-1} [M + Na] calculated 332.9964 found 332.9969.

Methyl-(2E,6E)-7-iodo-5-methoxy-2,6-dimethylhepta-2,6-dienoate (27)

To a solution of **26** (20 g, 64.5 mmol) in dry MeCN (120 mL), Ag$_2$O (37 g, 161 mmol) was added at room temperature, followed by methyl iodide (91 g, 645 mmol). Then, the reaction was stirred for 12 h at room temperature in a dark place. The reaction mixture was filtered through celite and concentrated to give a crude. The crude was purified by column chromatography (PE:EA = 20:1) to give methyl ether **27** (16 g, 49 mmol, 76%) as a yellow oil. ^{1}H NMR (400 MHz, CDCl$_3$) δ 6.69 (td, J = 7.2, 1.5 Hz, 1H), 6.27 (dd, J = 1.9, 1.0 Hz, 1H), 3.75 (dd, J = 7.6, 5.9 Hz, 1H), 3.74 (s, 3H), 3.21 (s, 3H), 2.53–2.42 (m, 1H), 2.41–2.31 (m, 1H), 1.83 (d, J = 1.4 Hz, 3H), 1.77 (d, J = 1.2 Hz, 3H). ^{13}C NMR (101 MHz, CDCl$_3$) δ 168.32, 147.10, 137.35, 129.45, 84.82, 79.73, 56.59, 51.82, 33.37, 29.71, 18.83, 12.70. IR(KBr)ν$_{max}$: 2949, 1715, 1435, 1273, 1099, 797, 744, 660 cm^{-1} [M + Na] calculated 347.0120 found 347.0124.

(2E,6E)-7-iodo-5-methoxy-2,6-dimethylhepta-2,6-dien-1-ol (28)

To a solution of methyl ether **27** (4.8 g, 14.8 mmol) in dry DCM (40 mL), DIBAL-H (20 mL, 1 M in DCM) was added at −20 °C dropwise. After stirring for 30 min, the reaction was quenched by water (0.8 mL) and 15% aqueous NaOH (0.8 mL). The temperature was allowed to warm to room temperature. After that, water (2 mL) and MgSO$_4$ (10 g) were added to the mixture, and it was stirred for 30 min and filtered through celite to give a crude. The crude was purified by column chromatography (PE:EA = 6:1) to give the product **28** (3.6 g, 82%) as a yellow oil. ^{1}H NMR (400 MHz, CDCl$_3$) δ 6.19 (s, 1H), 5.39–5.27 (m, 1H), 3.98 (s, 2H), 3.73–3.60 (m, 1H), 3.20 (d, J = 1.5 Hz, 3H), 2.36 (dt, J = 14.5, 7.1 Hz, 1H), 2.24 (dt, J = 14.6, 6.9 Hz, 1H), 1.94 (s, 1H), 1.76 (d, J = 1.4 Hz, 3H), 1.65 (s, 3H). ^{13}C NMR (101 MHz, CDCl$_3$) δ 147.49, 137.18, 120.77, 85.77, 79.20, 68.52, 56.46, 32.10, 18.83, 13.94. IR(KBr)ν$_{max}$: 3675, 2950, 1473, 1261, 1094, 1030, 801 cm^{-1} [M + Na] calculated 319.0171 found 319.0170.

4. Conclusions

In summary, we have achieved a 10-step (longest linear) total synthesis of nannocystin A on a four hundred milligram scale. Two steps were found problematic when scaled up, especially for the difficulty we met when we scaled up with the Kobayashi Mukaiyama aldol reaction to construct the carbon bond between C4 and C5. In order to overcome it, we employed a more convenient and cost-efficient Keck asymmetric vinylogous aldol reaction, and we finally obtained four hundred milligrams of nannocystin A. By starting from the synthesis of nannocystin A on a large scale, it should be possible, at least at the outset, to scale the production of any synthetic nannocystin analogue for further lead optimization and preclinical development.

Supplementary Materials: The following are available online at https://www.mdpi.com/article/10.3390/md19040198/s1, S1: conditions of direct epoxidation of compound **27**, S2: ^{1}H and ^{13}C NMR spectra for synthesized new compounds. S3. The e.e. value of Mukaiyama aldol reaction is > 66% shown in ^{1}H NMR of compound **29** and chiral HPLC data of compound **26**. S4. The determination of the absolute configuration by Mosher esters of compound **26**. S5. ^{1}H NMR for compound **17**; ^{1}H NMR and ^{13}C NMR for nannocystin A.

Author Contributions: Conceptualization, planning and designing of the research, L.W., T.Z. and Y.C.; synthesis and data collection, T.Z., S.M., W.L. and M.Z.; original draft preparation, L.W., T.Z. and S.M.; review and editing, L.W., T.Z. and M.Z. All authors have read and agreed to the published version of the manuscript.

Funding: We acknowledge financial support from the Natural Science Foundation of Tianjin (18JC-QNJC13900 to L.W); Fundamental Research Funds for the Central Universities; the National Natural Science Foundation of China (NSFC) (82073695 to L.W. and U1801288 to Y.C.); the National Science Fund for Distinguished Young Scholars (81625021 to Y.C.).

Institutional Review Board Statement: Not applicable.

Data Availability Statement: Not applicable.

Acknowledgments: We thank Lanshu Li for her helpful advisement.

Conflicts of Interest: The authors declare no conflict of interest. The founding sponsors had no role in the design of the study; in the collection, analyses, or interpretation of data; in the writing of the manuscript or the decision to publish the results.

References

1. Schäberle, T.; Goralski, E.; Neu, E.; Erol, Ö.; Hölzl, G.; Dörmann, P.; Bierbaum, G.; König, G. Marine Myxobacteria as a Source of Antibiotics-Comparison of Physiology, Polyketide-Type Genes and Antibiotic Production of Three New Isolates of *Enhygromyxa salina*. *Mar. Drugs* **2010**, *8*, 2466–2479. [CrossRef] [PubMed]
2. Albataineh, H.; Stevens, D. Marine Myxobacteria: A Few Good Halophiles. *Mar. Drugs* **2018**, *16*, 209. [CrossRef]
3. Höfle, G.; Bedorf, N.; Gerth, K.; Reichenbach, H. (GBF). German Patent DE 91-4138042, 1993. *Chem. Abstr.* **1993**, *120*, 52841.
4. Lee, F.; Borzilleri, R.; Fairchild, C.; Kim, S.; Long, B.H.; Reventos-Suarez, C.; Vite, G.; Rose, W.; Kramer, R. BMS-247550: A Novel Epothilone Analog with a Mode of Action Similar to Paclitaxel but Possessing Superior Antitumor Efficacy. *Clin. Cancer Res.* **2001**, *7*, 1429–1437. [PubMed]
5. Borzilleri, R.; Zheng, X.; Schmidt, R.; Johnson, J.; Kim, S.; DiMarco, J.; Fairchild, C.R.; Gougoutas, J.Z.; Lee, F.Y.; Long, B.H.; et al. A Novel Application of a Pd(0)-Catalyzed Nucleophilic Substitution Reaction to the Regio- and Stereoselective Synthesis of Lactam Analogues of the Epothilone Natural Products. *J. Am. Chem. Soc.* **2000**, *122*, 8890–8897. [CrossRef]
6. Kavallaris, M. Microtubules and resistance to tubulin-binding agents. *Nat. Rev. Cancer* **2010**, *10*, 194–204. [CrossRef]
7. Krastel, P.; Roggo, S.; Schirle, M.; Ross, N.T.; Perruccio, F.; Aspesi, P.; Aust, T.; Buntin, K.; Estoppey, D.; Liechty, B.; et al. Nannocystin A: An Elongation Factor 1 Inhibitor from Myxobacteria with Differential Anti-Cancer Properties. *Angew. Chem. Int. Ed.* **2015**, *54*, 10149–10154. [CrossRef]
8. Hoffmann, H.; Kogler, H.; Heyse, W.; Matter, H.; Caspers, M.; Schummer, D.; Klemke-Jahn, C.; Bauer, A.; Penarier, G.; Debussche, L.; et al. Discovery, Structure Elucidation, and Biological Characterization of Nannocystin A, a Macrocyclic Myxobacterial Metabolite with Potent Antiproliferative Properties. *Angew. Chem. Int. Ed.* **2015**, *54*, 10145–10148. [CrossRef]
9. Schoffski, P.; Guillem, V.; Garcia, M.; Rivera, F.; Tabernero, J.; Cullell, M.; Lopez-Martin, J.A.; Pollard, P.; Dumez, H.; del Muro, X.G.; et al. Phase II Randomized Study of Plitidepsin (Aplidin), Alone or in Association with L-carnitine, in Patients with Unresectable Advanced Renal Cell Carcinoma. *Mar. Drugs* **2009**, *7*, 57–70. [CrossRef]
10. Eisen, T.; Thomas, J.; Miller, W.H., Jr.; Gore, M.; Wolter, P.; Kavan, P.; Martin, J.A.; Lardelli, P. Phase II Study of Biweekly Plitidepsin as Second-line Therapy in Patients with Advanced Malignant Melanoma. *Melanoma Res.* **2009**, *19*, 185–192. [CrossRef] [PubMed]
11. Liao, L.; Zhou, J.; Xu, Z.; Ye, T. Concise Total Synthesis of Nannocystin A. *Angew. Chem. Int. Ed.* **2016**, *55*, 13263–13266. [CrossRef] [PubMed]
12. Huang, J.; Wang, Z. Total Syntheses of Nannocystins A and A0, Two Elongation Factor 1 Inhibitors. *Org. Lett.* **2016**, *18*, 4702–4705. [CrossRef]
13. Yang, Z.; Xu, X.; Yang, C.-H.; Tian, Y.; Chen, X.; Lian, L.; Pan, W.; Su, X.; Zhang, W.; Chen, Y. Total Synthesis of Nannocystin A. *Org. Lett.* **2016**, *18*, 5768–5770. [CrossRef]
14. Zhang, Y.; Liu, R.; Liu, B. Total synthesis of nannocystin Ax. *Chem. Commun.* **2017**, *53*, 5549–5552. [CrossRef]
15. Liu, Q.; Hu, P.; He, Y. Asymmetric Total Synthesis of Nannocystin A. *J. Org. Chem.* **2017**, *82*, 9217–9222. [CrossRef] [PubMed]
16. Poock, C.; Kalesse, M. Total Synthesis of Nannocystin Ax. *Org. Lett.* **2017**, *19*, 4536–4539. [CrossRef] [PubMed]
17. Meng, Z.; Souillart, L.; Monks, B.; Huwyler, N.; Herrmann, J.; Müller, R.; Fürstner, A. A "Motif-Oriented"Total Synthesis of Nannocystin Ax. Preparation and Biological Assessment of Analogues. *J. Org. Chem.* **2017**, *83*, 6977–6994. [CrossRef] [PubMed]
18. Wang, Z. The Chemical Syntheses of Nannocystins. *Synthesis* **2019**, *51*, 2252–2260. [CrossRef]
19. Zhang, W. From Target-Oriented to Motif-Oriented: A Case Study on Nannocystin Total Synthesis. *Molecules* **2020**, *25*, 5327. [CrossRef] [PubMed]
20. Liu, R.; Xia, M.; Zhang, Y.; Fu, S.; Liu, B. The journey of total synthesis toward nannocystin Ax. *Tetrahedron* **2019**, *75*, 1781–1794. [CrossRef]

21. Tian, Y.; Xu, X.; Ding, Y.; Hao, X.; Bai, Y.; Tang, Y.; Zhang, X.; Li, Q.; Yang, Z.; Zhang, W.; et al. Synthesis and Biological Evaluation of Nannocystin Analogues toward Understanding the Binding Role of the (2R,3S)-Epoxide in Nannocystin A. *Eur. J. Med. Chem.* **2018**, *150*, 626–632. [CrossRef]
22. Tian, Y.; Ding, Y.; Xu, X.; Bai, Y.; Tang, Y.; Hao, X.; Zhang, W.; Chen, Y. Total Synthesis and Biological Evaluation of Nannocystin Analogues Modified at the Polyketide Phenyl Moiety. *Tetrahedron Lett.* **2018**, *59*, 3206–3209. [CrossRef]
23. Tian, Y.; Wang, J.; Liu, W.; Yuan, X.; Tang, Y.; Li, J.; Chen, Y.; Zhang, W. Stereodivergent Total Synthesis of Br-Nannocystins Underpinning the Polyketide (10R,11S) Configuration as a Key Determinant of Potency. *J. Mol. Struct.* **2019**, *1181*, 568–578. [CrossRef]
24. Liu, Q.; Yang, X.; Ji, J.; Zhang, S.-L.; He, Y. Novel Nannocystin A Analogues as Anticancer Therapeutics: Synthesis, Biological Evaluations and Structure-activity Relationship Studies. *Eur. J. Med. Chem.* **2019**, *170*, 99–111. [CrossRef] [PubMed]
25. Shirokawa, S.-I.; Kamiyama, M.; Nakamura, T.; Okada, M.; Nazaki, A.; Hosokawa, S.; Kobayashi, S. Remote Asymmetric Induction with Vinylketene Silyl N,O-Acetal. *J. Am. Chem. Soc.* **2004**, *126*, 13604–13605. [CrossRef] [PubMed]
26. Keck, G.E.; Krishnamurthy, D. Pronounced Solvent and Concentration Effects in an Enantioselective Mukaiyama Aldol Condensation Using BINOL-Titanium(IV) Catalysts. *J. Am. Chem. Soc.* **1995**, *117*, 2363–2364. [CrossRef]
27. Xiang, J.; Ding, Y.; Li, J.; Zhao, X.; Sun, Y.; Wang, D.; Wang, L.; Chen, Y. Ovatodiolides: Scalable Protection-Free Syntheses, Configuration Determination, and Biological Evaluation against Hepatic Cancer Stem Cells. *Angew. Chem. Int. Ed.* **2019**, *58*, 10587–10590. [CrossRef]
28. Kakei, H.; Tsuji, R.; Ohshima, T.; Morimoto, H.; Matsunaga, S.; Shibasaki, M. Catalytic Asymmetric Epoxidation of a,b-Unsaturated Esters with Chiral Yttrium–Biaryldiol Complexes. *Chem. Asian J.* **2007**, *2*, 257–264. [CrossRef] [PubMed]
29. Candu, N.; Rizescu, C.; Podolean, I.; Tudorache, M.; Parvulescu, V.; Coman, S. Efficient Magnetic and Recyclable SBILC (Supported Basic Ionic Liquid Catalyst)-Based Heterogeneous Organocatalysts for the Asymmetric Epoxidation of Trans-Methylcinnamate. *Catal. Sci. Technol.* **2015**, *5*, 729–737. [CrossRef]
30. Wu, X.; She, X.; Shi, Y. Highly Enantioselective Epoxidation of α,β-Unsaturated Esters by Chiral Dioxirane. *J. Am. Chem. Soc.* **2002**, *124*, 8792–8793. [CrossRef] [PubMed]

MDPI
St. Alban-Anlage 66
4052 Basel
Switzerland
Tel. +41 61 683 77 34
Fax +41 61 302 89 18
www.mdpi.com

Marine Drugs Editorial Office
E-mail: marinedrugs@mdpi.com
www.mdpi.com/journal/marinedrugs

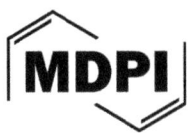

www.ingramcontent.com/pod-product-compliance
Lightning Source LLC
LaVergne TN
LVHW070628100526
838202LV00012B/758